METHODS OF BIOCHEMICAL ANALYSIS

Volume 34

METHODS OF
BIOCHEMICAL ANALYSIS

Series Editor

Clarence H. Suelter

Volume 34

BIOMEDICAL APPLICATIONS OF MASS SPECTROMETRY

Edited by

CLARENCE H. SUELTER
Department of Biochemistry
Michigan State University
East Lansing, Michigan

J. THROCK WATSON
Departments of Biochemistry and Chemistry
Michigan State University
East Lansing, Michigan

WILEY

An Interscience Publication
JOHN WILEY & SONS
New York • Chichester • Brisbane • Toronto • Singapore

An Interscience® Publication

Copyright © 1990 by John Wiley & Sons, Inc.

All rights reserved. Published simultaneously in Canada.

Library of Congress Catalog Card Number: 54-7232

ISBN 0-471-61303-7

Printed in the United States of America

10 9 8 7 6 5 4 3 2

SERIES PREFACE

Methods of Biochemical Analysis was established in 1954 with the publication of Volume 1 and has continued to the present with volumes appearing on a more or less yearly basis. Each volume deals with biochemical methods and techniques used in different areas of science. Professor David Glick, the series' originator and editor for the first 33 volumes, sensed the need for a book series that focused on methods and instrumentation. Already in 1954, he noted that it was becoming increasingly difficult to keep abreast of the development of new techniques and the improvement of well-established methods. This difficulty often constituted the limiting factor for the growth of experimental sciences. Professor Glick's foresight marked the creation of a unique set of methods volumes which have set the standard for many other reviews.

With Professor Glick's retirement from the series and beginning with Volume 34, I have assumed editorship. Because the rationale used in 1954 for the establishment of the series is even more cogent today, I hope to maintain the excellent traditions developed earlier. The format of Volume 34 and later volumes, however, is changed. Rather than cover a variety of topics as previous volumes did, each volume will now focus on a specific method or the application of a variety of methods to solve a specific biological or biomedical problem.

CLARENCE H. SUELTER

East Lansing, Michigan

PREFACE

Volume 34 focuses on mass spectrometry. The first chapter gives an overview of mass spectrometry, including a review of some of the recent advances that make this field of analytical biochemistry so exciting. The following chapters cover the topics of mass spectrometry of carbohydrates, peptide sequencing by mass spectrometry, mass spectrometry of nucleic acid components, and mass spectrometry in pharmacology. Each chapter is prepared by an authority in the field.

The expressed purpose of each chapter is to give the reader, both the novice and the authority, a meaningful presentation of the application of mass spectrometry to a variety of biological problems. The chapters are not a compilation of methods, but, rather, they provide insight into approaches that mass spectroscopists have used to solve these problems. Each chapter provides guidance in using appropriate methods for isolation and purification of the compound class prior to analysis or characterization by mass spectrometry. Each chapter also provides a "tutorial" on mass spectral interpretation based on the fragmentation pathways usually encountered for the particular compound type. In many cases, chemical modification of the parent compound and corresponding mass shifts in the spectrum are coordinated through reaction schemes and didactic descriptions. Modern approaches to analysis based on fast atom bombardment are described in conjunction with the more conventional analysis by electron impact and chemical-ionization mass spectrometry.

The editors have planned a compilation of chapters that could be used as a reference text for a course in mass spectrometry applied to biology.

CLARENCE H. SUELTER
J. THROCK WATSON

East Lansing, Michigan
February, 1990

CONTENTS

ABBREVIATIONS

5-FU	5-fluorouracil
abe	abequose
AIDS	acquired immunodeficiency syndrome
APCI	atmospheric pressure chemical ionization
AUC	area under concentration versus time curve
B	magnetic sector mass analyzer
B/E	linked scan at constant ratio of B to E
BCNU	N,N'-bis(2-chloroethyl)-N-nitrosourea
BEDU	5-(2-bromo-E-ethenyl)-2′-deoxyuridine
BEQQ	hybrid instrument (magnetic sector, electric sector and quadrupoles)
BSTFA	N,O-bis(trimethylsilyl)-trifluoroacetamide
CID	collisionally induced dissociation
CBZ	carbamazepine
cDNA	complementary DNA
CI	chemical ionization
CNBr	cyanogen bromide
CSF	cerebrospinal fluid
CZE	capillary zone electrophoresis
DBE	double bond equivalents (rings plus double bonds)
DCI	desorptive chemical ionization
DEI	desorptive electron-impact ionization
DES	diethylstilbesterol
DIP	direct insertion probe
DLI	direct liquid introduction (LC–MS interface)
DMS	dimethystilbesterol
DMSO	dimethyl sulfoxide
DOPA	dihydroxyphenylalanine
DTT	dithiothreitol
ECNI	electron-capture negative ionization
EI	electron impact or electron ionization
ESA or E	electronstatic analyzer

eV	electron volt (1 eV = 23.06 kcal/mol = 96.49 kJ/mol)
FAB	fast atom bombardment
FD	field desorption
FdUMP	2′-deoxy-5-fluorouridine monophosphate
fg	femtogram
FID	flame ionization detector
FUdR	2′-deoxy-5-fluorouridine
Ft	ftorafur
gal	galactose
GC	gas chromatography
GC–MS	gas chromatography–mass spectrometry
hex	hexose
HPLC	high-performance liquid chromatography
ICI 45, 673	an analog of propranolol with a tolyoxy rather than a naphthoxy ring
IR	infrared
IS	internal standard
ITD	ion trap detector
LC	liquid chromatography
LD	laser desorption
LSD	lysergic acid diethylamide
LSIMS	liquid SIMS
m/z	mass to charge ratio
man	mannan
MeNU	N-methyl-N-nitrosourea
MIKES	mass-analyzed ion kinetic energy spectra
MPTP	1-methyl-4-phenyl-1,2,3,6-tetrahydroxypyridine
MS	mass spectrometry
MW	molecular weight
NAPA	N-acetylprocainamide
NMF	N-methylformamide
NMR	nuclear magnetic resonance
NT	nortriptyline
OAc	acetyl
Pa	pascal (1 torr = 133 Pa)
PA	proton affinity
PD	plasma desorption
PDMS	plasma desorption mass spectrometry
pGlu	pyroglutamic acid

PITC	phenylisothiocyanate
PTH	phenylthiohydantion
PZQ	praziquantel
Q	quadrupole mass analyzer
QET	quasi-equilibrium theory
rDA	retro Diels–Alder reaction
RIA	radio-immune assay
RIMS	reaction-interface mass spectrometry
SDS	sodium dodecyl sulfate
SDS-PAGE	sodium dodecyl sulfate polyacrylamide gel electrophoresis
SFSU	specific functional structural unit
SIM	selected-ion monitoring
SIMS	secondary ion mass spectrometry
TBDMS	t-butyldimethylsilyl
TFA	trifluoroacetate
TFAI	trifluoroacetylimidazole
THC	tetrahydrocannabinol
TLC	thin-layer chromatography
TMAH	trimethylanilinium hydroxide
TMCS	trimethylchlorosilane
TMIPS	cyclotetramethylene isopropylsilyl
TMS	trimethylsilyl
TMTBS	cyclotetramethylene-t-butylsilyl
TOF	time of flight
TPCK	N-tosyl-L-phenylalanine chloromethyl ketone
TSP	thermospray
TSQ	triple-stage quadrupole
tyv	tyvelose
u	mass unit
UV	ultraviolet
VDMS	vinyldimethylsilyl
VPA	valproic acid

METHODS OF BIOCHEMICAL ANALYSIS

Volume 34

Mass Spectrometry: An Introduction

ROBERT J. ANDEREGG, *Department of Chemistry, University of Maine, Orono, Maine*

---

1. INTRODUCTION

When faced with a complex problem, there is a natural tendency to break it down into simpler, more manageable parts and to study these parts individually. Once the component parts are understood, one is a long way toward understanding the whole. It is no surprise to learn that when early chemists and biochemists sought to determine the structures of complex biomolecules, they frequently resorted to a "divide and conquer" strategy, chemically breaking the molecule down into smaller parts whose structures could be more easily deduced. This is the basic idea behind the technique of mass spectrometry (MS) as used for the structure determination of unknowns. If one can break a molecule down into smaller pieces, identify the fragments, and postulate how they fit together, the problem can be solved.

Since its discovery in 1912, MS has developed into one of the most powerful and versatile methods available for the study of biomolecules. Over the years, MS has been applied not only to problems of structure determination, but to everything from calcium metabolism to enzyme kinetics. It is unparalleled in its capacity to establish molecular weights of biomolecules, even those larger than 10,000 dalton. Analytical methods involving MS have been reported with detection limits in the femtogram (10^{-15} g) and attomole (10^{-18} mol) range. Of course, MS provides a superb method of gaining structural information, even to the extent of sequencing peptides (chapter 3) and complex carbohydrates (chapter 2).

This chapter will introduce this remarkable method, explain what it is and how it can be applied to so many diverse biochemical problems. Succeeding chapters will detail and illustrate some of these applications.

For the novice, the most basic question is, "What is MS?" MS can be defined as a spectrometric technique wherein one produces charged molecules and molecular fragments, and measures the mass (or mass-to-charge ratio) of each. The definition is deceptive, however, because by clever application of MS, one can obtain for more than molecular weight and structural information. MS is routinely used for the rapid identification or verification of structures. It is frequently used in quantitation. It can be used to study reactions in the gas phase, free from solvent effects. It can provide data on the physical properties of molecules, such as their ionization potentials and proton affinities, from which one can predict molecular reactivity.

How does MS work? Basically there are three important conditions that must be met. (1) The analyte molecules must be transferred to the gas phase at a relatively low pressure. This keeps them from colliding and reacting prematurely. (2) A charge must be placed on the molecule, a process called *ionization*. While uncharged, gaseous molecules move randomly and aimlessly through space. Once ionized, they have a "handle" by which their motion (and that of their charged fragments) can be controlled. (3) Finally, energy must be supplied to break some of the covalent bonds holding the molecule together. This is in excess of the energy required for ionization, but is essential to obtain the structural information desired. Mass spectrometers differ in the way they accomplish these goals, but all three conditions are generally met.

There are instrumental components common to all mass spectrometers, as shown schematically in Fig. 1. The basic design requires an *ion source*, where ionization, and sometimes fragmentation, take place. The ions then must be separated according to their mass or mass-to-charge ratio in the *mass analyzer*. The *detector* detects the ions, measuring the relative abundance of each. Usually a *data system* records, processes, and stores the information. The *vacuum system* maintains a low pressure in the instrument; the low pressure minimizes ion/molecule collisions so that the ions can move through the instrument in a well-defined path. To facilitate sample introduction, an *inlet system* provides a link between the outside world (including chromatographs) and the inside of the mass spectrometer. The sections that follow describe each of these components in more detail and discuss the basic approaches to spectral interpretation. Several monographs can be recommended that cover various aspects of mass spectrometry in detail. McLafferty's text (1) is perhaps the best available on mass spectral interpretation. Books by Watson (2), McFadden (3), and Chapman (4) deal with instrumentation and are extremely readable, even for the beginner.

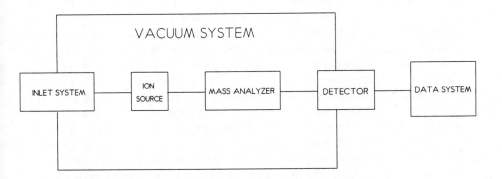

Fig. 1. Block diagram of a typical mass spectrometer.

2. INSTRUMENTATION

2.1. Ion Sources

2.1.1. ELECTRON IONIZATION

The ionization process is the most important step in the entire mass-spectrometric experiment; without it, nothing else can happen. Consider first the simplest and historically most popular ionization method—bombardment of the analyte molecules with a beam of energetic electrons. This is referred to as "electron ionization," "electron impact," or simply EI. Assume for the moment that the analyte molecules are in the gas phase at the appropriate pressure [typically 10^{-4}–10^{-3} Pa (1 Pa = 1 N/m^2 = 0.0075 Torr)]. Sample vaporization will be discussed subsequently. The goal in EI is twofold: to put a charge on the molecule so its path can be directed and to put sufficient energy into the molecule to break some of its chemical bonds. The energy of the electron beam accomplishes both objectives.

The process of ionization can be represented by Eq. 1,

$$M + e^- \rightarrow M^{\ddagger} + 2e^- \tag{1}$$

where M is the analyte molecule and e^- is an energetic electron. Upon collision, the analyte loses an electron and becomes a particle with an odd number of electrons and a positive charge. This is called a *radical cation*, and it has important consequences when one begins to consider fragmentation pathways and mechanisms. The $^+$ symbolizes the charge and the · represents the unpaired electron or *radical*.

The energy required for ionization is called the ionization energy or ionization potential. For most organic molecules, the ionization energy is between 7 and 15 electron volts (eV). A word about energy units is in order. Because of the way mass-spectrometric experiments are conducted, mass spectrometrists usually refer to energies in terms of eV, rather than kilocalories per mole or kilojoules per mole; 1 eV is equal to 23.06 kcal/mol or 96.49 kJ/mol. The ionization energy of a molecule is a function of a number of molecular parameters, including the molecular orbitals of the molecule and the capacity of the molecule to stabilize a positive charge. (The case of negative charges will be taken up in Section 4.2.)

If the energy of the electron that collides with the analyte molecule is less than the ionization energy, no ionization occurs. The energy of the electron beam must be at least 7–15 eV, just to cause ionization. Additionally, to break chemical bonds, there must be sufficient excess energy (called *excess internal energy*) available. Covalent bonds in organic molecules are of the order of 4–13 eV (100–300 kcal/mol). In early experiments in which the energy of the electron beam was varied, it was observed that the ion abundances became stable and reproducible at energies greater than about 35–40 eV. Most mass spectra found in spectral libraries have been recorded at an electron energy of 70 eV, an arbitrary value that has become the standard for EI methods.

The region of the mass spectrometer where ionization takes place is the ion source. A diagram of an EI ion source is shown in Fig. 2. As current passes through the filament (cathode), the temperature of the metal rises and electrons are emitted. These electrons are accelerated toward the target (anode) at energies determined by the voltage applied between the filament and the collector or the ion source. Analyte molecules introduced into this beam are bombarded by electrons, picking up sufficient energy for ionization and fragmentation to occur. Usually only a small fraction (less than 0.1%) of the analyte molecules are ionized in EI. The rest are pumped away into the vacuum system. Whenever an analyte molecule is ionized, it is quickly extracted from the ion-source region by a set of electric fields that accelerate and focus the ions. These electric fields, known as the *ion optics*, also guide the ions into the mass analyzer, where they are separated according to their mass-to-charge ratio. The time for the entire process is very short. Ionization itself occurs on the order of 10^{-16} sec, faster than the vibrations of the atoms that make up the molecule. There is sufficient time for the energy to redistribute itself throughout all of the vibrational modes of the molecule before fragmentation occurs. The excited molecule reaches a state of "quasi-equilibrium." The theory of the molecular decomposition was formulated in 1952 by Rosenstock et al. (5) using what is referred to as *quasi-equilibrium theory* (QET).

Because the pressure in the ion source is very low, ionized molecules do not usually collide with walls or other molecules before breaking apart. The decompositions that produce the fragments observed in EI–MS are, for the most

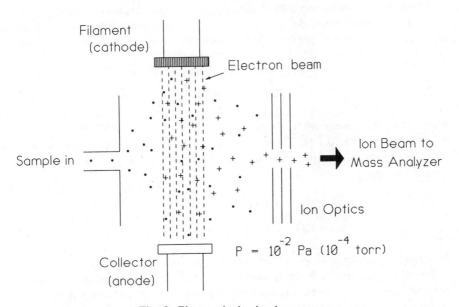

Fig. 2. Electron-ionization ion source.

part, *unimolecular*. Although ions spend only a few microseconds in the source, most of the fragment ions are produced by decompositions during that time.

EI continues to be a popular method of ionization for a number of reasons. Instrumentally, the ion source is simple, easy to heat, and easy to clean. One has good control of the ion beam and of the electron energy that is producing the ions. More importantly, the EI mass spectrum usually includes signals from at least some intact molecules and some fragments, so structural information is readily available, if one can interpret it. Finally, virtually all collections of standard mass spectra have been recorded under EI conditions, so if one wants to compare an unknown spectrum with those of standards, there is a common basis for comparison.

2.1.2. CHEMICAL IONIZATION

The ionization of a molecule by collision with a 70-eV electron is a little like cutting your fingernails with a chainsaw: it gets the job done, but may do a lot of damage in the process. Often, not enough of the molecule survives to indicate the molecular weight of the compound. As this is one of the most valuable pieces of information sought, it is not surprising that considerable effort has gone into the development of gentler methods of ionization. The foremost of these less energetic, or *softer* ionization modes, is *chemical ionization* (CI). As the name implies, ionization of the analyte in CI is a result of a gas-phase chemical reaction, rather than bombardment by energetic electrons. The reactions were first observed in EI mass spectrometers when the pressure became high enough for ion–molecule collisions (and reactions) to occur.

Chemical ionization using methane, one of the most popular of *reagent gases*, illustrates the principles. At low pressure in a mass-spectrometer ion source, methane bombarded with energetic electrons produces the expected fragments:

$$CH_4 + e^- \rightarrow CH_4^{\ddagger} + 2e^- \tag{2}$$

$$CH_4^{\ddagger} \rightarrow CH_3^+ + H\cdot \tag{3}$$

These are called *primary ions*. If the pressure in the ion source is allowed to increase to about 10–200 Pa (0.1–1.5 Torr), these primary ions will collide with neutral methane molecules. A series of chemical reactions takes place and a set of *secondary ions* is formed:

$$CH_4^{\ddagger} + CH_4 \rightarrow CH_5^+ + CH_3\cdot \tag{4}$$

$$CH_3^+ + CH_4 \rightarrow C_2H_5^+ + H_2 \tag{5}$$

This stable population of gas-phase ions and electrons is called a *plasma*.

In 1966, Munson and Field (6) observed that if a small amount of some other gas (the analyte) is present, a remarkably useful phenomenon occurs. Collisions of the secondary ions and the analyte molecules result in gas-phase acid–base chemical reactions. CH_5^+ is a very strong gas-phase Bronsted acid, and wants desperately to give up a proton to any likely acceptor. Most organic molecules can serve as proton acceptors:

$$CH_5^+ + M \rightarrow CH_4 + (M + H)^+ \tag{6}$$

The protonated molecule now carries a charge and is subject to all the forces we might want to apply. The energy of the ionization process is equal to the energy of the proton-transfer reaction. The analyte molecule is present at such low concentration relative to the methane that it rarely collides with a 70-eV electron.

The energy of the reaction depicted by Eq. 6 can be calculated by considering the relative tendency of the CH_5^+ to give up a proton and the tendency of the analyte M to accept the proton, a property known as *proton affinity* (PA). The

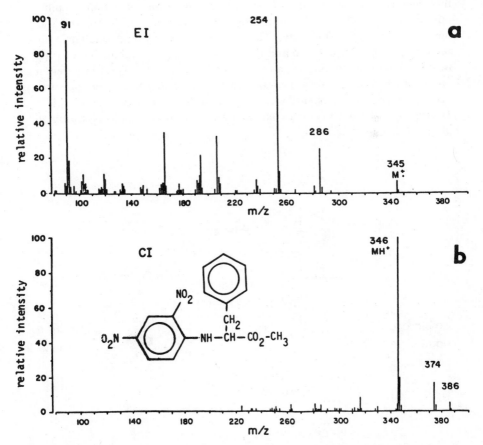

Fig. 3. (*a*) EI and (*b*) methane CI mass spectra of the 2,4-dinitrophenyl derivative of phenylalanine methyl ester (mol wt 345).

energy of the reaction is simply the difference between the PA of methane and the PA of the analyte, M. For example, acetone has a PA of 8.7 eV, compared to methane's PA of 5.5 eV. If a small amount of acetone is introduced into a CI plasma of methane, the proton transfer from CH_5^+ to acetone would generate 3.2 eV (8.7 eV − 5.5 eV) of "excess energy" that can go into the breaking of the covalent bonds (fragmentation) of the protonated acetone molecule. This is substantially less than the 15 eV or so of excess energy that result from the ionization of acetone by EI. The lower excess energy means that a larger proportion of the acetone will remain as $(M+H)^+$, with production of fewer fragment ions than in the corresponding analysis by EI–MS. Figure 3 compares the EI and methane CI mass spectra of the 2,4-dinitrophenyl derivative of phenylalanine methyl ester. Although the molecular ion (m/z 345) is of low abundance in the EI spectrum, the protonated molecule (m/z 346) is the most abundant ion, or *base peak*, of the CI spectrum.

Instrumentally, the CI ion source is much like the EI source. The major difference is that the pressure of reagent gas inside the ionization chamber is approximately 100 Pa (0.8 Torr), while the pressure outside (in the source housing) is 10^{-3} Pa (10^{-5} Torr). This is accomplished by using small holes to let the sample and electrons into and the ions out of the ionization chamber. [The mass analyzer is maintained at a pressure of 10^{-4} Pa (10^{-6} Torr) by differential pumping.] Figure 4 shows a diagram of CI ion source. The filament operates as before, ionizing the methane, which reacts to form the secondary ion plasma. Subsequent collisions of the secondary ions with analyte molecules ultimately protonate the analyte.

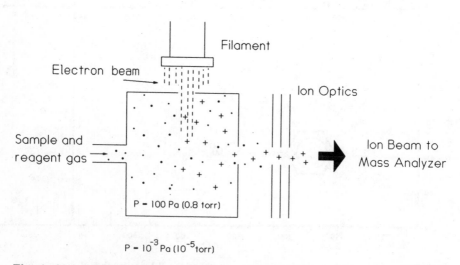

Fig. 4. CI ion source. Note that the pressure in the enclosed ionization chamber is approximately 10^5 times higher than that in an EI source.

2.1.3. DESORPTIVE IONIZATION

Although CI is an excellent method of soft ionization, it still requires that the analyte be in the gas phase. This restriction limits analysis to those compounds with an appreciable vapor pressure. A tremendous number of organic molecules, including some of the most interesting classes of biomolecules, are excluded. Amino acids, carbohydrates, nucleosides, and peptides all are relatively involatile. By the time one supplies sufficient heat to evaporate these molecules, enough energy is present to break the covalent bonds that hold the molecule together. Pyrolysis (thermal degradation) competes with evaporation.

Since the early 1970s, mass spectrometrists have sought to develop means to get molecules ionized and into the gas phase without extensive heating. This process is known as *desorptive ionization* (7). One of the early attempts was to place the involatile sample directly in the plasma of a CI ion source. *Desorptive chemical ionization* (DCI) produces CI-like ions, primarily $(M+H)^+$, from analytes that would normally decompose before evaporation. The soft ionization of CI is preserved, but the requirement of volatility is removed.

Another method of desorptive ionization is based on the presence of a strong electric field. In the presence of such a field, gas-phase molecules ionize in a process called *field ionization*. If an involatile sample is coated on a sharp point, a thin wire, or a blade and placed in the vicinity of a large electric potential (several kilovolts), desorptive ionization [*field desorption* (FD)] takes place. Both DCI and FD are more efficient if a small electric current is passed through the wire upon which the sample is coated. Although FD is effective for certain classes of molecules, it is often unpredictable. The analyte ion beam may be unstable, leading to problems of focusing the beam into the mass analyzer. For many compounds, FD does not give any signal at all from the sample.

Still another desorptive method comes from the field of surface science. If a solid surface is bombarded with a beam of energetic ions, material on the surface is sputtered into the gas phase. Beginning in the 1970s, *secondary ions MS* (SIMS) was used to study inorganic surfaces. The secondary ions observed were primarily derived from atoms of the metal making up the target. Benninghoven et al. (8) realized that there was great potential in SIMS for the study of involatile organic molecules as well. When amino acids were coated onto a surface and then bombarded with argon ions having an energy of several kilovolts, a range of molecular fragments, from intact molecules to small molecular debris, was observed.

By its very nature, SIMS is destructive to the surface being bombarded. If the mechanism for getting ions and molecules into the gas phase is by molecular sputtering under the impact of a beam of fast-moving particles, the surface will be abraded at the point of impact. Particularly for the case of an organic analyte coated on a solid support, the consequence of this is a strong secondary ion beam for a short time, but as the sample is worn away, the signal decreases and ultimately disappears. As this sample abrasion can be very fast (a few seconds), it is difficult to acquire a complete mass spectrum using a scanning instrument or to obtain precise mass measurements that require a more stable ion beam.

In 1981, Barber and coworkers (9) found a way to overcome the problem of signal transience. They reasoned that although a solid sample was worn away by the ion beam, the surface of a liquid target would be "refreshed" continuously. More precisely, as the surface of the liquid is abraded, other liquid flows back to replace it, presenting the impinging beam with fresh material. Barber used glycerol as the liquid *matrix* and dissolved or suspended the organic analyte in it. Glycerol, because of its low vapor pressure, is not readily evaporated by the vacuum system over the time period of sample analysis. When the glycerol surface is bombarded, ions from the glycerol and from the analyte are observed in a very stable secondary ion beam, lasting for many minutes. Barber also replaced the primary beam of ions (the beam impinging upon the surface) with a beam of energetic neutral atoms. Because of its simplicity and power, the technique, called *fast-atom bombardment* (FAB), continues to generate a great deal of excitement in the MS community.

The instrumental design of a FAB or SIMS ion source is diagrammed in Fig. 5. The analyte, either dry or dissolved in the liquid matrix, is coated on a surface of stainless steel, copper, or silver. The primary beam is introduced at right angles to the direction of the mass analyzer. As secondary ions are sputtered off the surface, they are accelerated and focused into the mass analyzer in the usual manner.

Nuclear physicists contributed yet another desorptive ionization method for MS. If the keV energies of SIMS and FAB work well for sputtering material into the gas phase, why not even more energetic beams? Nuclear-fission fragments, resulting from the spontaneous decay of radioactive nuclei, have energies of several MeV. When these particles hit a surface, all the momentum is transferred to the surface in an extremely short time, giving rise to local temperatures of several thousand degrees. This sets up a shock wave that vaporizes, ionizes, and sputters material even some distance away from the site of impact. The most commonly used element for this *plasma desorption* MS is ^{252}Cf, with a half-life of 2.64 years. Each fission event produces a burst of ions from the sample.

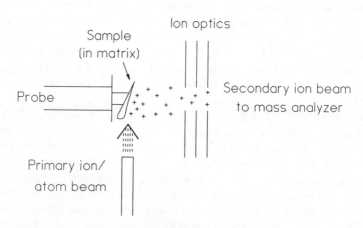

Fig. 5. SIMS/FAB ion source.

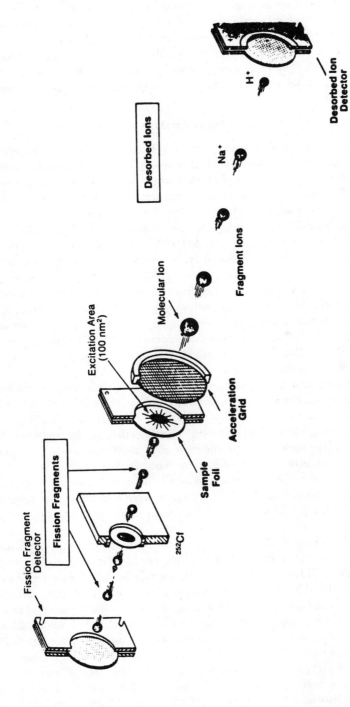

Fig. 6. Schematic of a ^{252}Cf plasma desorption experiment. (Reproduced with permission from Ref. 10.)

11

The instrumental setup (Fig. 6) is similar to that of SIMS, except that the ^{252}Cf is positioned behind a foil upon which the sample is coated. Because the ion beam comes in very short bursts (a few picoseconds), the system is ideal for time-of-flight mass analyzers (see subsequent discussion), the analyzer of choice for this ionization method. The mass spectra from ^{252}Cf plasma desorption resemble those of SIMS or FAB, with $M^{\ddagger}$, $(M+H)^{+}$, or $(M+\text{cation})^{+}$ ions dominating.

2.2. Mass Analyzers

Having generated the analyte ions by some mechanism, it is necessary to separate the ions and measure the mass of each. The ion optics focus and guide the beam into the mass analyzer. It is here that the charge placed on the molecules comes into play. It allows the particles to be manipulated in a number of ways. Although it is the mass of each molecular fragment that is of interest, it is generally the mass-to-charge ratio that is measured. It is impossible to differentiate between a fragment of mass 200 with a $+2$ charge and a fragment of mass 100 with a $+1$ charge. Fortunately, however, doubly charged species are not common for small molecules ($<m/z$ 2000), because it is energetically unfavorable to place two like charges so close together in space. The vast majority of the ions in MS are only singly charged, so whether one speaks of mass or mass-to-charge ratio becomes moot. Mass spectrometrists currently favor the notation m/z for this ratio, rather than the m/e seen in older works. The symbol e is reserved for the actual columbic charge on an electron, while z represents an integral number of these charges.

There are a variety of ways to separate ions by mass, depending on the forces used to direct them. For any mass analyzer, however, there are three important considerations to keep in mind: the *mass range*, the *scan speed*, and the *mass resolution*. Mass range is the workable range of masses that can be separated. This usually refers to the highest practicable mass, since most mass analyzers perform well for very low masses. Scan speed is, as the name implies, the rate at which the mass range can be swept. A fast scan speed is desirable if one is analyzing a rapidly changing system, for example, the eluate from a capillary gas chromatograph. A slow scan speed and a constant sample pressure might be used to obtain a very precise measurement of mass.

Mass resolution refers to the capacity to differentiate ions with very similar masses. Mathematically it is expressed as $m/\Delta m$. The usual definition of resolution is shown in Fig. 7. If two equally sized peaks are side-by-side, they are said to be resolved when the valley between them is 10% of the height of either one. *Unit mass resolution* means that one can differentiate between adjacent integral masses throughout the mass range. That is, one could distinguish m/z 100 from 101 and m/z 874 from 875. *High resolution* usually implies that one can differentiate ions that differ by only a small fraction (0.01) of a mass unit. As an example, ions with the formulas $C_{18}H_{36}O$ and $C_{17}H_{32}O_2$ have the same *nominal mass*, or mass expressed to the nearest integer, 268. If, however, the mass is expressed more precisely, the two ions have masses of 268.277 and 268.240, respectively. To

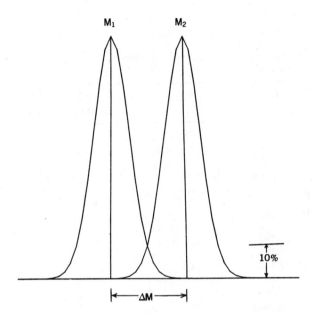

Fig. 7. Mass resolution to 10% valley definition; the "valley" or point of overlap is 10% of the maximal peak height. M_1 and M_2 are resolved adjacent masses.

differentiate these, a mass spectrometer would need a resolution of $R = 268/0.037$ ($R = m/\Delta m$), or about $R = 7200$. The precise mass values of some of the more common elements are listed in Table 1. These are based on the definition of the most abundant isotope of carbon as 12.00000.

2.2.1. MAGNETIC-SECTOR (AND DOUBLE-FOCUSING) MASS SPECTROMETERS

One of the forces that can be used to direct the motion of ions in the mass spectrometer is that of a magnetic field. When charged particles encounter a magnetic field perpendicular to their direction of motion, they begin to move in a circular orbit. Historically, the first mass spectrometers used magnetic fields to move the ions. A diagram of a simple *magnetic-sector* instrument is shown in Fig. 8a. The ions are accelerated out of the ion source with a kinetic energy ($mv^2/2$) supplied by the accelerating electric field V. Therefore,

$$zeV = mv^2/2 \qquad (7)$$

where e is the charge on an electron, z is the integral number of such charges on the ion of interest, v is the velocity, and m is the mass of the ion. When the ions enter the magnetic field (H), their trajectories bend. To describe a circular path,

TABLE 1

Accurate Masses and Natural Abundances of Common Elements[a]

Element	Mass	Percentage of Natural Abundance
Hydrogen		
^{1}H	1.007825	99.985
^{2}H	2.0140	0.015
Carbon		
^{12}C	12.00000	98.90
^{13}C	13.003355	1.10
Nitrogen		
^{14}N	14.003074	99.63
^{15}N	15.000108	0.37
Oxygen		
^{16}O	15.994915	99.762
^{17}O	16.999131	0.038
^{18}O	17.999160	0.200
Fluorine		
^{19}F	18.998403	100.0
Sodium		
^{23}Na	22.989767	100.0
Silicon		
^{28}Si	27.976927	92.23
^{29}Si	28.976495	4.67
^{30}Si	29.973770	3.10
Phosphorus		
^{31}P	30.973762	100.0
Sulfur		
^{32}S	31.972070	95.02
^{33}S	32.971456	0.75
^{34}S	33.967866	4.21
Chlorine		
^{35}Cl	34.968852	75.77
^{37}Cl	36.965903	24.23
Argon		
^{40}Ar	39.962384	99.60
Bromine		
^{79}Br	78.918336	50.69
^{81}Br	80.916289	49.31
Iodine		
^{127}I	126.904473	100.0

[a]Data from *CRC Handbook of Chemistry and Physics*, 66th ed., R.C. Weast, Ed., CRC Press, Boca Raton, FL, 1985–1986.

a

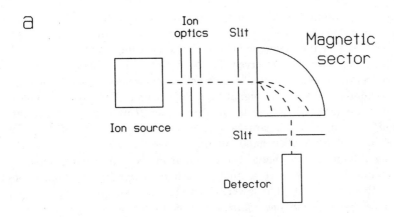

b

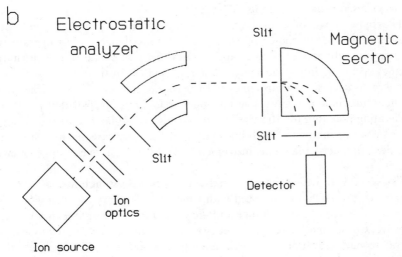

Fig. 8. (*a*) Diagram of a magnetic-sector mass analyzer and (*b*) double-focusing (electrostatic/magnetic-sector) mass analyzer.

the force the magnetic field exerts on the ion must exactly balance the centripetal force:

$$Hzev = mv^2/r \qquad (8)$$

where r is the radius of the circle described. Rearranging, one can show that

$$m/z = eH^2r^2/2V \qquad (9)$$

For any given magnetic field strength and accelerating voltage, only ions of a given mass-to-charge ratio will be allowed to traverse the flight tube and reach the detector. If either the magnetic field or the accelerating voltage is changed, ions of a different mass will be observed. To collect a complete mass spectrum, one wants to collect the ion current at all m/z values, so one would change H (or V) in a regular fashion and record the signal from the detector. This process is called *scanning* the mass range. It is possible to vary either H or V to obtain a mass spectrum. If H is varied in a linear fashion, the mass scale is nonlinear (m/z varies as H^2, see Eq. 9). On the other hand, all ions receive the same "push" from the accelerating voltage. If V is changed in a regular manner, the change in m/z is linear, but heavier ions receive a smaller push than lighter ions (m/z varies inversely with V, see Eq. 9). The lower the accelerating voltage for a given ion, the poorer will be its *transmission efficiency* (defined as the percentage of the ions formed that actually reach the detector). If the transmission goes down at high mass, there is an apparent decrease in sensitivity at high mass as well, a phenomenon known as *mass discrimination*. Each method of scanning has its advantages and disadvantages, but usually *voltage scanning* (vary V) is used if the mass range of interest is small (less than 20 mass units, or u), and *magnetic field scanning* is used if the mass range is large.

The mass range of a magnetic-sector instrument is limited by practical considerations in the choice of H, V, and r. It is dangerous to operate the accelerating voltage higher than about 10 kV because of the risk of discharge (arcing) occurring in the ion source. The radius of the instrument is usually less than 1 m to keep the spectrometer from becoming too unwieldy. Typically, a magnetic instrument might have an upper mass limit of 3500 daltons at full accelerating potential (4–10 kV). This mass range could be increased by using a lower V, but at the cost of high mass sensitivity. In any case, even with special high-field magnets, magnetic instruments rarely have a mass range of over 10,000.

The speed with which the mass analyzer can sweep through its mass range is determined primarily by the speed with which one can vary the magnetic field. Magnetic fields resist rapid change and are subject to hysteresis if scan speeds are excessive. Consequently, most magnetic-sector instruments are limited to scans of several seconds duration, although modern laminated-magnet technology is improving on this limit.

The mass resolution of magnetic-sector instruments is ultimately determined by the spread in kinetic energies of ions of the same m/z. This spread is the result of a number of factors including the range of kinetic energies that the analyte molecules had before ionization, the variation in energy imparted by electronic collisions, and the finite width of the region in space where ionization occurs. Small apertures, called *slits*, in the path of the ion beam can select a portion of the ion beam containing ions with similar energies. This selection causes a loss of sensitivity, however, because a large fraction of the ions, those that have the appropriate mass, but kinetic energies other than the ones selected, are discarded. Some compromise must usually be struck between acceptable sensitivity and acceptable mass resolution. For a single magnetic sector, a working mass resolution of 5,000–10,000 is typical.

If some way can be found to narrow the range of kinetic energies for ions of a given mass, the resolution can be greatly improved. This is frequently achieved by the addition of a second field, an electric field or *electrostatic analyzer* (ESA), which sends *isomass* ions (ions of the same m/z) of differing energy through compensating flight paths. Figure 8b shows one such arrangement. The ESA precedes the magnet, and focuses the ions based on their kinetic energy. Now a more uniformly energetic beam enters the magnetic sector, and higher mass resolution is possible. (If the ESA precedes the magnetic sector, the instrument is said to have "forward geometry"; "reverse geometry" indicates that the magnetic sector precedes the ESA. Both types have their own advantages.) With these types of *double-focusing* instruments (11), resolution of greater than 100,000 is not unusual. In practical terms, a resolution of 100,000 is equivalent to saying that at m/z 1000, one can still differentiate m/z 1000.00 from m/z 1000.01. Such precision is invaluable in helping to determine not only the mass, but also the elemental composition, of ions.

A variety of different arrangements of the ESA and magnetic field have been described for various purposes. The ESA can be placed before or after the magnet, or both before and after. For a complete discussion, the reader is referred to Ref. 11.

2.2.2. QUADRUPOLES

Another class of mass analyzer is based on the interaction of the ion beam with an oscillating (radio-frequency) electric field. The *quadrupole* mass filter is representative. As the name implies, the device consists of a set of four pencillike electrodes, arranged as in Fig. 9. Opposite pairs of the "rods" are electrically connected. Two electrical potentials, one dc and one ac, are applied to the rods. The total potential difference, V_{tot} is a function of time and can be expressed as

$$V_{tot} = U \pm V_0 \cos(\omega t) \tag{10}$$

where U is the applied dc potential, V_0 is the applied ac potential, ω is the angular frequency, and t is the time. As ions are accelerated into this varying electric field, their motion is influenced in a very complex way. With proper selection of U and V_0, only ions of one m/z will oscillate in a stable path and be transmitted through the quadrupole; all other ions will either collide with a rod and be lost or will have a unstable trajectory and will move out of the analyzer between the rods.

The quadrupole has a number of attractive features. The devices are compact (individual rods are usually about 1 cm in diameter and perhaps 10 cm long), relatively inexpensive, and very rugged. Because the ions must experience many cycles of the radio-frequency field for effective filtering, considerably less voltage is used for acceleration. With a magnetic sector, accelerating voltages of

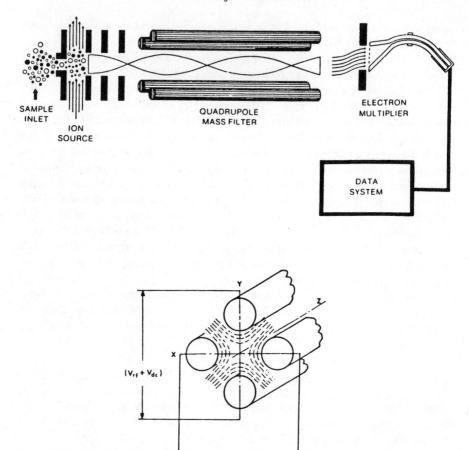

Fig. 9. Schematic diagrams of a quadrupole mass analyzer. (Reproduced with permission of Finnigan MAT and VG Instruments Corp., respectively.)

4–10,000 V are standard; with quadrupoles, acceleration is usually 5–30 V. Consequently, one does not have to be concerned with high voltages in the ion source. Transmission of ions through the mass analyzer is generally higher with a quadrupole than with a magnetic instrument.

One can scan the mass range of the quadrupole by either holding ω constant and varying U and V_0 or by holding U and V_0 constant and varying ω. In most cases, U and V_0 are varied, but in such a way that the ratio U/V_0 remains a constant. Because there are no magnetic fields, scan speeds can be very fast, requiring a second or less to scan the full mass range.

The mass range of a quadrupole is somewhat lower than that for magnetic instruments, as is the mass resolution. Mass resolution is determined by the number of oscillations an ion undergoes in its journey through the mass analyzer; the more oscillations, the greater the mass resolution. Lowering the accelerating voltage gives the ions lower velocities, so they take longer to traverse the analyzer and, consequently, undergo more oscillations. However, as with magnetic instruments, the smaller accelerating voltage also means poorer transmission of ions and a loss of sensitivity at high mass. Standard quadrupole instruments usually can achieve unit mass resolution up to mass 1000, although progress is being made with some quadrupole instruments for ions with masses up to 4000.

Early quadrupoles (prior to the mid 1970s) were built with rods of circular cross section because they were easier to machine. These quadrupoles suffered from severe mass discrimination. As the technology to manufacture rods with hyperbolic cross section matured, mass discrimination in quadrupoles became less of a problem, and, today, the mass spectrum from a properly tuned quadrupole is indistinguishable from one obtained on a magnetic instrument. Because of their relatively low cost and small size, quadrupole mass spectrometers are extremely popular in environmental and clinical laboratories. For a more complete discussion, the reader is referred to a recent review by Dawson (12).

Still another mass analyzer based on electric field interaction with the ion beam is the *ion trap detector* (ITD). This rather interesting device is diagrammed in Fig. 10. As in the quadrupole, an oscillating electric field, composed of dc and ac potentials, is applied to the cell, this time between the ring electrode and the end caps. A beam of electrons ionizes molecules in the cell. The ions move under the influence of the applied field, but their motion is confined to the dimensions of the cell. As the dc or ac component of the field is changed (or both are changed in concert), the motion of ions of some masses become unstable and half of these ions are ejected out the bottom of the cell. An electron multiplier detects the ions and produces the signal current. In the quadrupole mass analyzer, ions with stable trajectories are transmitted to the detector and ions with unstable trajectories are lost. In contrast, in the ion trap, ions with stable trajectories remain trapped in the cell, and ions are detected only when their trajectories are made unstable. Detailed reviews of the ion trap are available (13, 14).

The ion trap is similar in its performance characteristics to the quadrupole mass analyzer. Scan speeds can be very fast (< 1 sec). Transmission of ions, because there are no slits and few places for ions to get lost, is very high. Typical commercial ion traps achieve unit mass resolution up to about 650 daltons. The ion traps are simple and inexpensive, which should make them a popular choice for laboratories with a high volume of samples, such as contract environmental or clinical laboratories. At the present time, however, quadrupoles still outnumber ion traps in these settings.

Ion traps are closely akin to another class of mass analyzers, the ion cyclotrons and Fourier-transform mass spectrometers. Space does not permit their discussion here, but detailed information is available in recent reviews (15, 16).

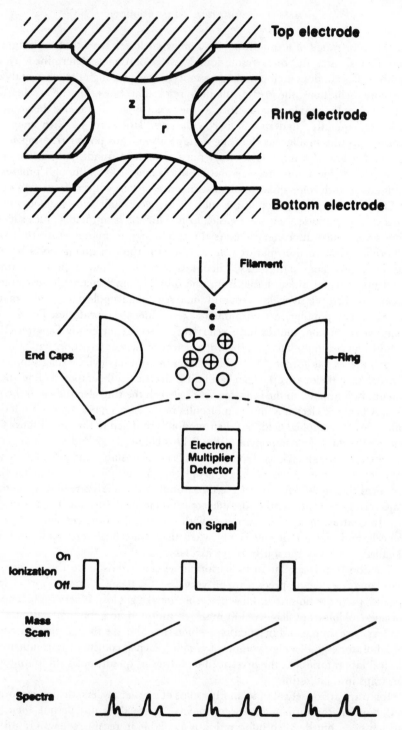

Fig. 10. Cross section and operation of the ion trap detector. (Reproduced with permission of Finnigan MAT Corp.)

2.2.3. TIME-OF-FLIGHT INSTRUMENTS

Perhaps the simplest type of force to act on an ion is no force at all. In the *time-of-flight* mass analyzer, after an initial acceleration out of the ion source, the ions are left to drift down a field-free tube. The basis of mass analysis is measurement of the time required for ions to reach the detector. If all ions carry a $+1$ charge, they will all receive the same kinetic energy when accelerated out of the source:

$$zeV = mv^2/2 \qquad (11)$$

The different masses will result in the corresponding ions traveling with different velocities:

$$v = (2zeV/m)^{1/2} \qquad (12)$$

The time required for an ion to reach the detector will depend only on the length of the *drift tube* (L) and the velocity:

$$t = L/v = (L^2 m/2zeV)^{1/2} \qquad (13)$$

By measuring this time for a known L, z, and V, it is a simple matter to calculate the mass of the ion.

In normal EI ion-source operation for a quadrupole or magnetic-sector analyzer, ions are being formed continuously and are leaving the ion source all the time. Clearly, that mode of operation is unacceptable for time-of-flight analyzers. The ions must all leave the ion source in a single, clean burst. That is, all ions must start the journey at the same, well-defined time. There are two methods of achieving this. One can turn the filament on for a very short period of time and then turn it off again. A pulse of ions is formed when the filament is on, and these ions are accelerated toward the detector as soon as they are formed. Alternatively, the filament can be left on all the time and the accelerating potential V can be turned on briefly and then turned off. In this fashion, ions are being formed all the time, but are only accelerated toward the detector in the brief interval when the accelerator is on.

Regardless of the method chosen, the pulsing can be repeated as soon as all ions from the first pulse have reached the detector. It is easy to calculate that this time period should be about 50 μsec for a typical set of instrument parameters: $L = 1$ m, $V = 2000$ V, $m = 1000$. This calculation means that if one measures the time of arrival of ions at the detector for 50 μsec after the initial pulse, one will collect all the ions formed up to mass 1000; a complete mass spectrum in 50 μsec! Scan speeds with the time-of-flight analyzer can be very fast.

The mass range for this analyzer is also impressive. The larger the mass of the ion, the more slowly it will travel. However, if one is willing to wait a sufficient length of time, all ions, regardless of mass, will reach the detector. To extend the mass range, one simply has to wait a little longer between pulses. There is, theoretically, no upper mass limit!

The mass resolution in the time-of-flight mass analyzer is determined by many factors (17) and is perhaps the greatest weakness of this device. Most commercial instruments have a mass resolution of only several hundred. This means that although ions of very high mass can be transmitted, the resolution is often too poor to resolve ions differing by several mass units.

Two additional features of the time-of-flight mass analyzer are worth noting. Nearly all ions formed are detected, that is, the *transmission* of ions from source to detector is very high, much higher than with magnetic or quadrupole instruments. Second, there is an inherent sensitivity advantage to the time-of-flight instrument. In a magnetic or quadrupole mass spectrometer, while some ions are being detected, other ions that are not transmitted through the mass analyzer are being lost. In contrast, ions in a time-of-flight analyzer reach the detector sequentially in time, and can be detected in their turn provided that a sufficiently fast data acquisition system is available (18). No ions are wasted during a mass scan, so potential sensitivity (detector signal/amount of sample ionized) is excellent. However, this sensitivity gain is partially offset because ion formation is not continuous.

It should be evident now why time-of-flight instruments are a logical choice for use with ^{252}Cf plasma-desorption ion sources (Section 2.1.3. and Fig. 6). Each nuclear fission event produces a narrow burst of sample ions that is accelerated and sent down the flight tube. By carefully measuring the time of arrival, a full mass spectrum can be recorded before the next burst of ions leaves the ion source.

2.3.   Detectors

MS detectors serve the function of converting the ion beam into an electrical signal (current or voltage) that can be measured, amplified, and recorded by whatever recording device or data system one happens to be using. Since the ion beam is composed of charged particles moving through space, it is already an electrical current (although not confined to a wire), so this is not a difficult task.

The most direct detector is simply to use an electrode to collect and measure the ion current. This is called a *Faraday cup*. The ion current inside a mass spectrometer is generally quite small (10^{-19}–10^{-12} ampere), so some sort of amplification is often necessary. The Faraday cup is used only in a few specialized types of instruments, when the measurement of ion current with high precision is desired. The precise measurement of isotope ratios is probably the most common application of such instruments.

More often, the amplification is incorporated into the detection using a device called an *electron multiplier*. This is shown diagrammatically in Fig. 11a. Ions arrive at the detector with a certain momentum, carried with them from their acceleration out of the ion source. This momentum is transferred to the first part of the detector as the ions strike it, causing several electrons to be ejected from the surface. The ejected electrons are accelerated by an electrical potential difference toward the next stage, or *dynode*, in a chain. In the acceleration, each electron gains sufficient momentum to eject two or three more electrons when it hits the

a

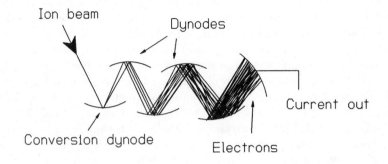

Ion beam

Dynodes

Conversion dynode

Current out

Electrons

b

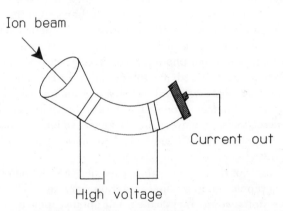

Ion beam

Current out

High voltage

Fig. 11. (*a*) Discrete-stage and (*b*) Channeltron electron multipliers.

next dynode. Electrons are thus cascaded down the chain, increasing in number at each stage. A popular design of this electron multiplier has 14 stages. If an average of three electrons are ejected for each particle impinging on each stage, the total number of electrons at the end of the detector will be 3^{14} or 4.8×10^6 for each ion that originally hit the first dynode. Electron multipliers are characterized by their *gain*:

$$\text{Gain} = \text{current out (electrons)}/\text{current in (ions)} \qquad (14)$$

For the example above, the gain would be simply 4.8×10^6 (electrons)/1 (ion) or 4.8×10^6. Gains of 10^4–10^7 are typical.

A second type of electron multiplier is shown in Fig. 11*b*. The principle of operation is the same as previously discussed, but rather than having discrete stages, the "horn"-type electron multiplier (also called a *Channeltron* multiplier) has a continuous surface. The surface is coated with a resistive material, so a large potential difference applied across it is distributed uniformly from one end to the other. The electron cascade moves from the front of the horn to the back. The horn multipliers are more compact and less expensive than the discrete-stage multipliers, and so are popular in the majority of commercial instruments.

A serious disadvantage of many of the mass analyzers described is that they are serial devices; ions of each m/z are transmitted through the analyzer one after the other. While ions of one m/z are transmitted to the detector, ions of all other m/z ratios are generally lost. (An exception to this is the time-of-flight analyzer.) It is obviously inefficient to be discarding most of the ions one generates, so considerable effort has gone into trying to develop both mass analyzers and detectors that can transmit and detect ions in parallel. These detectors would receive and record ions from a range of m/z simultaneously. Early detectors that did this were based on photographic detection.

Double-focusing mass spectrometers can be designed in such a way that the ions are all focused simultaneously in a plane, rather than sequentially on an exit slit. (This design is called *Mattauch—Herzog geometry*.) If a plate covered with a photographic emulsion is placed in the focal plane, ions impinging on the plate produce a darkening, much like photons in a camera. When the *photoplate* is developed, the lines can be observed, measured, and recorded. The distance of a line from some reference point is related to the m/z of the ions that impinged at that point; the darkness of the line is related to the number of ions of that m/z that were detected. The relationship between line darkness and ion abundance is not a simple one, however, and, usually, abundance information from a photoplate is only semiquantitative.

The resolving power of the photographic detector is a function of the size of grains in the photographic emulsion, but is generally very high. The efficiency of collecting all ions simultaneously is appealing, but photographic development of the photoplate makes it somewhat clumsy. Usually, only 10 or 12 mass spectra can be recorded on a single photoplate, and then the photoplate must be removed from the instrument and developed.

A modern electronic equivalent of the photoplate is the *array detector*. A series of tiny sensing elements are arranged side-by-side in the plane where ions from the mass analyzer are focused. The sensing elements are most often small Channeltron devices that perform in the same way as the electron multiplier previously described. Ions falling anywhere on this plane are detected, and the ion current is stored. The data system can then sample the output from each of the sensing elements sequentially to record the mass spectrum. After sampling an element, the output is reset to zero, and the process begins again. Ion current between sampling intervals is integrated, so no analyte ions are lost. Thus, the array detector can offer impressive sensitivity gains (19). The most serious disadvantage is that most mass analyzers are still designed to transmit ions serially, so the advantage of the array detector cannot be fully utilized.

2.4. Data Systems

The output from the detector is a continuously varying electrical current. It can be temporarily viewed on an oscilloscope, but eventually one would like some more permanent form of data output. While oscillographic chart recorders are sometimes used, the sheer volume of data generated—masses and abundances for hundreds of ions sampled every few seconds—makes a computerized data system almost a necessity. The speed and objectivity of the computer are ideally suited to the huge number of calculations required to convert the output of the electron multiplier into the graphs and tables useful to the analyst.

Figure 12 schematically shows some of the functions of the data system. For a complete discussion, the reader is referred to Chapman's outstanding monograph (4). The current from the electron multiplier is often filtered to remove high-frequency instrument noise, converted to an electrical voltage, and amplified. The baseline can be adjusted if necessary. The continuously varying (analog) signal is transformed to a digital signal (a series of discrete measured voltages) by an *analog-to-digital* (A/D) converter. Modern computers require digital data for all of their calculations. Next, the voltages corresponding to ions of a particular mass must be recognized as a peak. For each such peak, the time corresponding to the center of mass (*centroid*) and the peak area (abundance) must be determined. The time since the start of the scan will be directly related to the mass of the ion, the abundance is related to the number of ions of that mass detected.

In order to assign the proper mass to each peak located, the computer must refer to an internal reference table. This table is constructed by collecting the mass spectrum of a known *calibration compound*, usually a fluorinated alkane or amine. Because the masses of the ions in the calibration compound are known, the times assigned to those peaks can serve as a reference for measurement of peaks of unknown mass. The mass-assigned data are then ready to be stored along with other useful information about the analysis, for example, the total ion current for that spectrum or the retention time of the compound (the time elapsed since the beginning of the analysis). The computer then repeats the whole process on the next scan through the mass range. All of the calculations can be completed in a few milliseconds, so the calculations are performed in *real time*, that is, while the instrument continues to collect data.

In some applications, the analyst knows what he or she is looking for in the sample and simply wants to quantitate how much of that analyte is present. For this type of experiment, the mass analyzer can be set to transmit only one m/z throughout the course of the analysis. An ion is chosen that is characteristic of the analyte, perhaps the molecular ion or the base peak of the mass spectrum. This experiment is called *selected ion monitoring* (SIM). The advantage is that one does not waste time looking at ions not related to the analyte, so a higher proportion of the analysis time is used for recording relevant data. Consequently, the sensitivity of a SIM experiment is better than that of a scanning experiment. Because nonanalyte compounds usually do not have ions at the same m/z as the analyte, the signal-to-noise ratio is excellent.

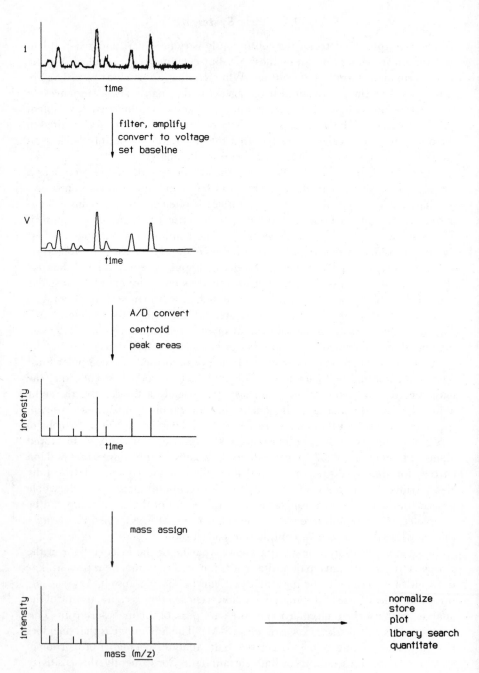

Fig. 12. Some of the functions of the data system.

The disadvantage of SIM is that without the confirming evidence of other analyte ions, one must assume that all observed signals come from the analyte. Compounds other than the analyte that have ions of the same mass as the one monitored can become serious interferants. Data systems can also be programmed to monitor two or more ions characteristic of the analyte. The mass analyzer transmits one m/z for a preselected time, then jumps to a new m/z for a timed interval, and so forth. Selected ion monitoring in this way reduces the likelihood detecting false positives, while still preserving many of the advantages of the technique, such as its high sensitivity.

Commercial mass-spectrometer data systems have a host of specialized programs for *data reduction*, as the processing of "raw" data is called. The most useful programs deal primarily with the data from GC–MS or LC–MS systems, because the volume of data from these experiments would otherwise be overwhelming. A continuously scanning mass spectrometer can collect many hundreds of mass spectra in the course of a 30-min analysis. Some of the software simply normalizes, tabulates, or displays the mass spectra, or sends them to a printer or plotter. If one needs to know where various compounds are eluting from the chromatograph, a *total ion profile* or total ion chromatogram can be reconstructed from a data base of consecutively-recorded mass spectra. This reconstructed total ion chromatogram is actually a plot of the sum of the intensities of all peaks recorded in each mass spectrum graphed as a function of scan number, as in Fig. 13b. When no material is in the ion source, the total ion current is low. As compounds elute from the chromatograph and enter the mass spectrometer, the total ion current increases to a maximum and then decreases again. The total ion chromatogram is analogous to the trace from a flame ionization detector (in GC) or a refractive index detector (in LC). It is *universal* in that it responds to any material that elutes from the chromatograph and is ionized.

More selective plots can be generated after an analysis is complete and the data have been stored in a computer data file. One of the most useful of these is called the *mass chromatogram* (20). This is a graph that shows the abundance of a particular m/z throughout the course of the analysis. It is analogous to the information that would be obtained if the mass analyzer was set to transmit only this m/z during the experiment, as is done in SIM. In contrast, however, the mass chromatogram is a selective display of a small subset of the stored data (one m/z of the many that were collected). Figure 13a shows a mass chromatogram of m/z 91 from an analysis of jet fuel. Although the reconstructed total ion chromatogram (Fig. 13b) is very complex, the mass chromatogram readily shows the location of compounds that have m/z 91 in their mass spectra. This ion is characteristic of toluene (scan 47), xylenes (scans 65, 67), ethyl benzene (scan 73), and several other alkylated benzenes. Mass chromatograms of other m/z values can also be generated to locate other classes of compounds.

The data system can help to improve the quality of the mass spectra. If contaminating ions are present, they can often be removed by *spectral subtraction* or *background subtraction*. For a detailed description of these and other procedures for spectral clean-up, see Ref. 4.

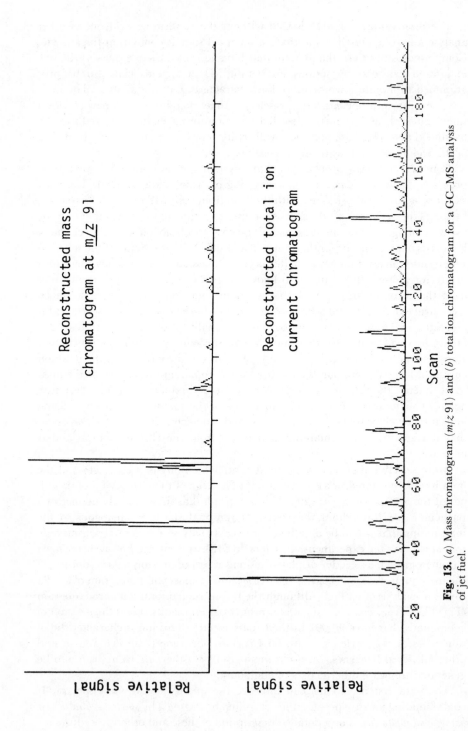

Fig. 13. (a) Mass chromatogram (m/z 91) and (b) total ion chromatogram for a GC–MS analysis of jet fuel.

A key feature of many mass-spectrometer data systems is the software designed to aid the analyst in the interpretation of results. Library searching and automated interpretation schemes fall in this category and are briefly described in Section 3.6.

2.5. Vacuum Systems

One of the most important and most neglected parts of any mass spectrometer is its vacuum system. The vacuum system keeps the pressure inside the instrument low; 10^{-3} Pa $(10^{-5}$ Torr) is typical. [The units of pressure used in mass spectrometry deserve comment. According to SI unit conventions, the proper unit of pressure is the *pascal* (Pa), 1 newton per square meter. One atmosphere is approximately equal to 10^5 Pa. Mass spectrometrists habitually use torr (mm Hg) instead of Pa; 1 Torr equals 133 Pa. Pa will be used in this chapter, but the reader should be warned that torr is far more common in the literature.] The low pressure in the mass spectrometer is necessary for a number of reasons. Electrical filaments can oxidize and burn out if heated in an appreciable pressure of oxygen. Electrical potentials, which can be in the kilovolt range, can cause a discharge in the ion source if the pressure exceeds about 10 Pa (0.1 Torr). The gas present in the mass-spectrometer ion source will contribute to the spectral background (for example, m/z 18, 28, and 32 from water, nitrogen, and oxygen, respectively), and can obscure the low-mass region of the spectrum. However, the most important reason for maintaining a low pressure in the mass spectrometer is to minimize collisions of the ions under analysis. All of the forces used to move the ions in a particular way are useless if the ion is continually colliding with other molecules and surfaces.

The average distance a molecule or ion travels without colliding with another gas molecule is called the *mean free path*. In mass spectrometry, the mean free path should be at least as long as the distance between the ion source and the detector. This ensures that few or no collisions occur. If the sample behaves as an ideal gas, the kinetic molecular theory can be used to show that at 25°C, the mean free path, L_f, in centimeters, is approximately

$$L_f = 0.66/P \tag{15}$$

where P is the pressure in Pa. For a mass spectrometer in which the ion source is 1 m from the detector, the pressure should be lower than 6×10^{-3} Pa $(5 \times 10^{-5}$ Torr). To get the instrument down to low pressure and keep it there, a number of types of vacuum pumps are used. The choice of pump depends to some extent on the applications of the instrument, but a few of the more common types are described below.

2.5.1. VACUUM PUMPS

The most efficient way to reduce the pressure from ambient to the 1 Pa (133 Torr) range is with a rotary mechanical pump, also called a *roughing pump* (see Fig. 14). At these relatively high pressures, the gas inside the vessel acts like a fluid.

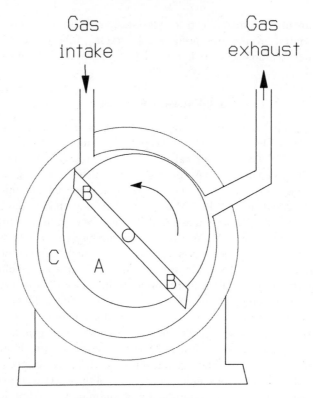

Fig. 14. Rotary pump diagram.

Molecules push each other along, and collisions are very common. (The mean free path is much less than 1 cm.) Movement of the gas under these conditions is referred to as *viscous flow* and is described by fluid dynamics. As the pressure decreases, the mean free path increases until it exceeds the average dimension of the chamber containing the gas. At this point, the gas is more likely to collide with a wall than with another gas molecule, and conditions of *molecular flow* become applicable. The pumping efficiency of the mechanical pump drops dramatically under these conditions, and to achieve lower pressure, some other type of vacuum pump must be used.

A common choice is the diffusion pump diagrammed in Fig. 15. A viscous liquid is heated at the bottom of the pump; the resulting vapor rises up through a central column and sprays out in a supersonic stream through a series of openings around the central column. The walls of the diffusion pump are water-cooled, so the hot fluid condenses on the walls and runs down to the bottom of the pump to begin the cycle again. Molecules of gas colliding with the relatively massive fluid vapor molecules are given a push toward the bottom of the pump where they are removed by a mechanical pump placed in series with the diffusion pump. In earlier times, mercury was used as a pump fluid, but its relatively high vapor

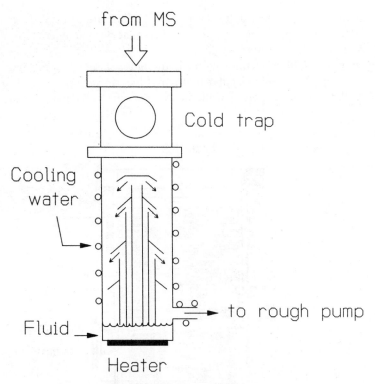

Fig. 15. Diffusion pump diagram.

pressure limited the pressure obtainable by the pump. In addition, mercury vapors can create a health hazard. Most diffusion pumps now use synthetic polymers as fluids. Polyphenyl ethers or silicone-based fluids have extremely low vapor pressures and can withstand the continual heating and cooling cycles for long periods without breaking down.

A serious concern with the use of a diffusion pump is the consequence of a sudden burst of pressure, as might be caused by a loss of vacuum. Under such circumstances, the fluid vapor is driven upward into the mass spectrometer, contaminating surfaces of the ion source, optics, and mass analyzer with which it comes in contact.

The ultimate pressure obtainable with an oil diffusion pump is determined in part by the fluid used and by the presence or absence of a *cold trap*. The cold trap serves the dual function of keeping the pump oil vapors from moving back up into the mass spectrometer (*backstreaming*) and keeping the bulk of the organic sample molecules from contaminating the pump oil. Although this sacrifices some pumping speed, a lower ultimate pressure is achievable, and the pump fluid lasts longer because it is not exposed to potentially reactive materials. Typical pressures obtained with oil diffusion pumps are 10^{-7}–10^{-5} Pa (10^{-9}–10^{-7} Torr) without a cold trap, and perhaps 10^{-9} Pa (10^{-11} Torr) with a cold trap. It should be stressed, however, that the elimination of leaks elsewhere in an operating mass spectrometer relieves much of the burden on the pump and provides the best ultimate pressure.

Another popular high vacuum pump is the *turbomolecular* pump. Figure 16 shows a diagram of a turbomolecular pump and its principle of action. If a gas molecule collides with a stationary wall, the angle of reflection equals the angle of

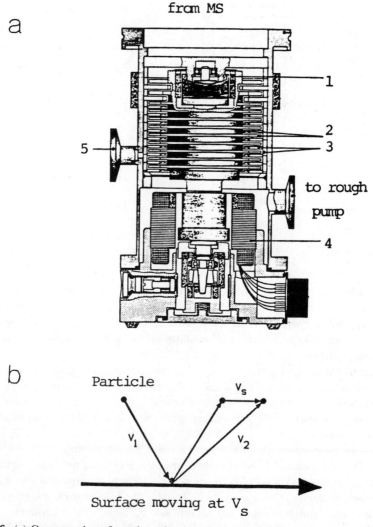

Fig. 16. (*a*) Cutaway view of a turbomolecular pump showing the intake (from MS), the magnetic bearing (1), the rotor (2) and stator (3), the motor (4), and vent connection (5). Gas is exhausted to the roughing pump. (*b*) The principle of operation of the turbomolecular pump. (Reproduced with permission of Balzer's, Inc.)

incidence. If the wall is moving, however, the molecule on reflection is given a slight push in the direction of wall motion. With a turbomolecular pump, a set of fast-moving (90,000 revolutions per minute, 400 m/sec) rotor blades provide moving surfaces with which the gas molecules collide. The motion of the molecules is directed toward the exit of the pump, where a mechanical pump removes gas from the system. The obtainable pressure range of the turbomolecular pump is comparable to that of a diffusion pump.

The turbomolecular pump is popular for several reasons. It has no pump fluid, so there is less mass-spectral background contributed from the pump than is the case with the oil diffusion pump. Additionally, because there is no fluid to heat up and cool down, the pump can start up faster and stop faster for venting than can the diffusion pump. There are disadvantages, as well, however. Because of the tremendous speeds of the rotors, they must be machined to extreme tolerances, making the turbomolecular pumps up to three to four times as expensive as a diffusion pump of comparable pumping speed. Also, the constant high speed wears the pumps out after several years, necessitating replacement. A diffusion pump, with no moving parts, can operate for many years with occasional fluid changes and replacement of the heater.

2.5.2. PRESSURE MEASUREMENT

Although pressure measurement seems like a simple task, 99% of mass spectrometrists have no idea of the exact pressure inside the ion source. In fairness, they have no need to know, as long as the instrument is performing properly, but the fact points out the difficulty of mass-spectrometric pressure measurement.

At pressures down to about 500 Pa (4 Torr), a simple mercury manometer is a suitable pressure-measuring device. The height of a column of mercury can be measured and will be proportional to the pressure of the system, regardless of what gas is present. This is known as a *direct pressure gauge*; pressure measurement is independent of the gas present. It becomes impossible to read precisely the height of a mercury column if pressures are less than 100 Pa, so alternate gauges are required.

The *thermal conductivity*, or *thermocouple* gauge, is one such device. If a small current is passed through a wire, resistance to the flow of current causes the wire to heat up. In air at atmospheric pressure, gas molecules colliding with the wire will carry away some of this heat, causing the temperature of the wire to decrease. As the pressure is lowered, the number of collisions is smaller, and there is less heat removed from the wire. The temperature of the wire is thus inversely related to the pressure of the gas surrounding the wire. The thermal conductivity gauge takes advantage of this phenomenon. It consists of a small wire and a thermocouple (a temperature-measuring device). As the pressure in the system is lowered, the thermocouple measures an increase in the temperature of the wire and displays it on a meter calibrated in units of pressure.

The response of the thermocouple gauge is dependent on the type of gas present. This is called a *relative pressure gauge*. The capacity of a gas to carry heat away from the wire will be a measure of its thermal conductivity, and will be a function of the molecular weight of the gas (and therefore its velocity and number of collisions with the wire per unit time) and the number of atoms in the gas molecule (and therefore the number of vibrational modes and the amount of heat removed by a single collision). If the gauge is calibrated for a pressure of nitrogen, as is usually the case, pressure readings for any other gas will be incorrect and must be corrected to reflect the difference in thermal conductivity of the gases.

The thermal conductivity gauge is useful for measuring pressures from atmospheric to about 0.1 Pa (10^{-3} Torr). These gauges are extremely rugged and long-lived. They are generally used to monitor the initial pump-down of the system or, occasionally, the pressure inside a CI ion source.

The *Pirani gauge* is a similar device, except that the heated wire makes up one arm of a Wheatstone bridge circuit. As the temperature of the wire increases, the resistance increases. This change in resistance is detected by the Wheatstone bridge and displayed on the meter in units of pressure. The Pirani gauge is also a relative pressure gauge and covers the same range of pressures as the thermocouple gauge.

For the low pressures inside an operating mass spectrometer, still another type of gauge is required. Often the choice is a *hot-filament ionization gauge*. One such design, called the inverted Bayard–Alpert gauge, is diagrammed in Fig. 17. Electrons are ejected from a heated filament and accelerated toward a grid by a large positive potential. As the electrons move through the intervening region,

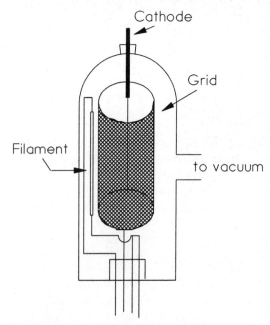

Fig. 17. Diagram of a Bayard–Alpert ionization gauge.

they collide with and ionize any gas molecules that might be present, just as they would in an EI ion source. The ions are collected at a wire cathode positioned down the center of the gauge. The current in this cathode is proportional to the pressure in the system.

As was the case with the thermocouple gauge, the hot-filament ionization gauge is a relative pressure gauge. The current in the cathode will depend not only on absolute pressure but also on the type of gas present. A more easily ionized gas (lower ionization potential) will have a higher apparent pressure than a less easily ionized one. As before, the gauge is calibrated for a particular gas, usually nitrogen or air, and must be corrected for use with any other gas.

The similarity between the ionization gauge and an EI ion source should not be overlooked. Ionization in the ion source of the mass spectrometer by collisions with energetic electrons shows the same dependence on compound class. That is, each type of analyte molecule will have its own relative sensitivity to ionization.

The hot-filament ionization gauge can be used to measure pressures from about 10^{-9} to 10^{-2} Pa. Operation at higher pressures dramatically shortens the lifetime of the gauge because of oxidation and eventual breakage of the filament.

2.6. Inlet Systems

Mass-spectrometer inlet systems serve two basic functions: to get the analyte into the gas phase and to reduce the pressure to a suitable range prior to ionization. If the sample is not completely pure, as is most often the case with biochemical samples, the inlet may be an interface between a separation device such as a chromatograph (GC or HPLC) and the mass spectrometer.

2.6.1 DIRECT INSERTION PROBE

The easiest samples to analyze are those that are gases or volatile liquids at room temperature. A significant fraction of the analyte is then already in the gas phase, and the inlet need only reduce the pressure from atmospheric to 10^{-3} Pa. A simple pin-hole leak or metering valve is sufficient in this case. The amount of analyte introduced can be controlled to match the rate of removal by the vacuum system, giving a constant low pressure of analyte.

For samples that are somewhat less volatile, heating may be required. The *direct insertion probe* (DIP) is designed for this type of sample. It consists of a long, heatable rod reaching into the mass spectrometer near the ion source. The sample is applied to the end of the rod or is placed in a glass capillary held in the end of the rod. As the temperature of the DIP is increased, analyte is evaporated into the ionization chamber. Even analytes with relatively high melting points can be analyzed with a DIP, because one needs only a partial pressure of 10^{-3} Pa of analyte to obtain a spectrum.

If the sample is impure, but the contaminants have vapor pressures sufficiently different from the analyte, some separation is possible by slowly increasing the temperature of the DIP. As the temperature is raised, the most volatile components of the mixture tend to evaporate first. The mass spectra of these components can be observed by scanning the mass range while the DIP is at low temperatures. Compounds with higher boiling points will evaporate from the DIP at higher temperatures, and their mass spectra are collected by scanning at later times. It should be pointed out, however, that the evaporation profiles of high and low boiling compounds overlap considerably and, thus, many scans taken at intermediate temperature will contain mixed spectra.

The DIP has rather well-defined limits. Meaningful mass spectra from samples that decompose upon heating are obviously inaccessible. This includes many interesting biochemical classes such as amino acids and carbohydrates. To obtain mass spectra of involatile compounds, one may need to make a chemical derivative or resort to one of the desorptive ionization methods described above. The DIP is also ineffective if the sample is a mixture of more than two or three components, or if the vapor pressures of the components are very similar. In these cases, one might choose to separate the sample via chromatography prior to mass spectrometric analysis.

2.6.2. GC–MS

A brute force approach to chromatography–MS is the so-called *off-line* method. The chromatograph is operated as usual, but fractions are collected at regular intervals (or whenever something is detected as eluting from the chromatograph). These samples are then carried over to the mass spectrometer and analyzed via the DIP as if they were pure materials. This approach places the fewest demands on the instruments, since both the chromatograph and mass spectrometer function independently. However, the off-line method places heavy demands on the analyst, particularly when samples are complex mixtures of tens or hundreds of components. Not surprisingly, *on-line* chromatographic–MS interfaces have been a fertile area for instrument development. The interfaces for gas chromatography–MS (GC–MS) were developed first, and are usually quite different from those designed for liquid chromatography–MS (LC–MS).

The direct coupling (on-line) of GC and MS provides the opportunity to analyze a tremendous variety of samples quickly and efficiently. It unquestionably stands as one of the milestones in MS development. [McFadden's book (3) is highly recommended for those wishing more detail.] To understand the interfaces used for GC–MS, one must consider the form of the analyte at the exit of the chromatographic column. By the nature of the separation, the analyte must necessarily be in the gas phase. In that regard, GC and MS are compatible. However, the eluate of the GC is at atmospheric pressure, and the MS must operate at 10^{-3} Pa (10^{-5} Torr). The major task of the interface, then, is to reduce the pressure to tolerable levels.

Early attempts at GC–MS interfaces sought to allow only a small portion of the GC eluate into the MS in a fashion similar to the inlets used for the analysis of pure gases. However, one should bear in mind that the analyte is present at trace concentration in a much greater volume of a neutral carrier gas (the GC mobile phase). In the so-called *split* interfaces, one discards a large portion of the analyte along with the carrier gas. To avoid "throwing away the baby with the bath water," a variety of interfaces were developed to discriminate against the carrier gas. In these devices, the partial pressure of the carrier gas is reduced to a greater extent than that of the analyte, resulting in an *enrichment* of the sample. By increasing the concentration of the analyte, one can achieve greater sensitivity in the mass spectrometer, while still allowing both the GC and the MS to function under their respective optimum conditions.

The most popular of the *molecular separators*, as the devices are called, is the *glass jet* separator, shown diagrammatically in Fig. 18. The eluate from the GC is expanded through a small orifice (0.1 mm) into a region of low pressure (0.1–1 Pa). The carrier gas, usually helium or nitrogen, has a lower molecular weight than the analyte, and so diffuses much faster into the region. (Diffusion rate varies as the inverse square of the molecular weight.) Consequently, the carrier gas radiates out from the orifice in a cone of larger diameter than that of the analyte. A small (0.25-mm) entrance (a *skimmer*) to the mass spectrometer is placed on the axis of the GC line a short distance (0.35 mm) from the GC outlet. The material sampled by this skimmer is enriched in analyte vapor relative to carrier gas. In other words, proportionately more of the carrier gas than the analyte is discarded in the pressure reduction. The pressure in the mass spectrometer is determined by the size of the skimmer opening. For typical packed-column GC, flow rates through the column are 25–30 mL/min; tolerable flows into the MS are typically a few hundred microliters per minute. For a greater degree of enrichment, two glass jets can be coupled in series. The glass jet separator is a nearly ideal GC–MS interface in that there are few surfaces for the sample to contact, minimizing the risk of adsorption or unwanted side reactions. However, the glass jet still results in loss of an appreciable fraction of the sample, and a concomitant loss in sensitivity.

The most dramatic change in GC over the past 15 years has been the shift from the use of packed GC columns to glass capillary columns. In these columns, the

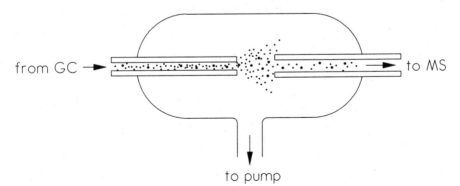

Fig. 18. Diagram of a glass jet separator for GC–MS. Large dots represent analyte molecules; smaller dots represent lower-molecular-weight carrier-gas molecules.

stationary phase is coated on or bonded to the inside wall of a long, narrow column (30 m × 0.25 mm is typical). This type of chromatography is characterized by superior chromatographic resolution in shorter times with lower carrier-gas flow rates. GC–MS interfaces for capillary GC are somewhat different and somewhat simpler than those for packed-column GC. Because the flow rates are much lower (0.5–2 mL/min), the entire eluate of the GC can be directed into the MS, so no sample is lost in the interface. If the vacuum system of the MS is designed properly, pressure in the ion source can still be maintained at tolerable levels for EI–MS. The only other requirement is that the transfer line between the GC and the MS be heated to avoid the condensation of sample components in the line. (This is also true of packed-column GC transfer lines.)

2.6.3. LC–MS

While many of the same considerations of GC–MS are also valid for LC–MS, the development of LC–MS interfaces has been much more problematical. The difficulty stems from the fundamental incompatibility of LC and MS. Usually the type of samples analyzed by LC are those that are not amenable to GC. They are often thermally unstable or very polar molecules. Vaporizing these molecules puts severe demands on the LC–MS interface. In addition, the problem of pressure reduction is more acute. Instead of a gas at atmospheric pressure, as at the outlet of a GC, in LC we have a liquid at atmospheric pressure. When the solvent is converted to a gas, it occupies far more volume than the liquid from which it came. (Remember, 1 mol of gas at standard temperature and pressure occupies 22.4 L of volume, while as a liquid, the same amount of material might occupy only a few milliliters.)

Nonetheless, the rewards for a successful LC–MS interface are high. HPLC is becoming the premier separation method for biological molecules, and an appropriate MS interface would extend the applicability of the method to many interesting classes of compounds.

One of the simplest types of LC–MS interfaces is *direct liquid introduction* (DLI). In this approach, a portion of the LC eluate is directed into the mass spectrometer through a pinhole leak. The pumping capacity of the vacuum system is usually increased to accommodate the increased burden of solvent. While some interesting applications have been reported, the DLI approach has a number of problems. Even with increased pumping capacity, the pressure in the ion source tends to be very high. This leads to CI-type spectra with correspondingly little fragmentation. Also, the ion source becomes covered with whatever involatile residues are left when the solvent evaporates. The use of involatile buffers in the LC solvents is intolerable, and frequent cleaning of the ion source is necessary. Since liquid flow rates into the mass spectrometer must be restricted to a few μL/min, the LC eluate is usually split, with a small fraction going to the mass spectrometer and the rest being discarded. As there is no enrichment of the analyte in this split, one is perforce discarding the bulk of the analyte along with the solvent.

The increasing use of microbore capillary LC columns has renewed interest in DLI techniques. With these columns, solvent flow rates are only μL/min, so the entire eluate can be directed into the mass spectrometer. While this improves sensitivity, it does little to address the other problems mentioned above.

If the volume of solvent is a major problem in LC–MS, it is reasonable to attempt selectively to remove the solvent, leaving behind the less volatile analyte. This is the idea behind a class of *transport* interfaces best characterized by the *moving belt*. A diagram appears in Fig. 19. The LC eluate is deposited on a belt, chain, or wire made of metal or some inert polymer (polyimide is often used). The belt continuously moves through a region where it is warmed with an infrared heater, evaporating the solvent. The well-behaved analyte remains as a residue on the belt. After a series of vacuum locks where the pressure is reduced to mass-spectrometric levels, the analyte on the belt moves into the region of the ion source. Here a flash heater quickly evaporates the analyte into the standard beam of energetic electrons or CI plasma. One can obtain EI or CI spectra at will. Next, a clean-up heater heats the belt to a still higher temperature to remove any residual sample, and the belt is cycled back to receive another load of eluate.

The moving-belt interface is among the most successful of LC–MS interfaces, as evidenced by the fact that, 10 years after its development, manufacturers still sell it. There have been some improvements, and some problems still remain. The most basic problem relates to the incompatibility mentioned earlier. If these compounds were easy to get into the gas phase, they would be analyzed by GC–MS. The fact that they are being separated by LC usually implies either a

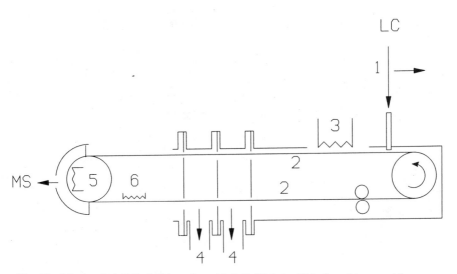

Fig. 19. Moving-belt LC–MS interface: (1) LC, (2) belt, (3) infrared heater, (4) vacuum pumps, (5) heater, and (6) clean-up heater. (Reproduced with permission from Finnigan MAT Corp.)

thermal fragility or an involatility. When strongly heated in the region of the ion source, the compounds often pyrolyze rather than volatilize. Also, there remain restrictions on the HPLC solvents, flow rates, and buffers that can be tolerated.

An exciting recent development in LC–MS is the interfacing of an LC to a FAB ion source, with or without the aid of a moving belt. As FAB is a desorptive ionization technique, the thermal stability or involatility of the analyte is of less importance. In fact, species that already carry a charge seem to be analyzed more efficiently than those that do not. In the case of a moving-belt FAB interface, glycerol may be included in the LC solvent, may be added to the belt after LC separation, or may be eliminated entirely. If glycerol is used, after removal of the LC solvents, what remains on the belt is a glycerol solution (or suspension) of sample. This is carried into the path of the atom gun, where sputtering and ionization take place as in normal FAB.

An alternative strategy is to combine a DLI-type interface with FAB in what is called a *continuous-flow FAB* probe (21). A few μL/min of the LC eluate is mixed with glycerol and allowed to ooze out onto the surface of an otherwise normal FAB probe. Sputtering and ionization occur as before. Time and more widespread use will be the judges of the success of these devices.

A very different type of LC–MS interface also has been quite successful. The *thermospray* interface (22) bears some resemblance to a DLI interface in that LC eluate is sprayed directly into a region of low pressure inside the vacuum system. However, in thermospray, the jet of liquid is heated to vaporize the solvent as it sprays into the vacuum region (see Fig. 20). A fine mist of solution droplets is

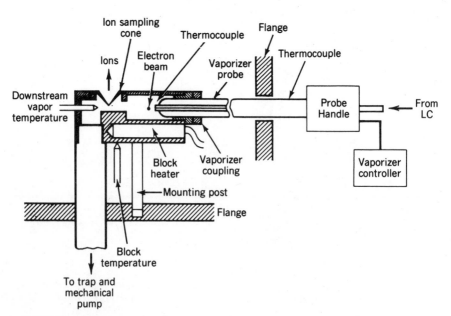

Fig. 20. Thermospray interface for LC–MS. (Reproduced with permission of Vestec Corp.)

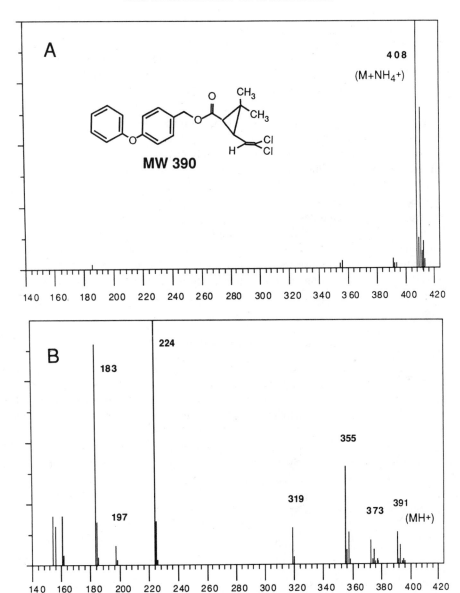

Fig. 21. Comparison of thermospray LC mass spectra of the synthetic pesticide *cis*-permethrin. (*A*) Filament-off spectrum and (*B*) filament-on spectrum. (Reproduced with permission from Ref. 23.)

formed, from which the solvent rapidly evaporates. If any ions are present in the solution (e.g., NH_4^+, H^+, Na^+), the droplets carry charges as they leave the nozzle. When the solvent evaporates, the less volatile analyte molecules find themselves in the gas phase, desolvated, and often in the company of a charge. This is exactly what is required for MS.

In order to keep the pressure low inside the mass analyzer, the ions in thermospray are directed through a small opening (skimmer) at 90° to the direction of the jet of liquid. The bulk of the uncharged particles are carried away by the pump without ever entering the mass spectrometer. Thermospray ionization, as the process of sample desolvation and ionization is called, is extremely gentle, with very little fragmentation being observed. The spectra are dominated by $(M+H)^+$ or $(M+cation)^+$, unless the sample itself already carries a charge, in which case M^+ is the major ion.

In addition to the thermospray ionization process, ions can be formed by another mechanism. Thermospray interfaces have a filament just downstream from where the jet of solution enters. If thermospray ionization is desired, the filament is not turned on. However, if the filament is turned on, the energetic electrons ionize molecules (predominantly solvent) in the stream. Since the pressure in this region is still relatively high, ion–molecule collisions take place, and the sample is ionized by a CI-like mechanism. The filament-on mode seems to produce more fragmentation than the filament-off mode, and thus is a useful complement for obtaining structural information. Figure 21 compares the mass spectra of a synthetic pesticide ionized by the two modes of operation.

3. DATA INTERPRETATION (EI)

Learning to interpret EI mass spectra can be compared to learning to play the harmonica. It is relatively easy to understand conceptually what is going on; with some practice, one can master the basics; but it takes years of work and a fair amount of luck to become proficient. When performed by an expert, it is truly a form of art.

The goal of the interpretation exercise is to identify the compound from which the spectrum was derived. By analyzing the pieces of a molecule, the interpreter seeks to reconstruct the whole. Even in cases where an unambiguous structure cannot be assigned, a surprising amount of information can be gleaned from a careful examination of the spectrum.

3.1. The Basics

The first step in the interpretation of an unknown is to collect as much information about the compound as is possible from sources other than the mass spectrum. Solubility data and IR, UV, or NMR spectra, if available, can provide important clues to assist in the interpretation. Knowledge of the source of the material is vital. If synthetic, what were the precursors? If natural, what were the separation steps leading up to the time the spectrum was collected? Although the mass spectrum must be collected in a vacuum, it should not be interpreted in one.

The mass spectrum is a summary of the experiment. If the data system has done its job correctly, the spectrum shows the masses of all of the fragment ions from the molecule along with their relative abundances. Spectra are usually plotted with m/z in the x direction and intensity in the y direction, with the intensity normalized so that the most abundant ion (the base peak) is 100% and all other ion abundances are expressed as a fraction of that. For each fragment ion, one would like to know the chemical formula and structure. Based on a wealth of experience stretching back at least 30 years, chemists have developed a set of rules to describe how molecules break apart under mass-spectrometric conditions. Several books on the subject can be recommended (1, 24, 25). Of course, a solid understanding of organic chemistry is invaluable to any interpretation effort.

The quasi-equilibrium theory (5) predicts that, because the ionization event is so fast, an electron can be lost from anywhere in the molecule, and there is sufficient time for the electron cloud to redistribute before fragmentation occurs. It is helpful to try to visualize where in the molecule the loss of electron density will appear. If one looks at the energy level diagram for various types of valence electrons, it is clear that the highest-energy electrons are in nonbonding orbitals on heteroatoms such as oxygen or nitrogen. Next highest are π-bonding electrons in double bonds or aromatic rings. Finally, the electrons in single (σ) covalent bonds are of lowest energy. After redistribution of the electron density following ionization, the loss of electron density will appear to be localized in the highest-energy levels.

The ion that remains is a radical cation. *Radical* means that the particle has an unpaired electron; *cation* means that it carries a positive charge. These two features can be considered as being formally localized in the ion in a *radical site*— the site of the unpaired electron—and a *charge site*—the site of the positive charge. These two sites start out at the same place in the molecule, the site of the lost electron, but they generally do not remain together as fragmentation occurs. Electrons in the bonds of the ion will move toward either the radical site or the charge site, causing bond cleavage. This can occur in two ways.

A single covalent bond between two atoms is a shared pair of electrons. When the bond breaks, the electrons can remain as a pair, staying with one or the other of the two atoms. This is called *heterolytic* bond cleavage. If, on the other hand, in the bond rupture one electron remains with each atom, the electron pair is separated and the cleavage is called *homolytic*. We will denote these types of bond cleavages using double-barbed arrows ($\rightarrow$) for heterolytic cleavage and single-barbed arrows ($\rightharpoonup$) for homolytic bond cleavage, as suggested by Budzikiewicz et al. (25).

As the ion breaks up, at least two fragments will be formed. One of these will carry the charge formerly borne by the parent ion (the charge site); the other will usually be neutral and may or may not carry the radical site:

$$M^{\ddagger} \begin{cases} \rightarrow A^+ + B\cdot \\ \rightarrow C^{\ddagger} + D \end{cases} \qquad (16)$$

Because the mass spectrometer only detects charged species, the charged fragments are the ones represented by peaks in the mass spectrum. The neutrals are pumped away, and their presence is inferred from the mass difference between molecular and fragment ions.

The abundance of any ion is the result of a balance between its rate of production and its rate of decomposition. The ease of production will depend on such factors as the ion's capacity to stabilize a charge, the number and strength of the bonds that were broken in forming the ion, and the stability of any neutral species that may have been formed simultaneously. Further decomposition will depend on the excess internal energy remaining in the ion, the availability of other easily broken bonds, and the stability of small neutral decomposition products.

Metastable Ions. One might well wonder how anyone knows that an ion arises by a particular pathway from a particular parent. One way to learn about these pathways is by the study of *metastable ions*. Most fragmentation observed in mass spectrometry takes place in the ion source. The ionization process itself is very fast (10^{-16} sec), and once an ion bears a charge, it is rapidly (a few microseconds) extracted out of the ion source toward the mass analyzer. Fragment ions are formed in the microsecond time interval between ionization and extraction. If ions survive the ion source, there is another time delay of a few microseconds while they travel through the mass analyzer toward the detector. "Stable" ions are those that reach the detector without further breakdown.

If an ion is accelerated out of the ion source with a mass m_p, but then decomposes to fragments on the way to the mass analyzer, it is called a metastable ion. If a magnetic sector is being used for the mass analysis, a curious phenomenon occurs. The initial kinetic energy of the metastable ion is divided between the fragments produced, and after the charged fragment travels through the mass analyzer, it is observed at an m/z that is neither that of the parent ion, m_p, nor that of the daughter ion, m_d. The m/z of this metastable ion, m^*, is given by

$$m^* = (m_d)^2/m_p \qquad (17)$$

For example, in the fragmentation of delta 9-tetrahydrocannabinol (THC), the active constituent of marijuana, the molecular ion, mass 314, loses a methyl group to form a major fragment ion of mass 299. A metastable ion might be observed for the transition at $m/z = (299)^2/314 = 284.7$.

How can one determine whether an observed peak represents a true fragment ion or a metastable ion? There are two clues. The measured m/z values of metastable ions are frequently an unusual fraction of a mass. (Note the 284.7 above.) Peaks representing stable ions are generally observed nearer to the integral nominal mass. Second, because there is a range of kinetic energies imparted to the fragment particles, the peaks representing metastable ions are always considerably broader than those for stable fragment ions, often extending over several tenths of a mass unit. It is interesting to note that peaks for metastable ions are only observed at $m/z = m^*$ in magnetic-sector instruments. They are not observed at all in quadrupole instruments.

3.2. Getting Started

3.2.1. ELEMENTAL FORMULAS

Some of the first information we seek in the interpretation process is the elemental formulas for the important ions in the spectrum. There are two basic clues to the formula of any ion in the spectrum: the mass of that ion and the *isotope pattern* of the peaks associated with it. It is easy to understand how the mass of an ion provides structural information. There are only a finite number of combinations of atoms that can be added together to give that mass. For example, what combinations of atoms constitute a mass of 30 daltons? If we are dealing with organic molecules, an ion of mass 30 could consist of two carbon atoms and six hydrogen atoms $[(2 \times 12) + (6 \times 1)]$; one carbon, four hydrogens, and one nitrogen $[12 + (4 \times 1) + 14]$; or one carbon, two hydrogens, and one oxygen $[12 + (2 \times 1) + 16]$. It is important to note that in theses calculations the atomic mass of the most abundant isotope of an element is used, not its *chemical average* mass. Carbon, therefore, has a mass of 12.0000, not 12.011 daltons per atom (see Table 1).

The mass of an ion limits the possible formulas that can be proposed. Of course, some good chemical sense also helps. One would not suggest that a formula of CH_{18} could be a likely candidate for m/z 30, because that violates our notion of chemical valence for carbon. Although the mass of an ion is very useful at low mass, as one considers ions of higher and higher mass, the number of reasonable combinations of atoms can become unwieldy.

It is evident now why the high-resolution mass measurement previously described is so valuable. If one knows the mass of an ion to an accuracy of several decimal places, most of the possible elemental combinations can be eliminated. For example, an ion of mass 128 could result from many elemental compositions, some of which are listed below:

$$C_{10}H_5, \quad C_9H_{20}, \quad C_5H_{18}N, \quad C_5H_{16}O, \quad C_7H_{16}Nz, \quad C_7H_{14}NO, \quad C_7H_{12}O_2,$$
$$C_6H_{14}N_3, \quad C_6H_{12}N_2O, \quad C_6H_{10}NO_2, \quad C_6H_8O_3, \quad HI \quad C_8H_{13}F$$

If, however, the mass of the ion is known to be 128.107 ± 0.002 u, most of the possibilities can be eliminated.

HI	127.912	$C_7H_{12}O_2$	128.084	$C_6H_{14}N_3$	128.119
$C_6H_9O_3$	128.047	$C_6H_{12}N_2O$	128.095	$C_7H_{16}N_2$	128.131
$C_{10}H_8$	128.063	$C_8H_{13}F$	128.100	$C_8H_{18}N$	128.144
$C_6H_{10}NO_2$	128.071	$C_7H_{14}NO$	128.108	C_9H_{20}	128.156
		$C_8H_{16}O$	128.120		

3.2.2. ISOTOPE PATTERNS

The other clue to an ion's formula is the pattern of isotope peaks that represent it. Many of the common elements have more than one stable isotope. Although the great preponderance of hydrogen is the ^{1}H isotope, a tiny fraction (0.015%) exists as the ^{2}H isotope (deuterium). As a consequence, whenever hydrogen appears in a molecular fragment, at least two ions will be observed in the mass spectrum: one for the ^{1}H form and one for the ^{2}H form. The relative abundances of these two ions will be determined on the basis of probability. If one H atom is present, 0.015% of the time it will be ^{2}H, so the intensity of the deuterium isotope peak will be 0.015% of the peak intensity representing the protium species. If five H atoms are present, each has a 0.015% probability of being ^{2}H, so the total intensity of the deuterium isotope peak would be 5 × 0.015 or 0.075% of the protium peak intensity. Table 1 shows the masses and natural abundances of some of the more common elements.

The isotope patterns of a few elements are very distinctive, and the presence of these elements can be recognized easily. Chlorine and bromine each have two abundant isotopes separated by two mass units: ^{35}Cl and ^{37}Cl, and ^{79}Br and ^{81}Br. The chlorine isotopes are in a ratio of approximately 3:1, leading to unusual doublets in the mass spectra of chlorinated compounds. If more than one chlorine atom is present in a fragment, the pattern of isotopes is more complicated, but still readily calculated. The mass spectrum of dichlorobenzene (Fig. 22) will serve as an example. The molecular ions are represented by peaks at m/z 146, 148, and 150; the intensity ratios of these peaks indicate that the molecular ions contain two chlorine atoms. If both of these are ^{35}Cl, the mass will be 146. If one of the two is ^{35}Cl and the other is ^{37}Cl, the ion will have a mass of 148. If both atoms are ^{37}Cl, the mass will be 150. The nominal mass (that

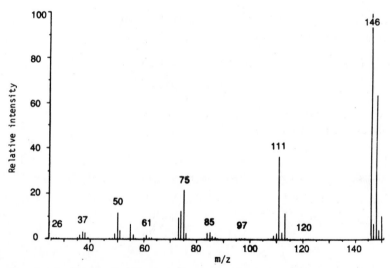

Fig. 22. Mass spectrum of dichlorobenzene showing chlorine isotope peaks beginning at m/z 146 for an ion containing two chlorine atoms and at m/z 111 for an ion containing one chlorine atom (26).

corresponding to the mass of the lightest isotopes) for the molecular ion of dichlorobenzene is 146.

The relative proportions of these ions reflect the statistical distribution of chlorine atoms in nature and can be calculated using the binomial expansion $(a + b)^n$, where a and b are the relative abundances of the ^{35}Cl and ^{37}Cl in nature and n is the number of chlorine atoms present in an ion. In the example above, $a = 0.75$ and $b = 0.25$, because 75% of the chlorine atoms observed in nature are ^{35}Cl and 25% are ^{37}Cl. Because dichlorobenzene has two chlorine atoms, $n = 2$. Expanding the binomial gives the relative intensity of the first peak (m/z 146) as $a^2 = (0.75)^2 = 0.5625$. The second peak has an intensity of $2ab = 2(0.75)(0.25) = 0.375$, and the third peak ($m/z = 150$) has an intensity of $b^2 = (0.25)^2 = 0.0625$. Normalizing these results in a relative intensity ratio of $100:67:11$, as observed in Fig. 22. The fragment ion represented by the peak at $m/z = 111$, corresponding to the loss of Cl from the molecular ion, contains only one chlorine atom. Its isotope peak intensity pattern is simply the 3:1 ratio (m/z 111 and 113) characteristic of a single Cl. The isotope peak patterns for several element combinations are shown in Fig. 23. More complete lists can be found in Ref. 1.

Unfortunately, most of the mass-spectral data encountered do not represent ions that contain elements with very distinctive isotope patterns. Carbon, hydrogen, oxygen, and nitrogen all have more than one stable isotope, but the

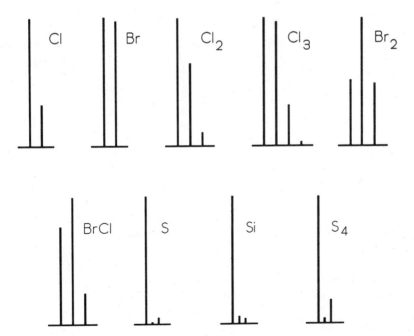

Fig. 23. Isotope peak intensity patterns for several common elements and combinations.

distribution is such that one isotope dominates all others. Still, some very useful information is contained in the intensity ratio of isotope peaks, particularly with regard to the number of carbon atoms present in an ion. The major isotope of carbon, ^{12}C, accounts for about 98.9% of the carbon in nature; ^{13}C adds most of the remaining 1.1%. Thus, an ion with nine carbon atoms will have a ^{13}C isotope ion abundance of $(9 \times 1.1\%) = 9.9\%$ relative to the all-^{12}C ion abundance. Of course, the heavy stable isotopes of hydrogen, oxygen, and nitrogen will also contribute to the abundance of this isotope ion, but the ^{13}C contribution is generally the most important. Consequently, when an ion is observed with an isotope ion abundance of around 10%, one can assume with some confidence that the ion contains *no more than* nine carbon atoms.

Two cautions should be expressed with regard to the interpretation of isotope ion abundances. Because of the limits of instrument precision, the abundances of *all* ions are subject to some experimental error. McLafferty (1) recommends that this error be estimated as 0.2% absolute abundance or 10% relative abundance, whichever is larger. Second, it is frequently impossible to determine whether ion abundance is derived solely from isotope contributions or from some interfering ion that coincidentally has the same mass as an isotope ion. As a result, the estimate of numbers of stable isotope contributors provides an upper limit, rather than an exact number. In the example above, one can assume that there are *no more than* nine carbon atoms, but there could be fewer than nine, if something else is contributing to the apparent isotope ion abundance.

3.2.3. DOUBLE-BOND EQUIVALENTS

After estimating the elemental composition of an ion from its mass and isotope ion abundance, one can calculate another useful bit of information—the number of rings or double bonds (*double-bond equivalents*, DBE) that the ion contains. This is readily computed for an ion of formula $C_wH_xN_yO_z$ using

$$DBE = w - x/2 + y + 1 \qquad (18)$$

Silicon atoms, if they are present, contribute like carbon and are included in w. Halogens (F, Cl, Br, I) behave like hydrogen and are included in x. Sulfur, like oxygen, makes no contribution to DBE. For example, the major fragment ion of THC at m/z 299 has a formula of $C_{20}H_{27}O_2$. Its DBE is simply $20 - 27/2 + 1 = 7.5$. When a fractional DBE is calculated, the fractional part is dropped, suggesting in this case an ion that contains seven rings or double bonds or both.

The DBE equation can be derived from the concept of *chemical valence*, that is, how many covalent bonds are generally formed between a particular atom and its neighbors. Carbon and silicon, for instance, usually have a valence of four, hydrogen and halogen atoms a valence of one, and nitrogen a valence of three.

In addition to the number of rings or double bonds or both in an ion, the DBE can help to determine whether an ion is even-electron or odd-electron. When the

DBE calculation yields a fractional value, as in the THC ion above, the ion is even-electron. When the DBE has an integral value, the ion is odd-electron. Molecular ions are *always* odd-electron.

3.2.4. NITROGEN RULE

The concept of chemical valence results in one more useful principle. Most of the common elements that have even masses also have even valence: ^{12}C, valence = 4; ^{28}Si, valence = 4; ^{16}O, valence = 2; ^{32}S, valence = 2. Most of the common odd-mass elements have odd valence: ^{1}H, valence = 1; ^{19}F, valence = 1; ^{35}Cl, valence = 1. The exception to this generality is nitrogen. ^{14}N has an even mass, but an odd valence (valence = 3). The consequence of this is the *nitrogen rule*: If an odd-electron ion has an odd mass, it has an odd number of nitrogen atoms. There are corollaries that can be summarized as in Table 2.

This rule is most often applied to candidate molecular ions. Because all molecular ions are odd-electron species, an odd mass indicates an odd number of nitrogen atoms; an even mass indicates an even number (or zero) of nitrogens. Fragment ions are usually, but not always, even-electron. In the THC example cited, the fact that the DBE calculated to be 7.5 indicates that an even-electron ion is involved, and therefore it is a fragment ion. The corollary to the nitrogen rule specifies that an even-electron fragment ion with an odd mass must have an even number of nitrogens (or, as in this case, zero).

3.2.5. MOLECULAR ION IDENTIFICATION

A good next step in the interpretation process is to try to identify the molecular ion, from which all fragment ions arose. McLafferty (1) identifies three criteria for recognizing the molecular ion. (1) It must be the ion of highest mass in the spectrum (excluding isotope peaks). This is so because only unimolecular decompositions are likely at the low pressures associated with EI–MS. There is no easy way for atoms from some other substance to get attached to the molecule of interest. (2) It must be an odd-electron ion. All stable organic molecules start

TABLE 2

The Nitrogen Rule[a]

Mass	Number of Electrons	
	Even	Odd
Even	Odd number of N	Even number of N
Odd	Even number of N	Odd number of N

[a]Even number of N includes zero.

out with paired electrons. Loss of one electron in the ionization event will result in an odd-electron ion remaining. (This also means that the DBE will be an integer, not a fraction.) (3) It must reasonably account for the observed fragment ions. Losses of 4–14 and 21–25 mass units are unlikely to occur; there are no ready combinations of atoms whose composite atomic weights add up to these masses. A fragment ion at, for example, 9 u lower than the mass of a purported molecular ion is evidence for an incorrect assignment of $M^{+\cdot}$ or the presence of a contaminant.

The molecular ion is not always represented in a mass spectrum. Its absence is frustrating, in that the molecular weight is then difficult to deduce, but the absence of M^{+} provides some useful information, in that it indicates that the molecule is very unstable, or contains at least one very facile fragmentation pathway. Aliphatic alcohols are notorious in this regard. They very readily lose 18 u, the elements of water. If M^{+} is observed at all, it is of very low abundance.

3.2.6. SPECTRAL APPEARANCE

Finally, in the initial stages of the interpretation of a mass spectrum, the overall "shape" of the spectrum should be noted. If there are few peaks, it is a sign that there are relatively few easily cleaved bonds in the molecule. Aromatic compounds are representative of this class, often displaying only one or two peaks of appreciable intensity. If the spectrum has many fragment ion peaks, one knows that there are many bonds of approximately equal strength, any of which can be cleaved with equal facility. Long-chain hydrocarbons or fatty acids are typical of this case.

3.3. Fragmentation Mechanisms

Having determined the possible elemental compositions for prominent ions in the spectrum, calculated DBE's, proposed a molecular ion, and observed the general appearance of the spectrum, the next step in the interpretation process is to begin to explore the relationship of ions to one another. Bond fragmentation can be thought of as resulting from electron movement toward either the radical site or the charge site of the parent ion. Sometimes, in order to explain the appearance of a particular fragment ion, one must invoke more than one bond cleavage, but these processes follow a logical sequence. Often, new bonds are formed in the highly energetic parent ion during unimolecular decomposition, leading to rearranged products. Some of the more important mechanisms are considered below.

3.3.1. σ CLEAVAGE

If a molecule contains no heteroatoms and no double or triple bonds, the electron lost in the ionization process must come from a sigma (single) bond. This obviously weakens that bond; it is left with only one shared electron instead of two. This is now likely to be the weakest bond in the molecule and so is the preferred site for cleavage. Saturated hydrocarbons are characterized by this type of σ *cleavage*, illustrated with decane below (Scheme 1).

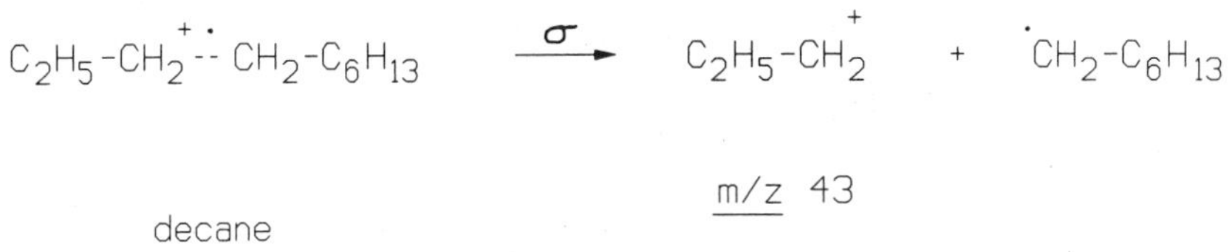

$$C_2H_5-CH_2^{+\cdot}--CH_2-C_6H_{13} \quad \xrightarrow{\sigma} \quad C_2H_5-CH_2^+ \quad + \quad {}^{\cdot}CH_2-C_6H_{13}$$

<u>m/z</u> 43

decane

Scheme 1. Decane.

Because all of the single bonds in the decane molecule are approximately equally likely to lose the electron, a rather nonspecific cleavage results. This often results in a series of ions differing by 14 u. For hydrocarbons, this series occurs at m/z 29, 43, 57, 71, 85, 99, etc. The presence of such a series is a good clue to the presence of a particular functional group (in this case, an alkyl chain) in the molecule. If branching occurs in the chain, the secondary or tertiary carbon atom provides a good site for stabilization of the charge. As a result, ions associated with cleavage near the branch point are of somewhat greater abundance than ions originating elsewhere in the chain.

3.3.2.   RADICAL SITE-INITIATED CLEAVAGE

Recall that the radical site is the place in the ion where the unpaired electron is localized. A major class of fragmentations occurs as a result of a drive to re-pair this lone electron. These are called *radical site-initiated* processes. Since all other electrons in the molecule occur in pairs, matching the electron at the radical site with another electron must result in the separation of some other pair of electrons. If the electron moving toward the radical site comes from a covalent bond, the bond is homolytically cleaved (see Scheme 2). Homolytic bond cleavage is characteristic of radical site-initiated processes.

When heteroatoms are present in the analyte, the initial electron loss will often be from a nonbonding electron pair. The radical site will then be localized at that point. For example, in amines, the radical site may occur initially on nitrogen, an electron being lost from the nitrogen nonbonding pair. An electron from a bond one carbon away (the α position) may move toward the radical site to pair up with the free electron on nitrogen. Propyl amine produces an abundant ion of mass 30 by this mechanism (Scheme 2).

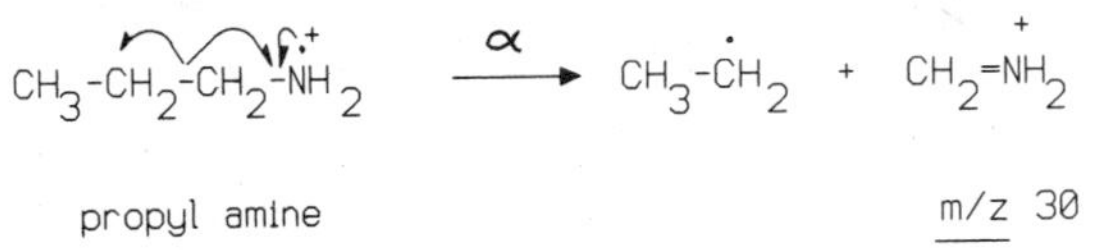

$$CH_3-CH_2-CH_2-NH_2^{\cdot+} \quad \xrightarrow{\alpha} \quad CH_3-{}^{\cdot}CH_2 \quad + \quad CH_2^{+}{=}NH_2$$

propyl amine   m/z 30

Scheme 2. Propyl amine.

There are several things to note about this mechanism that are common to all radical site-initiated processes. Two fragments are formed, a neutral (uncharged) radical and a fragment ion. The charge site has remained where it was in the

52

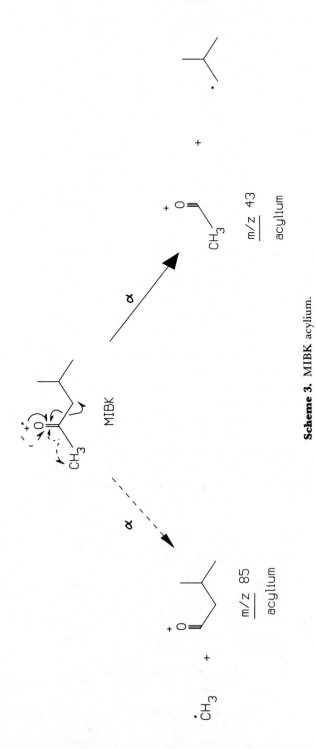

Scheme 3. MIBK acylium.

parent ion, the radical site has moved to a new position. Finally, although the parent ion was an odd-electron ion, the new fragment ion has all its electrons paired and is now an even-electron product. In all subsequent fragmentations that this ion undergoes, the products will be even-electron species. The electron migration cleaves the carbon–carbon bond homolytically. A new radical site is formed on the carbon atom in the neutral ethyl fragment and the unpaired electron on nitrogen forms a new π bond between carbon and nitrogen. Because the bond cleaved is α to the site of electron loss, this type of fragmentation is referred to as α *cleavage.*

Other heteroatoms such as oxygen and sulfur can also undergo radical site-initiated α cleavage. In fact, these are represented by some of the most prominent peaks observed in many mass spectra. In carbonyl compounds, α cleavage leads to a special ion called an *acylium* ion, as shown in Scheme 3 for methyl isobutyl ketone (**MIBK**).

The parent ion can lose either the methyl group or the isopropyl group, depending on which bond is broken. Usually, the extent to which each of these occur is determined by the size of the alkyl group lost. A larger alkyl group often can better stabilize the new radical site, and so loss of the larger alkyl group may be preferred. The relief of steric strain is greater with the loss of the larger alkyl group as well. Although acylium ions of both mass 43 and mass 85 are possible in methyl isobutyl ketone, the ion of mass 43 ion is represented by the base peak (loss of the larger alkyl), while the ion of mass 85 ion (loss of methyl) has a relative abundance of about 20%. α cleavage is a prominent fragmentation mechanism in ketones, aldehydes, and carboxylic acid derivatives, often producing the base peak of the spectrum and allowing the location of the carbonyl group in a hydrocarbon chain.

The electron initially lost from a molecule may also be from a π bond rather than from a nonbonding pair on a heteroatom. In this case, the radical site and charge site start out at the position of the double bond. 4-Octene can serve as an example. Once an electron is lost, α cleavage may occur to pair up the unpaired electron, leaving an allylic cation (Scheme 4):

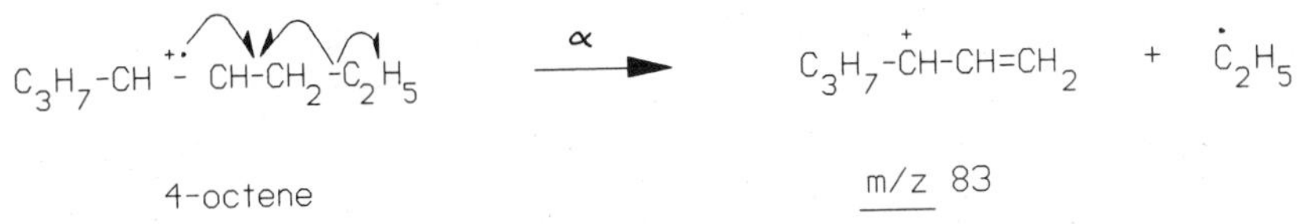

4-octene   m/z 83

Scheme 4. 4-Octene.

This can be stabilized by two resonance forms (Scheme 5):

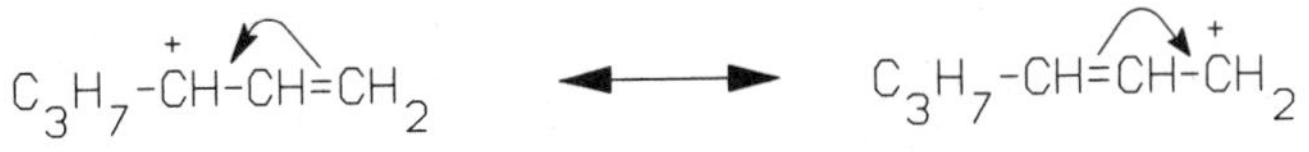

Scheme 5. Resonance forms.

Unfortunately, because the radical site can also move along the carbon chain (through hydrogen transfers), several isomeric forms of the radical molecular ion are formed, each leading to the formation of an allylic ion of different mass. Thus, the mass spectra of olefins rarely provide a discrete set of peaks that indicate the location of the double bond in the original molecule.

If the double bond is part of an aromatic system, cleavage occurs α to the aromatic ring. In the case of monosubstituted benzene rings, this leads to a very characteristic ion at m/z 91, the *tropylium* ion, produced from propyl benzene by the following mechanism (Scheme 6):

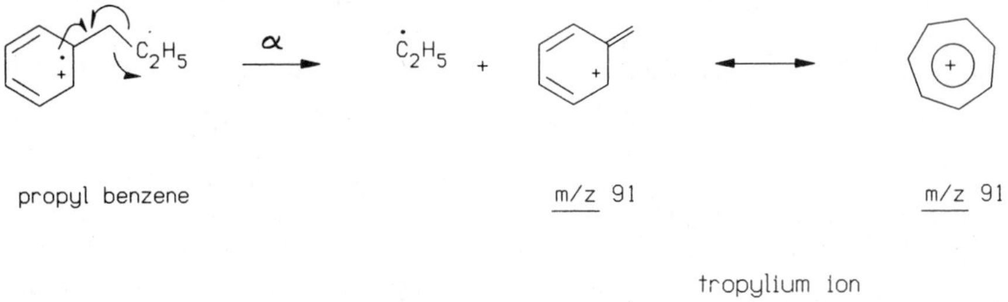

propyl benzene   m/z 91   m/z 91

                                                                                    tropylium ion

Scheme 6. Tropylium ion.

When more than one type of functionality is present in a molecule, α cleavage may be possible at more than one site. The relative ease of cleavage will depend on the stabilities of the radical and cation formed. In general, the order will be determined by the tendency of each functional group to share its electrons. That order is approximately N > O, S, π, R > Cl, Br, H, where π represents a double bond or aromatic system and R represents an alkyl group (1). One might predict from this that in the case of amphetamine, with both a nitrogen and an aromatic ring, α cleavage will be more likely near the amine than near the aromatic ring (Scheme 7 on page 55).

This is borne out by the fact that in the mass spectrum of amphetamine, the ion of mass 44 (α cleavage near N) is represented by the base peak. α cleavage near the benzene ring produces an ion of mass 91 that has less than 10% relative abundance.

3.3.3.   CHARGE SITE-INITIATED CLEAVAGE

Another type of fragmentation is initiated by electrons moving toward the charge site of the parent ion. Bond cleavage in this case is heterolytic (the electrons move as a pair as the bond breaks), rather than homolytic, as was the situation with radical site-initiated fragmentation. The driving force for these cleavages is the attraction of electrons to the electron-deficient site where the positive charge is localized. This type of cleavage is also called *inductive* cleavage. The loss of bromine from ethylene dibromide (the base peak of the spectrum) can be explained by this mechanism (Scheme 8 on page 55).

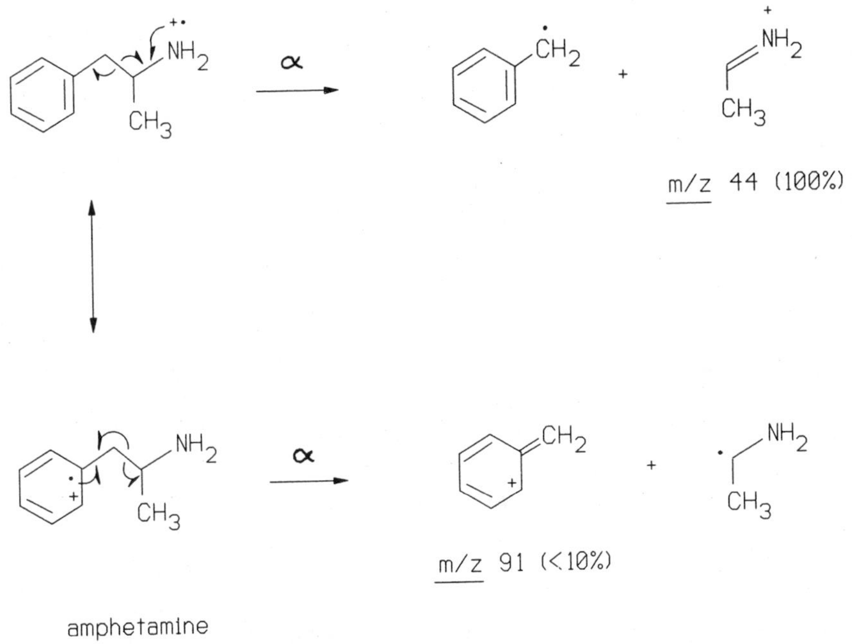

m/z 44 (100%)

m/z 91 (<10%)

amphetamine

Scheme 7. Amphetamine.

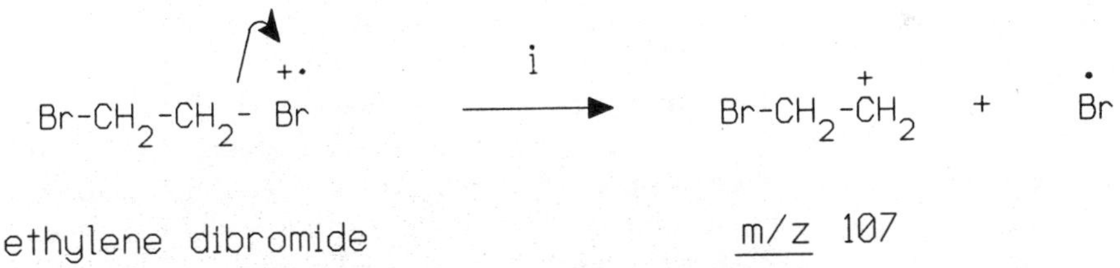

ethylene dibromide   m/z 107

Scheme 8. Ethylene dibromide.

The initial electron is lost from one of the nonbonding pairs on Br, leaving the charge site and radical site there. The pair of electrons forming the C–Br bond migrates toward the positive charge. In so doing, the C–Br bond is broken heterolytically and a new charge site develops on the carbon atom. In charge site-initiated cleavage, the radical site remains where it is and the charge site moves.

In many cases both charge site and radical site-initiated processes could conceivably occur in the same ion. When diethyl ether is ionized, the charge and radical sites are localized initially on oxygen (Scheme 9 on page 56).

Charge site-initiated cleavage breaks the bond adjacent to the oxygen, while radical site-initiated cleavage would break the C–C bond in the α position. Both of these processes will occur to some extent, the degree will be determined by the

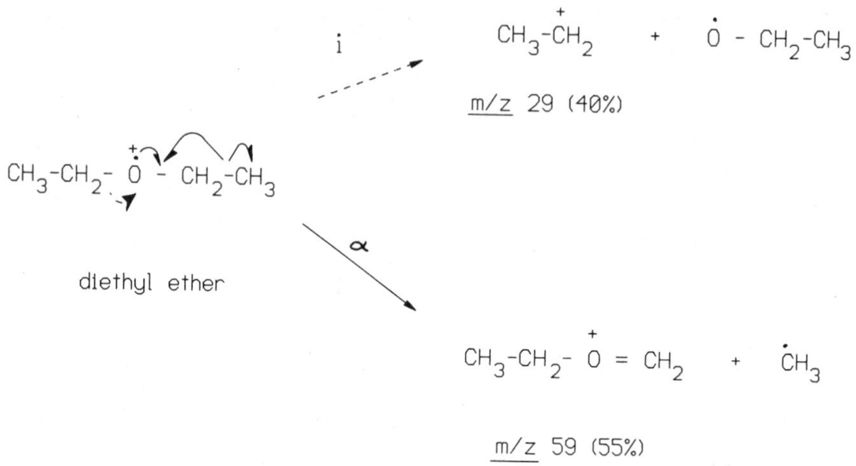

$$CH_3 \overset{+}{-}CH_2 \quad + \quad \overset{\cdot}{O} - CH_2 - CH_3$$

$$\underline{m/z} \ 29 \ (40\%)$$

$$CH_3 - CH_2 - \overset{+\cdot}{O} - CH_2 - CH_3$$

diethyl ether

$$CH_3 - CH_2 - \overset{+}{O} = CH_2 \quad + \quad \overset{\cdot}{C}H_3$$

$$\underline{m/z} \ 59 \ (55\%)$$

Scheme 9. Ether.

stability of the ion and radical formed. In the case of ethers, radical site-initiated cleavage will usually predominate unless a particularly stable radical is formed by the charge site-initiated reaction. In the fragmentation of diethyl ether, the α-cleavage fragment ion of mass 59 has a relative abundance of 55%, compared to the inductive cleavage product of mass 29 with a relative abundance of 40%.

Carbonyl compounds can undergo charge site-initiated cleavage, but usually it occurs as a two-step process. This is illustrated with methyl isobutyl ketone in Scheme 10 on page 57.

The bond broken is the same one as in α cleavage, but now the charge is retained on the alkyl group rather than the carbonyl group. Again, both processes may occur in ketones and aldehydes, the extent of each determined by the relative stability of the products formed. In methyl isobutyl ketone, α cleavage produces ions of mass 43 (100%) and of mass 85 (20%). The inductive cleavage products of masses 15 and 57 have relative abundances of 28% and 39%, respectively.

Charge site-initiated fragmentation is generally less important than radical site-initiated cleavage when both are possible. However, in many circumstances there is no radical site present, so charge site-initiated processes become the primary mode of fragmentation. It has been noted that in any odd-electron ion, cleavage of a single bond results in the formation of a neutral radical and an even-electron ion. If the even-electron ion is to break down further, it must be by way of charge site-initiated pathways. There is no longer any radical site present. Subsequent fragmentation will only result from charge site-initiated cleavages or rearrangements (see subsequent discussion). Similarly, soft ionization techniques like CI produce even-electron protonated molecules, $(M+H)^+$. These ions usually undergo charge site-initiated fragmentation, if they fragment at all. There is no radical site in the molecule.

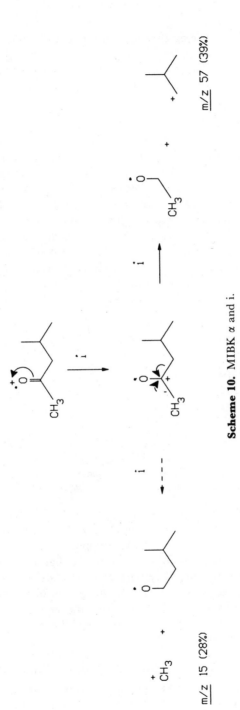

Scheme 10. MIBK α and i.

Inductive cleavage, being driven by attraction of electrons to an electron-deficient site, will depend in large part on the electronegativity of the charge site. In general, the order of ease of undergoing inductive cleavage follows the electronegativity: F > Cl > Br, I > O,S ≫ N,C (1).

3.3.4. REARRANGEMENTS

There is an important group of fragmentation processes in which not only are bonds broken, but new bonds are formed. The product from such a rearrangement can be misleading, in that the structure of the fragment ion will contain bonds not present in the original molecule. The analyst must be constantly aware that these processes occur, and must not be fooled by them. The rearrangements are also useful, in that they frequently indicate something about the proximity of atoms within a molecule. Certain rearrangements are very isomer-specific, and therefore useful in differentiating isomers, a task not generally possible by MS.

The simplest of rearrangements is the transfer of a H atom from one part of the molecule to another, often followed by the elimination of a small neutral molecule. The loss of water from aliphatic alcohols, such as cyclohexanol, is a good example (Scheme 11).

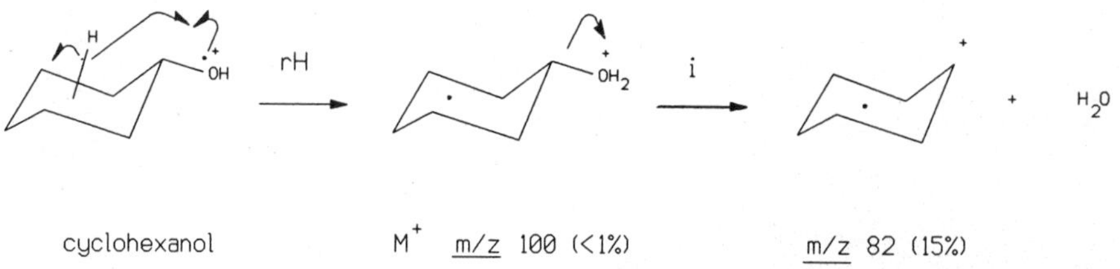

cyclohexanol   M$^+$ m/z 100 (<1%)   m/z 82 (15%)

Scheme 11. Cyclohexanol.

The initial transfer is probably radical site-initiated, with a H· transferred to the oxygen from somewhere in the ring. The electron on hydrogen pairs with the free electron on O, forming a new bond and developing a new radical site somewhere in R (presumably on the atom from which the H migrated). The second step of the rearrangement is the inductive (charge site-initiated) cleavage of the C–O bond, liberating water and moving the charge site to the ring carbon. This rearrangement is so facile in cyclohexanol that the molecular ion is of extremely low abundance (<1%), while the $(M-H_2O)^+$ has a relative abundance of 15%. Alkyl halides also undergo this type of rearrangement to liberate HCl, HBr, HF, etc.

It is interesting to note that when an odd-electron ion, such as the cyclohexanol molecular ion, rearranges, the product is another odd-electron ion. Similarly, if the starting ion has all electrons paired, rearrangement will lead to another ion with an even number of electrons.

Methyl esters of carboxylic acids will often undergo α cleavage to yield ions corresponding to $(M-31)^+$. However, in some circumstances, transfer of a hydrogen atom and loss of methanol (a rearrangement process) is preferred. The most notable case of this type is with ortho-substituted benzoic acids, as in methyl salicylate (Scheme 12), a phenomenon known as the *ortho effect*.

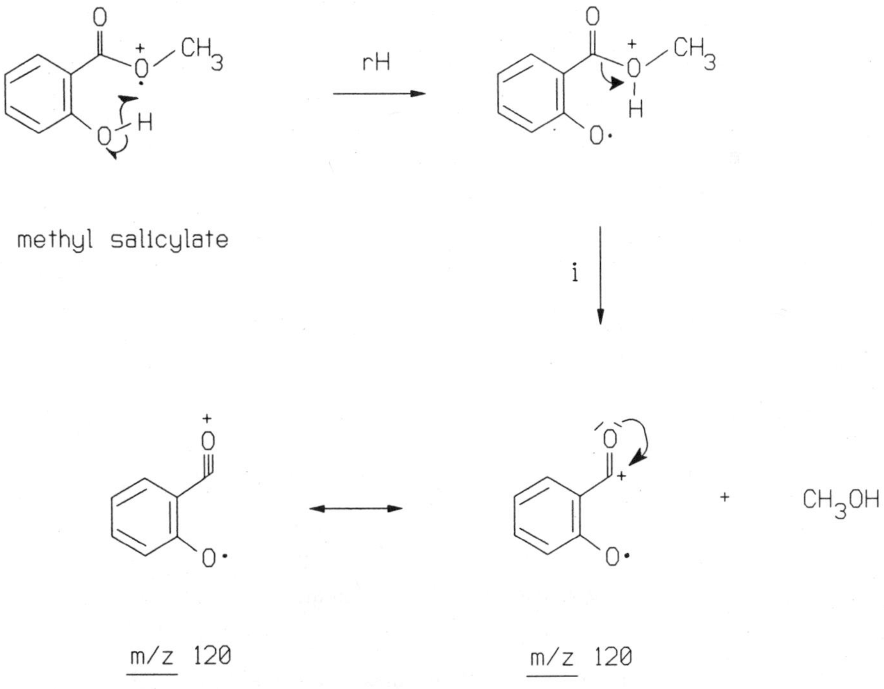

methyl salicylate

Scheme 12. Methyl salicylate.

If the hydroxyl is in the meta or para position, H transfer is not favorable, and loss of 31 u occurs. With the hydroxyl in the ortho position, loss of 32 u is seen. The driving force for this rearrangement may be the formation of the very stable neutral, methanol.

Another well-characterized rearrangement is the so-called *McLafferty rearrangement*. This rearrangement also has some very specific configurational requirements, so when it occurs, the analyst gains further insight into the molecule's structure. The cleavage produces the base peak in the mass spectra of fatty acid methyl esters (Scheme 13 on page 60).

The rearrangement starts with the transfer of an H atom from the γ position to the oxygen. This is a radical site-initiated transfer, with the new radical site forming on the γ carbon. Two possible products can now be formed by a series of

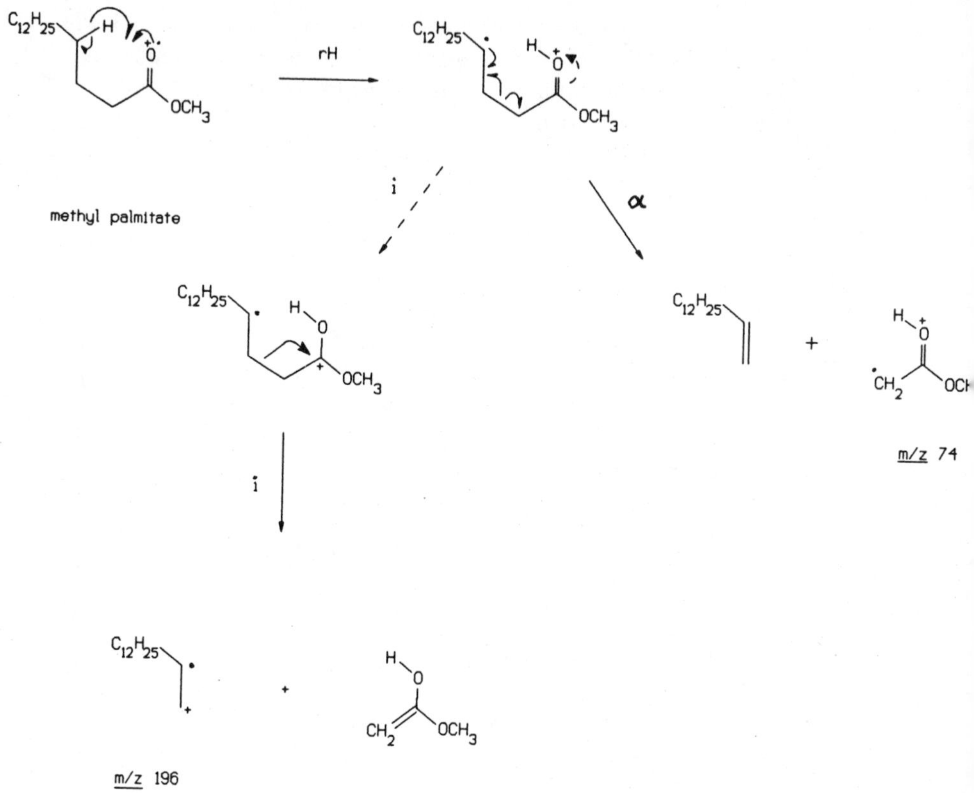

methyl palmitate

m/z 74

m/z 196

Scheme 13. Methyl palmitate.

either charge or radical site-initiated bond cleavages. The bond between the α and β position is broken in either case, but the charge can be retained on the carbonyl portion or on the alkyl portion of the molecule, depending on the relative stabilities. The six-membered cyclic transition state is key to this rearrangement, so participating hydrogens must be attached to the γ position. Double bonds in the α or β positions will distort the transition state and reduce the likelihood of rearrangement.

Other heteroatoms may take the place of oxygen, or the heteroatom can be absent entirely, as with the case of alkyl benzenes, of which pentyl benzene is illustrative (Scheme 14 on page 61).

The rearrangement leads to an ion of mass 92 that will appear along with the inevitable tropylium ion of mass 91 (see previous discussion). The presence of the peak at m/z 92 is a good indicator that the alkyl chain attached to benzene is at least three atoms long, in order for the six-membered transition state to be achieved.

Aromatic rings tend to be very stable; ions retaining them are very abundant. The rings do break down, however. Usually the driving force for this decompentyl benzene

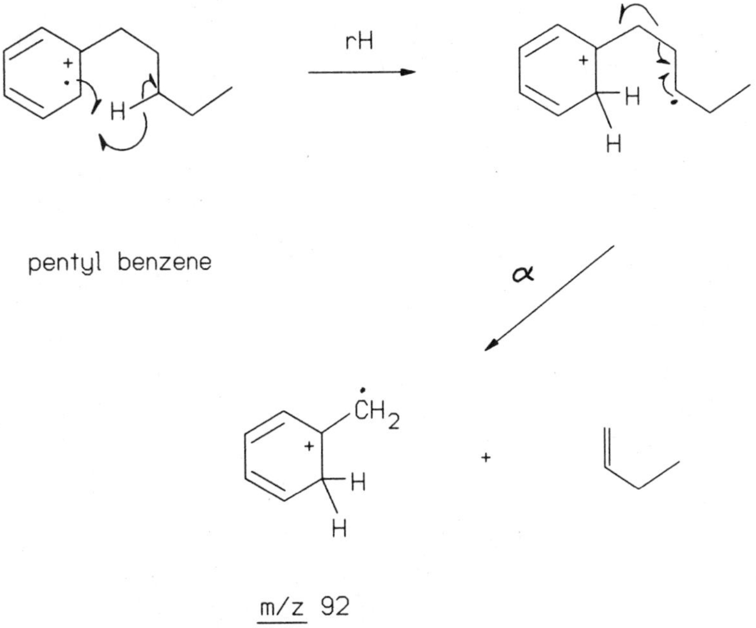

α

m/z 92

Scheme 14. Pentyl benzene.

position is the formation of a very stable small neutral molecule like C_2H_2 or CO. The ring probably closes back together after ejection of the neutral, so this process is a rearrangement. The mass spectrum of phenol (C_6H_5OH) has a very abundant molecular ion peak at m/z 94. The actual structure of this ion is likely to be a seven-membered ring including the oxygen (Scheme 15).

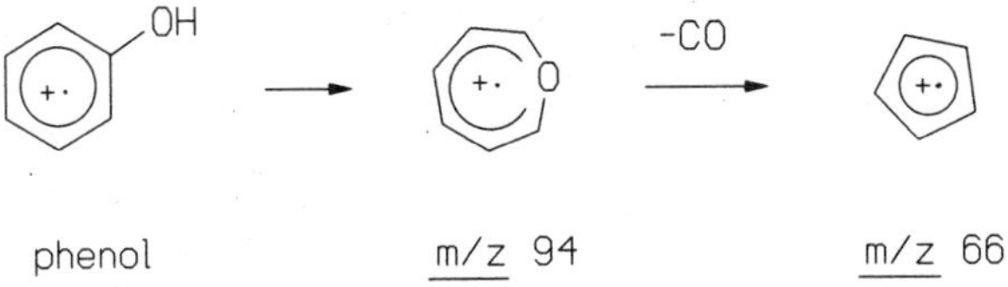

phenol   m/z 94   m/z 66

Scheme 15. Phenol.

This already involves some rearrangement, since new bonds are being formed. Little fragmentation of the molecular ion is observed, but a minor fragment ion peak appears at m/z 66, corresponding to the loss of CO, presumably with ring closure again as in Scheme 15. This involves still more bond rearrangement. Such complicated series of rearrangements make interpretation of spectra of compounds with substituted aromatic rings tricky. The substitution pattern is often

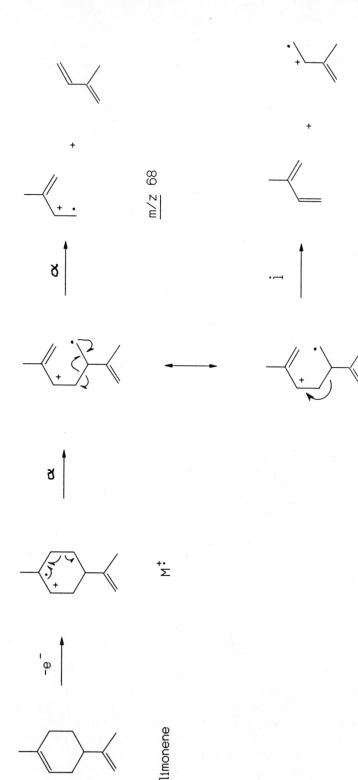

Scheme 16. Limonene.

m/z 68

m/z 68

M$^{+\cdot}$

limonene

$-e^-$

α

α

i

62

difficult or impossible to determine, except in unusual circumstances, such as the ortho effect mentioned previously.

Another rearrangement is observed in the mass spectra of molecules containing a substituted cyclohexene group, as illustrated with the terpene, limonene (Scheme 16 on page 62).

Ionization involves loss of an electron from the π system of the double bond, leaving the charge and radical sites at that position. As before, a series of electron migrations can occur, this time leading to products that look like an olefin and a conjugated diene.

This rearrangement is the reverse of a powerful reaction in organic synthesis, the Diels–Alder reaction. For that reason, this mass spectrometric rearrangement is known as the *retro-Diels–Alder* (rDA) rearrangement. As before, the charge can be retained on either fragment of the molecule, depending on relative stabilities. In the case of limonene, the molecule is split exactly in half and the two fragments have the same mass. The utility of this rearrangement in mass spectrometry is that it allows one to locate where on the cyclohexene ring substituents are attached. Different isomers will produce dienes and olefins with different masses. Cyclopentene or cycloheptene rings do not undergo this rearrangement to any great extent; the six-membered ring is again important. The class of molecules for which the rDA rearrangement is probably most important is the terpenoids, including the related steroids. These often contain cyclohexene moieties, and the pattern of substituents can sometimes be deduced.

Although there are many other types of fragmentation processes, space does not permit their discussion here. McLafferty's text (1) is highly recommended. Using combinations of the basic reactions previously described, the origins of the major ions in most mass spectra can be postulated.

3.4. Strategy for Interpretation

Each person must develop his or her own systematic strategy for interpreting unknown mass spectra. The key is to be systematic, considering all of the information one has or can glean from the spectrum. Care must be exercised to keep an open mind, as one of the most common pitfalls in interpretation is to try to fit the interpretation to a preconceived idea about what the result *should* be. McLafferty (1) suggests a series of steps that appear below in modified form:

1. Collect as much information as possible about the compound from sources other than the mass spectrum. Other spectral information or a knowledge of the source of the material are good places to start.

2. Using the masses and stable-isotope peak intensity patterns, try to postulate elemental compositions for the major ions in the spectrum. Calculate DBE; decide if ions are odd-electron or even-electron.

3. Identify the molecular ion using the following three criteria: the suspected ion must be the highest mass ion in the spectrum, it must be odd-electron, and it must reasonably account for the fragment ions represented in the spectrum.

4. Look for spectral features that are characteristic of particular functional groups. These might include characteristic losses, series of ions at low mass, or characteristic ions (e.g., tropylium ion). From the overall "shape" of the spectrum, decide if it might be aromatic or might contain many or few easily cleaved bonds.

5. Using the functional groups indicated in step 4, postulate molecular structures that might account for the ions observed. (Open-mindedness is especially important at this step to be sure to include all possible structures and isomers!)

6. Predict some of the major fragment ions that would be expected for each of the structures postulated in step 5. See how well these match the ions represented in the spectrum. Narrow the possibilities by eliminating structures that do not fit.

7. If possible, obtain standard spectra of the remaining structures. Compare these with the unknown to verify identity.

Even with the best systems, interpretation may be difficult or impossible. Practice interpreting a variety of unknown spectra is the best way to sharpen one's skills. A few simple examples are presented below.

3.5. Examples

Example 1. The spectrum in Fig. 24 seems quite simple. The base peak is at m/z 43, with an isotope peak at m/z 44 of 2.4% relative intensity, indicating a maximum of two carbons. Chlorine, bromine, sulfur, and silicon can be eliminated because nowhere are their unusual isotope peak patterns in evidence.

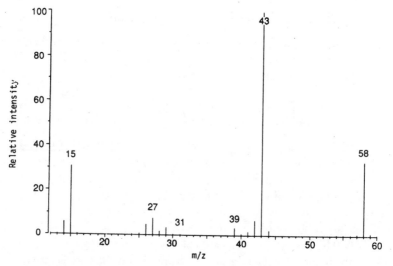

Fig. 24. EI mass spectrum considered as Example 1 (26).

Likely compositions for the ion of mass 43 are C_2H_3O or C_2H_5N. The peak at m/z 15 almost certainly represents CH_3. It is rarely anything else.

The molecular ion peak appears to be at m/z 58. This ion fits all of the criteria for a molecular ion. It should be noted that the two most abundant fragment ions, represented by peaks at m/z 43 and 15, add up to 58. Apparently a single bond is cleaved and the charge can be retained on either fragment. The even mass of the molecular ion indicates an even number of nitrogen atoms, probably none, because there is no evidence of nitrogen elsewhere in the spectrum. If we assume the compositions C_2H_3O and CH_3 for the ions of mass 43 and 15, respectively, the molecule must have a formula of C_3H_6O. The number of DBE is easily calculated to be $3 - 6/2 + 1 = 1$. There is one double bond.

We can begin to propose possible structures based on the data so far. Three structures suggest themselves:

$$CH_2{=}CH{-}CH_2{-}OH \qquad CH_3{-}CH_2{-}\overset{\overset{\displaystyle O}{\|}}{C}{-}H \qquad CH_3{-}\overset{\overset{\displaystyle O}{\|}}{C}{-}CH_3$$

Allyl alcohol   **Propanal**   **Acetone**

Of these, allyl alcohol has no CH_3 group to lose, but might be expected to lose 18 (H_2O) instead. We can eliminate this possibility. Propanal would be expected to undergo α cleavage to produce ions of mass 57 and 29. Neither of these ions is represented in the spectrum. Acetone, the remaining structure, fits the spectrum best. α cleavage on either side of the carbonyl group gives the ion of mass 43. Inductive cleavage can form the ion of mass 15. Comparison of the "unknown" spectrum with authentic spectra of acetone and propanal would verify the conclusion that acetone is the correct answer.

Example 2. The spectrum in Fig. 25 shows some rather unusual clusters of peaks, one beginning at m/z 248 and another beginning at m/z 169. These peak clusters should immediately alert the analyst to check for elements with multiple abundant stable isotopes. Comparing the spectrum in Fig. 25 with the examples in Fig. 23 suggests that the peak at m/z 248 represents an ion containing two bromine atoms and that the ion of mass 169 contains one bromine atom. (The mass difference between these two ions, $248 - 169 = 79$, also indicates a loss of one bromine atom.) Subtracting the mass of the bromine atoms (2×79) from 248 leaves 90 u for the rest of the molecule. The other stable isotope peaks, for example at m/z 249 or 251, offer little additional information. The relative abundance of the ion of mass 251 is 10% of that of mass 250, allowing for a maximum of nine carbon atoms. Combinations of atoms adding up to 90 u are not very plentiful, with C_7H_6 being a likely possibility.

One can suggest that the peak at m/z 248 represents the molecular ion. The formula $C_7H_6Br_2$ has a DBE of $7 - 8/2 + 1 = 4$. (Recall that Br is calculated as H in the DBE equation.) The fact that the DBE is an integer indicates that the ion of mass 248 is an odd-electron ion. It is the ion of highest mass represented in

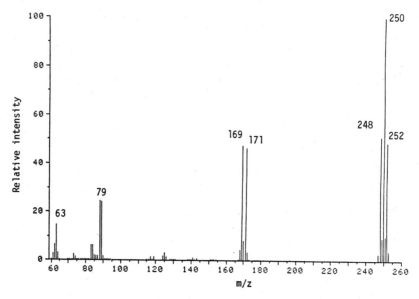

Fig. 25. EI mass spectrum considered as Example 2 (26).

the spectrum (neglecting isotope peaks), and reasonable fragmentation (loss of Br) is observed.

A useful feature of the spectrum is the *lack* of extensive fragmentation. The abundance of M^+ is high, indicating a very stable molecule. With DBE = 4, one should consider the presence of a benzene ring. Postulating structures, one arrives at a set of isomers of dibromotoluene:

Upon impact with a 70-eV electron, all of these are likely to adopt a seven-membered ring structure, analogous to a dibromotropylium ion. Consequently, the mass spectra of the various isomers will be very similar or indistinguishable. At this point, one should resort to IR, or especially NMR, spectroscopies to differentiate among the possibilities.

Example 3. The mass spectrum in Fig. 26 is much more complicated, with many ions throughout the mass range. High-resolution mass spectral data were used to assign the formula $C_6H_{12}O_2$ to the ion of nominal mass 116. Knowing the elemental composition facilitates data interpretation by constraining the number of formulas that must be considered. There are no Cl, Br, Si, or S isotope peaks in the spectrum, so those elements can be excluded from consideration. The major

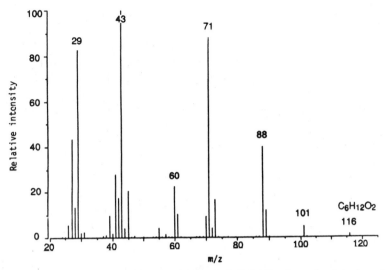

Fig. 26. EI mass spectrum considered as Example 3 (26). The formula of the ion of mass 116 was determined by high-resolution mass spectrometry.

ions, of mass 43, 71, and 29, have a maximum of three, four, and two carbon atoms, respectively, as evidenced by the relative intensities of the isotope peaks at m/z 44, 72, and 30. Because the high-resolution data show no nitrogen, elemental formulas can be restricted to C, H, and O. The peak at m/z 43 likely represents either C_3H_7 or C_2H_3O. The peak at m/z 71 cannot represent C_5H_{11}, because the isotope peak intensity indicates a maximum of four carbon atoms. C_4H_7O or $C_3H_3O_2$ are reasonable guesses. The peak at m/z 29 probably represents C_2H_5 or CHO. All of these ions are even-electron species; their DBE all calculate to fractional values.

Although the ion of mass 116 is of low abundance, it satisfies all the criteria for a molecular ion. The loss of 15 u (a methyl group) as indicated by the peak at m/z 101 is always an encouraging sign. The low abundance of M^+ indicates that the molecule has several facile fragmentation pathways available.

Most of the abundant fragment ions in the spectrum are of odd mass (e.g., m/z 71, 43, 29). The nitrogen rule states that these must be even-electron ions, and they probably result from single-bond cleavage. However, there are two ions represented in the spectrum by peaks with even masses, m/z 88 and 60. These must be odd-electron fragments, and must be formed by rearrangement of the molecular ion. Knowing this increases the importance of these two ions, as rationalizing their formation may help later in determining the arrangement of atoms in the molecule. The first rearrangement results in the loss of 28 u from the molecular ion: $116 - 88 = 28$. The second ion may be formed by loss of 56 u from M^+ or from a second loss of 28 u from the ion of mass 88. Losses of 28 u generally correspond to C_2H_4 or CO neutrals.

To summarize the characteristics deduced thus far: the molecular ion has a nominal mass of 116 and a formula of $C_6H_{12}O_2$. There is one DBE. The molecule has a methyl group, possibly a C_2H_5 fragment, and can rearrange to lose at least one 28-u moiety. Retro Diels–Alder rearrangements can be eliminated from consideration, because there is only one DBE, and a cyclohexene system must have at least two. The McLafferty rearrangement is another class of likely rearrangements. These might result if the single DBE were in the form of a carbonyl moiety. This is consistent with the molecular formula, and, thus, it will be used as a working hypothesis. The loss of 28 u in a McLafferty rearrangement involves a structure of the form:

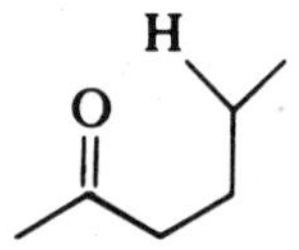

To determine if the α position carries an alkyl group, one can look for α-cleavage products that would come from either side of the carbonyl. The major peak at m/z 71 represents a likely candidate. It corresponds to a loss of 45 u from the $M^{\ddagger}$, presumably $(M - C_2H_5O)^+$. This seems to indicate an ethyl ester functionality:

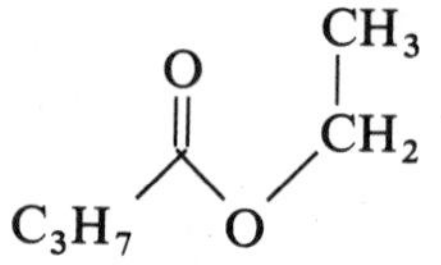

The presence of the C_3H_7 is confirmed by the peak at m/z 43 and a small $(M - C_3H_7)^+$ at m/z 75.

The second of the rearrangement ions becomes important at this stage. It is difficult to rationalize a loss of 56 u from the working model of the unknown. However, a loss of a second 28 u from the ion of mass 88 is readily explained if the C_3H_7 group can undergo a second McLafferty rearrangement. In order for this to occur, the propyl group cannot be branched, but must be linear. The required six-membered transition state can only be achieved with one arrangement of atoms:

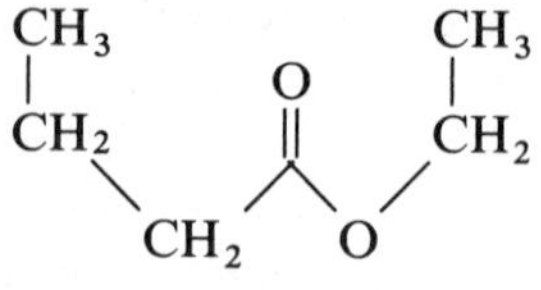

The spectrum must be that of ethyl butyrate. The formation of fragment ions is summarized in Scheme 17.

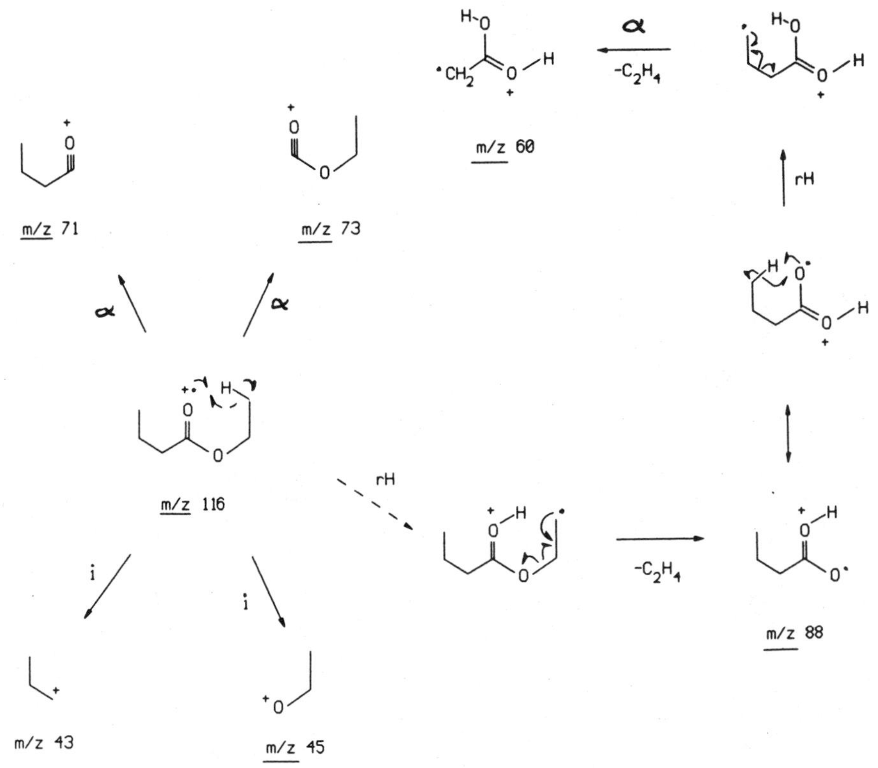

Scheme 17

Example 4. The spectrum in Fig. 27 is dominated by a peak at m/z 30, with other important peaks at m/z 107–108 and m/z 137. The isotope peak at m/z 31 has an intensity of 3% relative (to m/z 30), and could represent one or two carbon atoms. Possible formulas are C_2H_6, CH_2O, or CH_4N. The ion represented by the peak at m/z 108 has an isotope peak about 9.5% relative intensity, allowing a maximum of eight carbon atoms. One can postulate formulas of C_8H_{12}, C_7H_8O, $C_7H_{10}N$, or C_6H_6NO as likely possibilities. The elements with unusual distributions of stable isotopes (e.g., Cl, Br, S, Si) can be eliminated from consideration because their isotope peak patterns are not in evidence. Most of the other ions are of sufficiently low abundance that little can be learned from their isotope ion peaks.

A probable candidate for $M^{\ddagger}$ is the ion at mass 137. It fits the three previously listed criteria. If the peak at m/z 137 does represent the molecular ion, and therefore an odd-electron species, the nitrogen rule requires that the molecule have an odd number of nitrogen atoms. The very intense peak at m/z 30 is further evidence of nitrogen. Amines readily undergo α cleavage, and the even-electron

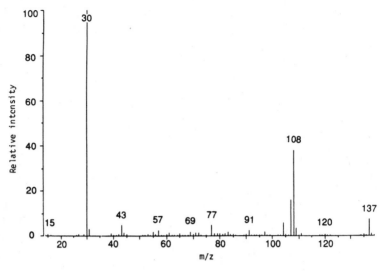

Fig. 27. EI mass spectrum considered as Example 4 (26).

fragment ions so produced are very stable. An intense peak at m/z 30 often represents an ion of the form $CH_2{=}NH_2$, arising from α cleavage of a primary amine (see Scheme 2).

Interestingly, the loss of 30 u from the molecular ion (mass 137) would give rise to an ion of mass 107, and the spectrum does have a peak corresponding to such an ion. The peaks at m/z 30 and m/z 107 probably represent complementary pieces of the molecule. If the ion of mass 30 contains the nitrogen atom, the ion of mass 107 cannot.

A reasonable assumption for the ion of mass 108 is that it contains one more hydrogen atom than the ion of mass 107. This being true, the ion of mass 108 is also unlikely to contain nitrogen. A fragment ion with an even mass (108 u) and with no nitrogen must be an odd-electron species, and therefore must result from a rearrangement process. Of the formulas suggested earlier, only C_8H_{12} and C_7H_8O are still possible. These ions have DBE's of 3 and 4, respectively, indicating a high degree of unsaturation or perhaps an aromatic ring. The minor peaks at m/z 91 and m/z 77 are also indicative of a benzene ring, so C_7H_8O (4 DBE) seems slightly more likely than C_8H_{12} (3 DBE).

Once again, the rearrangement ion (mass 108) takes on special significance. If the ion of mass 107 results from single-bond cleavage and contains an aromatic ring and if the ion of mass 108 involves a hydrogen rearrangement to the aromatic ring, the system is reminiscent of the pentyl benzene example in Scheme 14. In pentyl benzene, the ions of interest have masses of 91 and 92; in Fig. 27, the peaks are at m/z 107 and 108. The difference seems to be the presence of an extra 16 u (probably an oxygen atom) in the ions represented in Fig. 27. However, the presence of the rearrangement ion suggests that an alkyl chain at least three atoms long is attached to the aromatic ring in order for a cyclic six-membered transition state to be possible (see Scheme 18). The alkyl chain must also be the site of the primary amine.

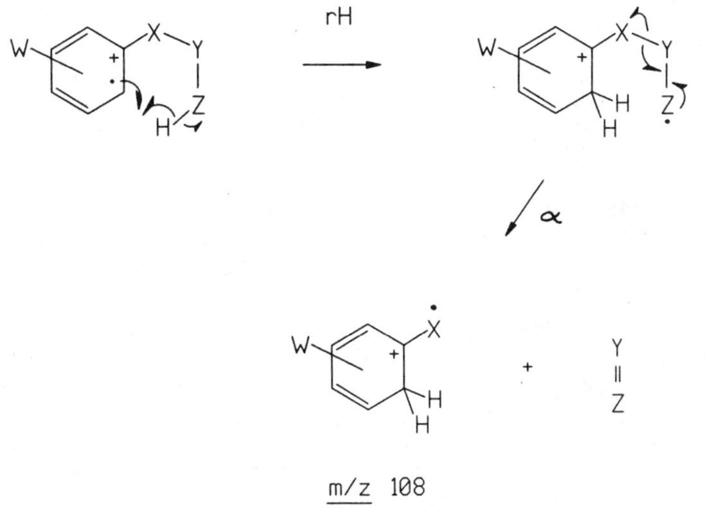

Scheme 18

There still remain a number of possible isomers:

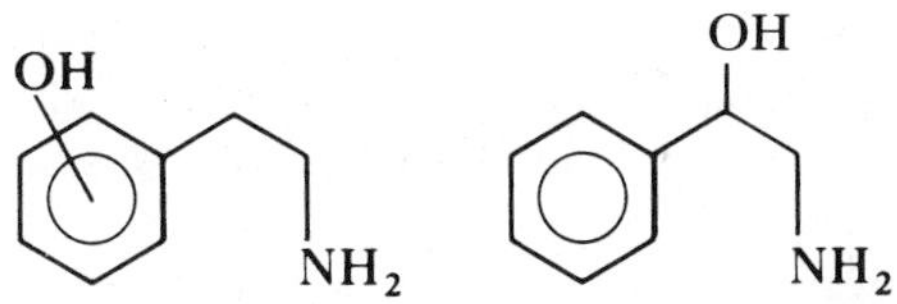

Structure **B** is unlikely, because it would be expected to lose 18 u (water) and produce an ion of mass 119, and no such ion is represented in Fig. 27. The other isomers would be difficult to differentiate without reference to the mass spectra of standard compounds. (The spectrum is actually that of tyramine.)

3.6. Computerized Aids to Interpretation

Anyone who has interpreted many mass spectra will attest that it can be a long and frustrating labor. Not surprisingly, people have long sought to utilize computers to aid in the interpretation process. Computers can do repetitive calculations with extreme speed and are not subject to the interpretive bias that might influence the human interpreter. Finally, if computers can aid in the identification of samples, less training is required for routine data interpretation. There is no question but that computers can be of tremendous assistance in compound identification, if a healthy distrust is maintained by the analyst.

There are two approaches to computer-aided interpretation: *library searching* or *retrieval* methods and *artificial intelligence* or interpretive programs. The first of these is widely available on most commercial mass-spectrometer data systems, and is routinely used in most laboratories. The second usually requires more sophisticated software and careful interpretation, so is primarily used by a few specialized labs. The artificial intelligence methods will not be considered further here, but have been reviewed recently (27).

Since the mid-1950s, the mass spectra of tens of thousands of organic compounds have been collected. Many of these have been compiled into libraries of reference spectra; these spectra represent known compounds analyzed under standard conditions. A spectrum-by-spectrum visual comparison of an unknown mass spectrum with several thousand reference spectra is obviously unworkable, but with computer assistance, such a search can be completed in a few minutes or even seconds.

Different algorithms have been developed to perform the comparison between the unknown and the reference spectra. Ideally, one seeks from the calculation a number, or *metric*, that represents the quality of the match between the two. On many commercial systems, the calculation is designed to provide a number between 0.0 and 1.0, with 0.0 being a very poor match and 1.0 being a perfect match. The library search result is a list of the (usually 10) best matching compounds from the reference library, that is, those with the comparison metric closest to 1.0.

Most search routines perform acceptably well when the unknown compound is pure and a standard spectrum of that compound exists in the reference library. The more usual (and more difficult) situation occurs when either the sample spectrum is impure or when none of the reference spectra exactly match the unknown. Under these circumstances, one would like the search routine to retrieve those spectra from the library that most closely match the unknown. The assumption is made that compounds with similar mass spectra will be chemically similar. The performance of commercial library search routines on these more difficult unknowns is somewhat variable, and a careful analyst will always check the computer's result by visually inspecting the unknown and reference spectra to verify that they are indeed similar.

Two serious considerations with regard to library searching must be kept in mind. The storage of tens of thousands of mass spectra in a computerized database requires a substantial amount of computer storage space. Additionally, the number of calculations involved in comparing an unknown mass spectrum to those thousands of reference spectra is tremendous, even with the aid of a computer. Good library searches take time. A number of shortcuts have been proposed to alleviate one or both of these problems. Most often the shortcuts involve some sort of spectral *abbreviation*, rather than storing and comparing the full mass spectra. The compromise is in the quality of the reference information and the quality of the search results, both of which must suffer to some extent with spectral abbreviation. In the end, the analyst must choose between a very fast search and a slower, but perhaps more satisfactory search. Chapman (4) has reviewed many of the more common spectral abbreviation and retrieval algorithms.

One final note regarding library searching deals with the reference library itself. There is some benefit to having a very large spectral database, in that one is less likely to miss unusual compounds that might turn up in an unknown sample. Even the largest commercial databases, however, are biased in their coverage of compound classes. Historically, the easiest compounds to study by MS, and hence the compound classes that are best represented in reference libraries, are those molecules that are reasonably volatile and of relatively low molecular weight ($< m/z$ 500). Many classes of biological molecules do not fit into these categories. Consequently, spectral databases include hundreds of spectra of hydrocarbons and small lipids, but frequently have few or no peptide or nucleotide spectra. Many laboratories choose to generate their own spectral libraries, representing the compound classes most likely to be encountered in analyses in that lab. These smaller, more tailored databases, often provide more accurate and speedier search results.

4. SPECIAL TECHNIQUES

As powerful as EI–MS is, there are many instances in which it cannot provide complete information satisfactorily. Other mass-spectrometric techniques, including those listed subsequently, can be used in conjunction with or in place of EI–MS to accomplish the desired analytical goal.

4.1. Chemical Ionization

Unlike EI–MS, little needs to be said about the interpretation of CI mass spectra. CI is a soft-ionization technique, chosen because it causes less fragmentation than EI. Still, CI continues as an active research area, primarily because of the capability to study gas-phase chemistry.

In its usual mode, ionization in CI results from proton transfer from a reagent ion to the analyte molecule (see Section 2.1.2). The dominant analyte ion is often $(M + H)^+$. Excess internal energy for fragmentation comes from the difference in proton affinities between the reagent and analyte. The fragments observed in CI are often somewhat different than those in EI. For example, the $(M + H)^+$ is an even-electron ion; there is no radical site. For that reason, the radical site-initiated fragmentation mechanisms found in EI–MS are of less consequence in CI. CI fragmentation is dominated by charge site-initiated loss of small neutral molecules (inductive cleavage) and low-energy rearrangements.

Figure 28 shows the mass spectra of a methoxime-trimethylsilyl derivative of prostaglandin E_1 (MW = 599) under EI and several different CI conditions (28). In the EI spectrum (Fig. 28A), a variety of fragment ions result from radical site-

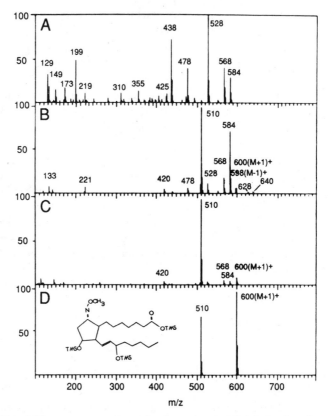

Fig. 28. EI and CI mass spectra of a methoxime-trimethylsilyl derivative of prostaglandin E_1 (mol wt 599) using various reagent gases. (*A*) EI, (*B*) methane CI, (*C*) isobutane CI, and (*D*) ammonia CI. (Reproduced with permission from Ref. 28.)

initiated processes. For example, the base peak of the spectrum at m/z 528 represents α cleavage and loss of a C_5H_{11} fragment from the alkyl side chain. In the CI spectrum using methane as a reagent gas (Fig. 28*B*), some fragmentation is observed, but the fragments are now primarily the result of charge site-initiated processes. The base peak at m/z 510 represents a hydrogen migration and inductive cleavage (rearrangement and loss of TMSOH).

Fragmentation in CI mass spectra is decreased by decreasing the excess energy available to the analyte molecules. This is accomplished by selecting a reagent gas that has a proton affinity closer to that of the analyte. Isobutane (PA = 8.5 eV) and ammonia (PA = 9.0 eV) have higher proton affinities than methane (PA = 5.5 eV), so CI with these reagent gases will produce spectra with less fragmentation than those in methane CI. Figures 28*C* and 28*D* compare the spectra of the prostaglandin derivative ionized by reaction with isobutane and ammonia, respectively. Fragmentation is reduced until, in the ammonia CI spectrum, the $(M+H)^+$ ion becomes the base peak of the spectrum.

Care must be exercised, however, in assuming that the base peak of the CI mass spectrum represents $(M+H)^+$. There are a number of circumstances when this will not be the case. Saturated alkanes have very low proton affinities, and hence are poor proton acceptors in CI reactions. Often, rather than seeing proton transfer, one will observe transfer of a hydride (H^-) from the alkane to the reagent ion:

$$M + C_2H_5^+ \rightarrow (M-H)^+ + C_2H_6 \qquad (19)$$

$(M-H)^+$ will be a prominent ion, rather than $(M+H)^+$. There is no way of knowing for an unknown sample if this is occurring, so caution is always advised.

In other circumstances, although $(M+H)^+$ does form, it so readily undergoes fragmentation that it is not seen. The base peak of the spectrum may be $(M+H-\text{small neutral})^+$. Aliphatic alcohols are a case in point. The isobutane CI spectrum of 2-hexanol (mw = 102) has its base peak at m/z 85, $(M+H-H_2O)^+$; the peak for $(M+H)^+$ at m/z 103 is only about 2.5% relative intensity.

As the difference between the PA of the analyte and the reagent gas becomes small, adduct formation increases. One can think of the collision of a reagent ion and an analyte molecule as forming a transient complex that subsequently breaks apart:

$$M + C_2H_5^+ \rightarrow [M + C_2H_5]^+ \rightarrow (M + H)^+ + C_2H_4 \qquad (20)$$

The less excess energy the intermediate complex has (the closer the PA's of the reactants), the more likely that this complex will be stable enough to be observed. In methane CI spectra, in addition to $(M+H)^+$ ions, one frequently sees $(M+29)^+$ and $(M+41)^+$ ions. These are probably the result of collisions of the analyte with $C_2H_5^+$ and $C_3H_5^+$ reagent ions, both of which have higher PA than CH_5^+. These adduct ions are represented in Fig. 28B at by peaks at m/z 628 for $(M+29)^+$, and at m/z 640 for $(M+41)^+$.

Adduct ions can be particularly prominent in CI mass spectra if ammonia is used as the reagent has. Figure 29 shows the ammonia CI mass spectrum of a trimethylsilyl derivative of prostaglandin F_1 (mol wt 644). The $(M+NH_4)^+$ adduct ion is represented by the base peak, while the $(M+H)^+$ is not observed at all. This again is reason to be wary, in that it is difficult to know if the peak one observes represents $(M+H)^+$ or $(M+NH_4)^+$. This is not a serious problem if peaks are observed for both species, as they can be recognized by their mass difference of 17 u.

Because CI tends to produce little fragmentation, it is a popular choice for quantitation of analytes by mass spectrometry. If all of the ion current for the analyte is represented by a single m/z, there will be greater sensitivity (signal produced per unit weight of analyte added) than if the ion current is spread out over tens or hundreds of fragment ions, as in EI. For example, Weisberger et al. (29) used CI with ammonia as a reagent gas for the determination of the drug

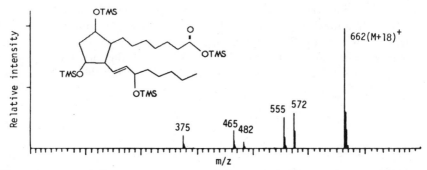

Fig. 29. Ammonia CI mass spectrum of a trimethylsilyl derivative of prostaglandin F_1 (mol wt 644). (Reproduced with permission from Ref. 28.)

albuterol in blood plasma. The CI mass spectrum of the trimethylsilyl derivative of albuterol is shown in Fig. 30. The simple spectrum provides a diagnostic peak at m/z 456 that was used for quantitation down to 250 pg/mL.

If the conjugate base of the reagent ion has a higher proton affinity than the analyte, the reaction in Eq. 6 will be endothermic, that is, energy will have to be supplied in order to make the reaction proceed. In a CI source, only two-body collisions take place. No mechanism exists for adding energy to force a reaction to proceed. Exothermic reactions will proceed spontaneously upon collision of the ion and molecule. Endothermic reactions will not proceed at all. Even though analyte may be present in the ion source, if the proton affinity of the analyte is lower than that of the reagent gas, proton transfer does not occur and the analyte is not ionized (protonated) or observed. This can lead to selectivity in the ionization process. If a reagent gas is chosen that has a proton affinity higher than

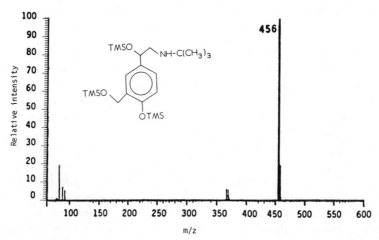

Fig. 30. Ammonia CI mass spectrum of the trimethylsilyl derivative of albuterol (mol wt 455). (Reproduced with permission from Ref. 29.)

some of the components in a mixture and lower than others, only those compounds with a proton affinity higher than the reagent gas will be observed. The other components will not be ionized or detected (30).

Chemical ionization need not always involve the transfer of a proton. A variety of reagent gases have been proposed that promote other gas-phase chemistry for specific analyses. Hunt and Sethi (31) have discussed several of these.

4.2.　Negative Ion Formation

To this point, only positively charged ions have been considered. Negative ions are also formed in the ion source. However, because of the electric fields used to extract, accelerate, and analyze positive ions, the negative ions are not observed. If the polarity of the electric fields in the instrument are changed, however, these negative ions can be detected. Under electron impact conditions, the negative ions tend to be low-mass "molecular debris"—ions like Cl^-, OH^-, O^-. This is because collisions of an analyte molecule with energetic electrons promote two fragmentation processes: *ion-pair formation* (Eq. 21) and *dissociative capture* (Eq. 22):

$$M + e^- \rightarrow A^+ + B^- + e^- \tag{21}$$

$$M + e^- \rightarrow A^- + B \tag{22}$$

Which of these two reactions takes place will depend on the energy of the electron. Ion-pair formation predominates at electron energies above 15 eV; dissociative capture occurs when the electron energy is 2–15 eV. The negative ions formed will be those parts of the molecule that can best stabilize the negative charge. This usually turns out to be the electronegative elements present, such as halogens or oxygen.

The molecular debris carries little structural information and no information at all about the molecular weight, so is generally of limited value. If the energy of the electron is lowered still further, however, negative-ion MS can be extremely useful. Under these conditions, when the energy of the electron approaches 0 eV (so-called *thermal electrons*), certain sample molecules can capture and retain the electron in a process known as *resonance capture*:

$$M + e^- \rightarrow M^{\overline{\cdot}} \tag{23}$$

Those molecules that are ionized best in this process are, not surprisingly, molecules that have a high affinity for electrons and can best stabilize an excess negative charge. Halogenated compounds (those containing F, Cl, Br, I), nitro compounds, and highly conjugated aromatic systems are among the best analytes. The difference in ionization efficiency between these compounds and others that are not good electron capturers is often dramatic. Molecules that are good electrophiles may be detected at 1000-fold higher sensitivity than the same compound analyzed with EI or positive ion CI (32).

Instrumentally, the major requirement for electron-capture negative-ion MS is a source of thermal electrons. Usually this is achieved in a CI-like experiment. Recall that in CI, methane at a pressure of 100 Pa is bombarded with energetic electrons. Referring to Eq. 2, one observes that in addition to the ionized methane atom, two electrons are products of the reaction. These electrons have less energy after colliding with methane than before, and continue to lose more energy with each successive collision. After a very short time in the ion source, the electrons have lost all of their excess energy; they are said to have been "thermalized." At this stage they are available for capture by an electrophilic analyte.

The negative-ion mass spectra of electron-capturing molecules are generally quite simple. Because there is little excess energy imparted in the ionization process, fragmentation is minimal. The molecular anion often dominates the spectrum. When fragmentation does occur, only relatively weak bonds are broken and the negative charge is retained where it is best stabilized. Figure 31 shows the negative-ion mass spectra of two representative compounds. The

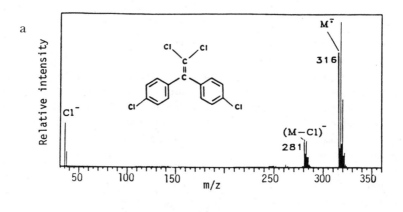

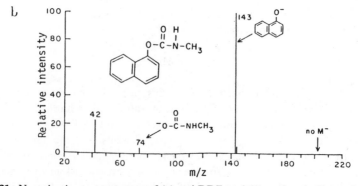

Fig. 31. Negative-ion mass spectra of (a) p,p'-DDE and (b) carbaryl. (Reproduced with permission from Refs. 33 and 34, respectively.)

spectrum of p,p'-DDE is dominated by $M^{\cdot}$, with few significant fragment ions. In the mass spectrum of the pesticide carbaryl, on the other hand, the base peak represents a fragment ion, the naphthoxyl ion. This ion is particularly stable because the negative charge can be delocalized from the oxygen through a series of resonance structures involving the aromatic ring.

There are three benefits to using negative-ion MS; the greatest of these is the remarkable sensitivity. Compounds that are good electrophiles, such as the polychlorinated dibenzo-p-dioxins, can be detected down to the picogram level, even in very complex tissue samples. For compounds that are not naturally electrophilic, the formation of a suitable chemical derivative can make them so. Amino acids are not particularly good electrophiles. If, however, they are reacted with fluorodinitrobenzene (Sanger's reagent), the resulting 2,4-dinitrophenyl amino acids are excellent electron capturers and can be detected at the femtomole (10^{-15} mol) level. The drug amphetamine, when reacted with perfluorobenzoyl chloride to make an electrophilic derivative, can be detected at the 10 attomole (10^{-17} mol) level (35).

A second benefit of negative-ion MS is the selectivity of the ionization process. Biological samples are often very complex mixtures, but rarely are many electrophilic species present. A method that can selectively detect some components in the mixture while ignoring all others can offer significant gains in signal-to-noise levels. The *chemical noise*, caused by compounds in the sample that are not the analyte, is decreased markedly, and the detection limit for an electrophilic analyte is correspondingly better.

When analyte molecules do undergo fragmentation in negative-ion MS, the third benefit can be realized. Negative-ion fragments are those that can best stabilize a *negative* charge, ions observed in positive-ion MS are those that can best stabilize a positive charge. This difference means that the two types of spectra will offer complementary information about the molecule. Figure 32 shows the positive- and negative-ion mass spectra of a permethylated tetrapeptide, Met-Gly-Met-Met. One can see that different ions are formed by each ionization method, and the two sets of ions taken together provide a more complete picture of the molecule than either set alone (36).

Negative-ion MS does seem to be somewhat more dependent on instrumental conditions than other modes of ionization. Spectra obtained on different mass spectrometers in different laboratories can look quite different, both with regard to the extent of fragmentation and to overall sensitivity. Particular care must be given to the ion-source temperature and pressure of reagent gas (usually methane). As the source temperature increases, the amount of fragmentation generally increases. The amount of sample used is also critical. Because of the extreme sensitivity of the technique, the ion source can be easily overloaded. If the population of thermal electrons in the ion source becomes depleted, further increase in analyte concentration produces no further increase in signal, but may lead to changes in the appearance of the mass spectrum, particularly evident in the relative abundance of the ions. The theory and applications of negative-ion MS have been the subject of several excellent reviews (37, 38).

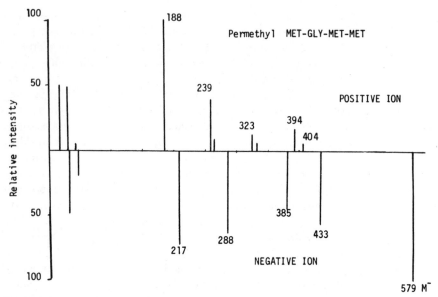

Fig. 32. Positive-ion and negative-ion mass spectra of the permethylated tetrapeptide Met-Gly-Met-Met (mol wt 579). (Reproduced with permission from Ref. 36.)

4.3. Desorptive Ionization

The various desorptive ionization methods (FD, SIMS, FAB, ^{252}Cf-PD; see Section 2.1.3) were developed to be soft-ionization processes for large, nonvolatile molecules. Consequently, the mass spectra of the compounds desorbed tend to be rather simple, with few fragment ions. The $(M+H)^+$ or $(M+Na)^+$ or both are the dominant ions; sodium is a ubiquitous contaminant and is difficult to eliminate. Fragment ions are usually of low abundance unless the analyte is very fragile or is heavily loaded into the ion source.

In all of the desorptive methods, some general similarities are apparent. Analytes that already carry a charge, so-called *preformed charge* molecules, seem to be detected with relative ease. Tetraalkyl ammonium salts like choline or charged detergents are ready examples. It is thought that upon bombardment, these molecules can be sputtered directly into the gas phase where, because of their charge, they are readily extracted and analyzed.

Molecules that do not carry a charge but are easily protonated are next most readily observed. Peptides might fall into this class. The proton may come from the matrix, so the acidity of the matrix is important. Additionally, traces of some other acid, often formic or trifluoroacetic acid, may be added to the sample or matrix to ensure analyte protonation, thus improving ionization efficiency. Molecules that neither carry a charge nor are readily protonated are generally detected with poorest sensitivity under desorptive ionization conditions. This order, preformed charge > polar noncharged > nonpolar noncharged, is just the opposite of that expected when samples must be heated and vaporized prior to ionization as in EI. In EI–MS, one might form a chemical derivative to decrease the polarity of a molecule and make it more volatile. In desorptive-ionization MS, one might prepare a chemical derivative that actually *increases* the polarity by adding a permanent charge to the analyte.

Some investigators have used SIMS in the analysis of drug mixtures (39). Under normal SIMS conditions, $(M+H)^+$ ions are observed for each drug in a mixture if sufficient sample is applied to the probe. However, if the drug mixture is derivatized to place a charge on certain components in the mixture without affecting the other components, a degree of selectivity can be achieved. The derivatized drugs that carry a charge are detected with much greater sensitivity than those that are neutral. Figure 33 shows the SIMS mass spectrum of a drug mixture after derivatization to place a charge on one of the components, acetaminophen. As a result of derivatization, one compound carries two charges (mol wt 410, m/z 205) and is not readily detected; another compound carries no charge (mol wt 235) and is not detected. Only acetaminophen, derivatized to form a singly charged species (mol wt 305), is observed in the secondary-ion mass spectrum.

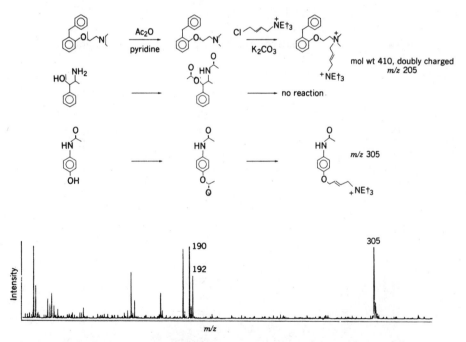

Fig. 33. Secondary-ion mass spectrum of a drug mixture. The three active ingredients in a Sin-U-Tab tablet were derivatized to observe only the acetaminophen. Ions at mass 90 and 92 result from excess derivatizing reagent. (Reproduced with permission from Ref. 39.)

In FAB–MS analysis the sample is nearly always dissolved or suspended in a liquid matrix. This may be glycerol, thioglycerol, dithiothreitol/dithioerythritol mixtures, or one of many other choices. Upon bombardment with the atom beam, this matrix, as well as the analyte, is ionized and detected. Consequently, the low-mass region of a FAB mass spectrum is dominated by peaks representing clusters of the matrix: protonated and natriated (sodium adducts) dimers, trimers, and higher oligomers. Figure 34 shows a FAB mass spectrum of an underivatized oligopeptide from the epithelial cell growth factor, prostatropin (40). The strong signal for the $(M+H)^+$ is obvious at m/z 1540. There is little fragmentation of the peptide, and the low-mass end of the spectrum is obscured by peaks related to the matrix. Peptides are generally amenable to analysis by FAB–MS, probably because of the large number of basic sites in the molecules (see Chapter 3).

The presence of the matrix has another important consequence in FAB–MS. It is observed that molecules with a high surface activity are more easily detected in FAB–MS. This is thought to be a result of the clustering of surface-active molecules at the surface of the glycerol droplet. Because these molecules are close to the surface, they are more readily sputtered into the gas phase. Glycerol is a hydrophilic matrix; compounds that are hydrophobic tend to migrate to the glycerol–vacuum interface. Hydrophilic compounds dissolve well and are distributed in the bulk of the droplet. This can lead to problems when mixtures are analyzed by FAB. If hydrophilic and hydrophobic peptides are present in the same sample, signals from the hydrophobic peptides dominate, suppressing the

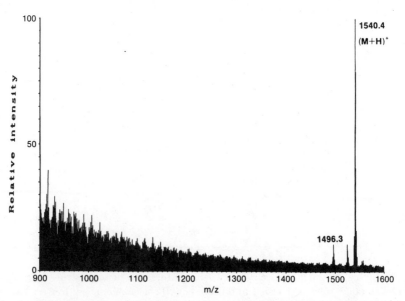

Fig. 34. FAB mass spectrum of an underivatized tetradecapeptide from prostatropin (mol wt 1539). (Spectrum courtesy of Dr. S. A. Carr, Smith Kline and French Labs.)

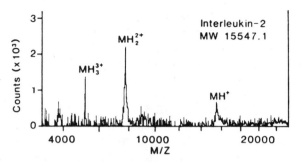

Fig. 35. ^{252}Cf plasma-desorption time-of-flight mass spectrum of interleukin-2. (Reproduced with permission from Ref. 42.)

signals from the hydrophilic peptides. Similarly, if peptides and glycopeptides are present in the same sample, the more hydrophilic glycopeptides may be overlooked because their signals are suppressed by those of the free peptides.

^{252}Cf plasma-desorption MS is popular for the analysis of large proteins because of its sensitivity and extreme mass range (41). The largest proteins that have been analyzed by mass spectrometry (>mol wt 25,000!) have been analyzed by PD–MS with a time-of-flight mass analyzer. Figure 35 shows the PD mass spectrum of interleukin-2 (42). In addition to the protonated molecules, abundant doubly and triply charged ions are observed. Although the mass resolution is poorer than that of SIMS or FAB using a double-focusing mass analyzer, it is still adequate to determine the molecular weight of the protein with an accuracy of plus or minus a few mass units. The PD–MS technique is an excellent way to monitor the progress of a large peptide synthesis, where at each step, one would like to know if the desired amino acid residue has been incorporated. Furthermore, in separating peptide and protein mixtures by HPLC, the application of PD–MS as a monitor of collected fractions allows the investigator to know instantly the molecular weights of each peptide in the fraction.

Schiebel and Schulten (43) compared 10 desorptive-ionization methods for a set of biomolecules and noted some general trends. The FD mass spectrum of vitamin B_{12} showed a prominent M^+, $(M+H)^+$, and $(M+Na)^+$ with little fragmentation until late in the analysis, when thermal degradation began to appear. SIMS analysis of B_{12} showed $(M+H)^+$, $(M+Na)^+$, and $(M+Ag)^+$ (a silver target was used). At higher mass, cluster ions appeared corresponding to $(2M+H)^+$ and $(2M+Ag)^+$. The only significant fragment ion was $(M-CN)^+$. The FAB mass spectrum of B_{12} showed $(M+H)^+$ and a few fragment ions.

4.4. Tandem MS

An exciting and relatively recent development in mass spectrometry is the use of a mass spectrometer as a separation device prior to a second mass spectrometer. This technique, *tandem MS* or *MS/MS*, opens up a wide range of analyses and experiments that would be difficult or impossible by any other method (44). Figure 36 shows a conceptual representation of the processes accomplished in one type of tandem MS experiment.

Ionization of the analyte can occur by any of the methods discussed so far. Ions are accelerated and analyzed as before. The mass analyzer allows ions of one particular mass to be transmitted into a *field-free region* of the instrument, where no electric or magnetic fields interfere with the ion's motion. In this region, the ion decomposes to form fragments, either unimolecularly or after collision with an inert gas. [The reader will recognize that ions that decompose in the field-free region of their own accord are simply metastable ions, which were described earlier (see Section 3.1). The use of a collision gas to provide additional energy for

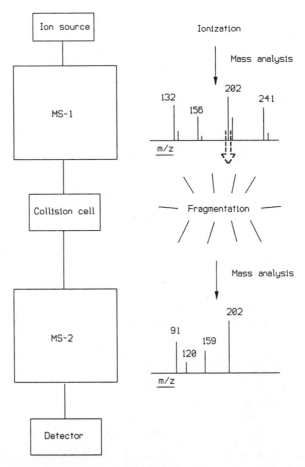

Fig. 36. Conceptual schematic of one type of MS–MS experiment. After ionization and mass analysis by MS-1, a particular *m/z* ratio is transmitted to the collision cell for fragmentation. The daughter ions are analyzed by scanning MS-2.

the decomposition leads to what is called *collisional activation* (CA) or *collision-induced decomposition* (CID).] The ions formed by decomposition of the *parent ion* are generally referred to as *daughter ions*. The second mass analyzer separates these daughter ions, transmitting them in turn to the detector.

Almost any of the mass analyzers discussed in Section 2.2 can be used as the first or second components of a tandem instrument. The first such experiments used a double-focusing mass spectrometer, with each sector providing one level of analysis. Commercial instruments are now available with various combinations of mass analyzers. As a shorthand notation, the arrangement is usually specified by a series of letters, Q representing a quadrupole; E, an electric sector; and B, a magnetic sector. Thus BEQ would signify an instrument with a double-focusing mass spectrometer (BE) as the first mass analyzer (MS-1) and a quadrupole (Q) as the second mass analyzer (MS-2). When two quadrupoles are linked together, the "field-free" region is usually encompassed by a third set of quadrupole rods. Because there are actually three quadrupoles in succession, these instruments are known as *triple quads* or *triple stage quadrupoles* (TSQ), but only the first and third quadrupoles are used for mass analysis. Combinations of magnetic sector instruments and quadrupoles are called *hybrid instruments*.

A variety of experiments can be performed on a tandem instrument. The technique of selecting a parent ion with MS-1 and analyzing the daughter ions with MS-2 is *daughter ion scanning*. MS-1 is held fixed at the m/z of the parent, MS-2 is scanned through the mass range. This type of experiment is useful if MS-1 is being used as a separation device. With samples that are complex mixtures, a soft-ionization method can produce molecular ions (or protonated molecules) for each component in the mixture. MS-1 can then select the parent ion of interest for CID, ignoring ions from all other compounds, provided that they have different masses. MS-2 separates and detects fragment (daughter) ions transmitted from the collision cell following CID. Interpretation of the daughter ion spectrum provides the structural information on the selected parent. Figure 37 shows a typical daughter ion spectrum from the peptide methionine enkephalin. Because of the MS/MS technique, the investigator can assume with confidence that all of the peaks in this daughter ion mass spectrum represent fragment ions that originate from the parent ion of mass 574. The fragments in the daughter ion spectrum allow the determination of the sequence of amino acids in this peptide (see Chapter 3). Very little sample clean-up is required, and the only interferants of concern will be compounds that have precisely the same molecular weight as the analyte.

In other circumstances, one might wish to know what components in a mixture were producing a given daughter ion. In this case, one would set up a *parent ion scan*. MS-2 is fixed to transmit the daughter ion of interest and MS-1 is scanned to analyze all higher masses that might be possible parent ions. Only when a true parent traverses MS-1 and the appropriate daughter ion is transmitted through MS-2 is a signal obtained at the detector. Parent ion scanning is used when determining what components of a mixture are chemically related or when tracing an ion's genealogy, that is, the fragmentation mechanisms that lead to the formation of a given daughter ion.

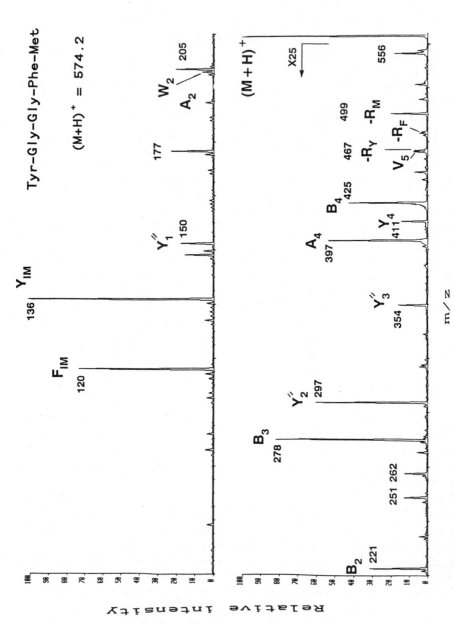

Fig. 37. Daughter ion spectrum of Met-enkephalin. The protonated parent (*m/z* 574) was produced by FAB–MS. Letters indicate sequence ions in standard MS nomenclature (see Chapter 3).

Finally, both mass analyzers in a tandem experiment may be scanned, but in such a way that a constant mass difference is maintained between them. This is *neutral loss scanning* and is used to locate compounds in a mixture that belong to a particular compound class. For example, alcohols are known to readily lose 18 u (water). A neutral loss scan in which MS-1 is scanned through the mass range and MS-2 is scanned to transmit ions 18 mass units lower than those transmitted by MS-1 will allow the identification of all the alcohols in a sample.

Regardless of the scan mode of tandem MS or the choice of mass analyzers, one thing is clear. A tandem MS experiment is more instrumentally complex and expensive than analysis using a single mass analyzer. Under what circumstances might tandem MS be worth the added complications? An important example was described in the preceding paragraphs in which CID was used to stimulate dissociation of a protonated peptide and a daughter ion scan provided fragment ion peaks derived from $(M + H)^+$ for purposes of determining the amino acid sequence in the peptide.

Fatty acids provide a second example. Many naturally occurring fatty acids contain one or more double bonds. EI–MS is of little value in locating the position of these double bonds because the high-energy process of EI ionization causes the double bond to migrate up and down the alkyl chain. The EI mass spectra of various isomers of fatty acids differing only in the position of the double bonds are quite similar. Adams and Gross (45) have shown that tandem MS can be used to locate branch points and double bonds in fatty acids. If the fatty acids are ionized by FAB in the presence of a lithium salt, ions for $(M + Li)^+$ and $(M - H + 2Li)^+$ are observed. MS-1 can select either of these ions, and collisional activation provides a series of daughter ions useful in determining the structure of the alkyl chain. Figure 38 shows the daughter-ion mass spectra of ions derived from linolenic acid. The positions of the double bonds can be assigned unambiguously (45).

Another example illustrating the specificity and sensitivity of MS/MS is described in Chapter 5, Section 5.5.3.4. in the context of analyzing hair for morphine content. Yet another exciting application lies somewhere in the future of tandem MS. A simple EI mass spectrum is a two-dimensional data set. It can be (and usually is) represented as a plot of m/z in one dimension and relative intensity of the peaks in the other dimension. Imagine if that same material were analyzed by tandem MS in such a way that ion current at each m/z of the original spectrum were selected sequentially by MS-1, collisionally activated, and the daughter ions recorded. For each m/z, one would now have a daughter-ion spectrum that could serve as a fingerprint of the parent ion, in the same way that EI spectra are currently used to characterize chemical compounds. The data set would now have a third dimension and would carry much more information about a compound than the current two-dimensional spectrum. A more unique three-dimensional fingerprint would provide a far greater degree of specificity than is currently possible, and would likely prove as successful in structural analysis as modern two-dimensional NMR techniques. This kind of MS/MS

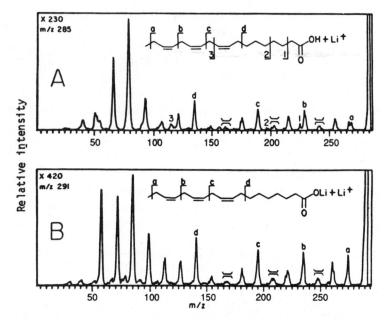

Fig. 38. Daughter-ion spectra of (A) $(M+Li)^+$ and (B) $(M-H+2Li)^+$ ions derived from linolenic acid (mol wt 278). (Reproduced with permission from Ref. 45.)

experiment is beyond current instrumental capabilities in terms of spectral collection, storage, and retrieval, but is certain to develop in the not-too-distant future.

References

1. F. W. McLafferty, *Interpretation of Mass Spectra*, 3rd ed., University Science Books, Mill Valley, CA, 1980.

2. J. T. Watson, *Introduction to Mass Spectrometry*, 2nd ed., Raven, New York, 1985.

3. W. H. McFadden, *Techniques of Combined GC—MS*, Wiley, New York, 1973.

4. J. R. Chapman, *Computers in Mass Spectrometry*, Academic Press, New York, 1978.

5. H. M. Rosenstock, M. B. Wallenstein, A. L. Wahrhaftig, and H. Eyring, *Proc. Natl. Acad. Sci. USA* **38**, 667–678 (1952).

6. M. S. B. Munson and F. H. Field, *J. Am. Chem. Soc.* **88**, 2621–2630 (1966).

7. R. J. Cotter, *Anal. Chem.* **52**, 1589A–1606A (1980).

8. A. Benninghoven, D. Jaspers, and W. Sichtermann, *Appl. Phys.* **11**, 35–39 (1975).

9. M. Barber, R. S. Bordoli, R. D. Sedgwick, and A. N. Tyler, *J. Chem. Soc. (London) Chem. Commun.* 325–327 (1981).

10. R. D. Macfarlane, *Anal. Chem.* **55**, 1247A–1264A (1983).

11. H. E. Duckworth, R. C. Barber, and V. S. Venkatasubramanian, *Mass Spectroscopy*, 2nd ed., Cambridge University Press, London, 1986, pp. 84–108.

12. P. H. Dawson, *Mass Spectrom. Rev.* **5**, 1–37 (1986).

13. J. Allison and R. M. Stepnowski, *Anal. Chem.* **59**, 1072A–1088A (1987).

14. G. C. Stafford, Jr., P. E. Kelley, J. E. P. Syka, W. E. Reynolds, and J. F. J. Todd, *Int. J. Mass Spectrom. Ion Proc.* **60**, 85–98 (1984).

15. M. V. Buchanan, Ed., *Fourier Transform Mass Spectrometry: Evolution, Innovation, and Applications*, American Chemical Society, Washington, DC, 1987.

16. D. A. Laude, Jr., C. L. Johlman, R. S. Brown, D. A. Weil, and C. L. Wilkins, *Mass Spectrom. Rev.* **5**, 107–166 (1986).

17. R. B. Opsal, K. G. Owens, and J. P. Reilly, *Anal. Chem.* **57**, 1884–1889 (1985).

18. J. F. Holland, C. G. Enke, J. Allison, J. T. Stults, J. D. Pinkston, B. Newcome, and J. T. Watson, *Anal. Chem.* **55**, 997A–1012A (1983).

19. J. S. Cottrell and S. Evans, *Anal. Chem.* **59**, 1990–1995 (1987).

20. R. A. Hites and K. Biemann, *Anal. Chem.* **42**, 855–860 (1970).

21. A. E. Ashcroft, J. R. Chapman, and J. S. Cottrell, *J. Chromatogr.* **394**, 15–20 (1987).

22. C. R. Blakley, J. J. Carmody, and M. L. Vestal, *J. Am. Chem. Soc.* **102**, 5931–5933 (1980).

23. D. A. Garteiz and M. L. Vestal, *LC Magazine* **3**, 334–346 (1985).

24. K. Biemann, *Mass Spectrometry: Organic Chemical Applications*, McGraw-Hill, New York, 1962.

25. H. Budzikiewicz, C. Djerassi, and D. H. Williams, *Interpretation of Mass Spectra of Organic Compounds*, Holden-Day, San Francisco, CA, 1964.

26. Spectra are reprinted with permission from the EPA/NIH Mass Spectral Database (currently called NIST/EPA/MSDC Mass Spectral Database), courtesy of Dr. S. Lias, NIST Mass Spectrometry Data Center, Gaithersburg, MD 20899.

27. D. P. Martinsen and B. H. Song, *Mass Spectrom. Rev.* **4**, 461–490 (1985).

28. T. Ariga, M. Suzuki, I. Morita, S. Murota, and T. Miyatake, *Anal. Biochem.* **90**, 174–182 (1978).

29. M. Weisberger, J. E. Patrick, and M. L. Powell, *Biomed. Mass Spectrom.* **10**, 556–558 (1983).

30. I. Dzidic and J. A. McCloskey, *Org. Mass Spectrom.* **6**, 939–940 (1972).

31. D. F. Hunt and S. K. Sethi in *High Performance Mass Spectrometry: Chemical Applications*, M. L. Gross, Ed., American Chemical Society, Washington, DC, 1978, pp. 150–178.

32. J. R. Hass, M. D. Friesen, D. J. Harvan, and C. E. Parker, *Anal. Chem.* **50**, 1474–1479 (1978).

33. E. A. Stemmler and R. A. Hites, *Anal. Chem.* **60**, 787–792 (1988).

34. S. Safe and O. Hutzinger, *Mass Spectrometry of Pesticides and Pollutants*, CRC Press, Cleveland, OH, 1973, p. 17.

35. D. F. Hunt and F. W. Crow, *Anal. Chem.* **50**, 1781–1784 (1978).

36. D. F. Hunt, G. C. Stafford, Jr., F. W. Crow, and J. W. Russell, *Anal. Chem.* **48**, 2098–2105 (1976).

37. J. G. Dillard, *Chem. Rev.* **73**, 589–643 (1973).

38. H. Budzikiewicz, *Angew. Chem. Int. Ed. Engl.* **20**, 624–637 (1981).

39. D. A. Kidwell, M. M. Ross, and R. J. Colton, *Biomed. Mass Spectrom.* **12**, 254–260 (1985).

40. J. W. Crabb, L. G. Armes, S. A. Carr, C. M. Johnson, G. D. Roberts, R. S. Bordoli, and W. L. McKeehan, *Biochemistry* **25**, 4988–4993 (1986).

41. B. Sundqvist and R. D. Macfarlane, *Mass Spectrom. Rev.* **4**, 421–460 (1985).

42. I. Jardine, G. F. Scanlan, A. Tsarbopoulos, and D. J. Liberato, *Anal. Chem.* **60**, 1086–1088 (1988).

43. H. M. Schiebel and H. R. Schulten, *Mass Spectrom. Rev.* **5**, 249–311 (1986).

44. K. L. Busch and R. G. Cooks, in *Tandem Mass Spectrometry*, F. W. McLafferty, Ed., Wiley, New York, 1983, pp. 11–39.

45. J. Adams and M. L. Gross, *Anal. Chem.* **59**, 1576–1582 (1987).

Mass Spectrometry of Carbohydrates

CARL G. HELLERQVIST, *School of Medicine, Vanderbilt University, Nashville, Tennessee* and
BRIAN J. SWEETMAN, *School of Medicine, Vanderbilt University, Nashville, Tennessee*

1. INTRODUCTION

Complex carbohydrates are recognized as important components in specific molecular interactions that govern a multitude of important biological phenomena. Cell–cell adhesion, cell–substrate adhesion, cell motility, metastases of tumor cells, hostile and symbiotic microbial adhesion to eucaryotes and procaryotes, and viral absorption are some of these now generally recognized areas. Detailed structural information about specific carbohydrate epitopes is needed in order to understand the molecular events underlying these phenomena.

The development of gas-chromatography phases capable of separating the many isomeric sugars derived from complex bacterial and plant poly- and oligosaccharides was a major factor in developing modern analytical carbohydrate chemistry. Another development came in the combination of the separatory power of the gas chromatograph with the specificity of a mass spectrometer, as pioneered by Dr. Ragnar Ryhage at the Karolinska Institute in Stockholm, Sweden. These developments set the stage for a quantum leap in analytical chemistry, which made possible, for the first time, the analysis of milligram quantities of complex carbohydrates. The first polysaccharide subjected to this now standard technique, an arabinogalactan, is the subject for the thesis of Dr. Bouveng in 1964. The structural elucidation required more than 100 g of material and three years of work to isolate and characterize the compound. By contrast the new GC–MS methodology made it possible to quantitatively and qualitatively confirm the work of Bouveng over a period of only two weeks with the procedures devised for hydrolyzing (1), separating (2), and analyzing (3) 5 mg of the arabinogalactan and its corresponding partially methylated alditol acetates. Since this time, further methodological advances have been introduced using open tubular gas-chromatographic columns, which have resulted in dramatic improvements in the capacity to resolve compounds by gas chromatography. More recently, innovations in mass-spectrometer design, such as an extended mass range, and new ionization techniques, such as fast-atom bombardment, have increased dramatically the diversity of problems that are amenable to analytical carbohydrate chemistry.

The first polysaccharide subjected to this analytical procedure was the O-antigenic side chain from *Salmonella typhimurium* (4). This paper and a paper by Björndal, Hellerqvist, Lindberg, and Svensson (5) became Citation Classics, which reflect the enormous interest in and the importance of the field of analytical carbohydrate chemistry. During the following years this basic methodology was utilized for sequence analysis. Dr. K. A. Karlson showed that analysis by GC–MS of fully methylated glycolipids could yield partial sequence information of heterosugars in the oligomer (6). Combined with linkage analysis, substantial structural information could be obtained (7). Recent technological advances in both gas chromatography and mass spectrometry have also resulted in substantial improvements in this methodology for elaborating the partial structures of both native and derivatized oligosaccharides (8–11).

The recent work by Angel et al. (11) has added a sophisticated dimension to sequence analysis of complex oligosaccharides derived from glycoproteins and glycolipids. The methodology combines the established analytical tool of periodate oxidation with reduction, methylation, and structural analysis using FAB–MS. Their procedure (11) was modified by our laboratory (12, 13) to take advantage of known preferences for fragmentation around functional groups in alditol derivatives (5) to sequence polysaccharides and oligosaccharides.

The intent of this chapter is to provide the reader with a general, practical strategy for elucidating complex carbohydrate structures using mass spectrometry. It is, therefore, neither intended nor is it appropriate, in this context, to attempt a broader review or evaluation of the numerous approaches that have been taken in elaborating carbohydrate structures. The format of this chapter will be to introduce the reader to practical hints relevant to (a) preliminary sample evaluation; (b) sample preparation; (c) quantitative and qualitative sugar analysis; (d) qualitative and quantitative linkage analysis; (e) anomeric configuration determination; and (f) sequence analysis using mass spectrometry as the primary analytical tool.

2. SAMPLE EVALUATION

2.1. Polysaccharides

The isolation of a structurally homogeneous polysaccharide from any biological source, be it from plant, bacteria, or mammalian cells, is hampered by the fact that biosynthetic principles rule out the existence of polysaccharides with homologous structures of the same size. Furthermore, structural modifications are made to the basic polysaccharide after its initial synthesis.

Bacterial polysaccharides in general, be they lipopolysaccharides or capsular polysaccharides are polymerized repeating units synthesized by polymerases with limited specificity for structural features beyond a basic backbone structure (14). The polymer is then subjected to "posttranslational modifications" with the addition of substituents that can be glycosides (15), acyl groups (16), pyruvates, cyclic acetals (17), phosphates (18), sulfates (19), taurine moieties (20), and so forth. Many of these functional groups are readily detectable by NMR spectroscopy, which is often used to obtain structural information without consuming valuable sample. It should be noted also that the Division of Research Resources of the National Institutes of Health operates several service centers that can provide assistance in the areas of NMR spectroscopy and mass spectrometry.

The biosynthesis of both mammalian and plant polysaccharides may well depend on similar polymerization mechanisms, which are not yet fully understood. At present, chain elongation in mammalian polysaccharides is assumed to involve the sequential addition of glycosides from specific nucleotide donors (21). In addition to the types of posttranslational modifications described above, these types of polysaccharides may also be subject to isomerization after polymerization. The formation of L-iduronic acid residues (22) and subsequent N- and O-sulfation in mammalian proteoglycans, for instance, serve to illustrate that this apparent random conversion of D-glucuronic acid to iduronic acid residues is, in fact, carefully regulated in order to give rise to specific oligomeric structures within the polymer to control certain highly specific biological functions (21–24).

2.2. Oligosaccharides

Investigators interested in the structure of complex oligosaccharides derived from mammalian glycoproteins and glycolipids are urged to acquire a mastery of the known biosynthetic pathways and enzyme specificities governing the synthesis of the compound of interest, be it glycolipid, ganglioside (25), O-linked (26) or N-linked oligosaccharide (27).

Polysaccharides can be isolated, usually with substantial effort, in reasonable amounts for structural analysis. Oligosaccharides, associated with biological function in mammalian systems, however, are rarely obtainable in amounts sufficient for absolute structural determination. For instance, cell–substrate (28) and cell–cell adhesion (29) are triggered by the specific interaction of only one or a few molecular structure conformations out of approximately 10^5 possible structural conformations. The biologically or pathophysiologically active carbohydrate substructure of interest is most likely a small epitope within a structure (23, 30). Knowledge of known biosynthetic pathways can often be used to deduce significant tentative structural information about both the core structure and the substituents. The investigator can then often plan an analytical approach to the particular problem based on this preliminary information that will yield maximum structural information from any given amount of material. Significant knowledge can often be obtained without resolving the complete structure.

3. SAMPLE PURIFICATION

Because of the complex mechanisms involved in the biosynthesis of polysaccharides, the term homogeneity is hardly applicable to a polysaccharide of interest. Microbial as well as mammalian polysaccharides are most often composed of repeating structural entities varying from disaccharides in proteoglycans (21) to decasaccharides in bacterial polysaccharides (31). In addition, the degree of polymerization of the repeating units is highly variable. As a consequence, a biologically active polysaccharide may have a molecular weight range that differs by thousands of daltons.

A diverse range of methodology is available for the purification of poly-saccharides. The choice of an appropriate methodology for a particular poly-saccharide depends, in part, on the biological origin of the compound of interest because specific biosynthetic factors may restrict both composition and structural variations. The biological function of a polysaccharide, however, is associated usually with a specific functional structural unit (SFSU), which may range in size from a pentasaccharide to an octasaccharide. An SFSU by extrapolation from our knowledge of immunology (30) need not be larger than a hexasaccharide. Specific degradation procedures may therefore be used to isolate and purify to homogeneity intact SFSUs from polysaccharides or complex oligosaccharides (32, 33).

To the uninitiated analytical carbohydrate chemist, it may seem surprising that the unrestricted biosynthesis of a simple hexasaccharide from the eight most common sugars can yield more than 4.76×10^9 distinct possible structures. Thus, even with the SFSU isolated to homogeneity, the elucidation of its structure could still be a formidable task. Fortunately, as discussed, biosynthesis of polysaccharides in both mammalian and microbial systems follow very well-defined rules that yield polysaccharides with repetitive structures, and oligosac-charides with cautiously predictable core structures. Figure 1 illustrates the magnitude of the analytical problem of resolving the structure of a triantennary N-linked oligosaccharide, and the consequences of different analytical approaches.

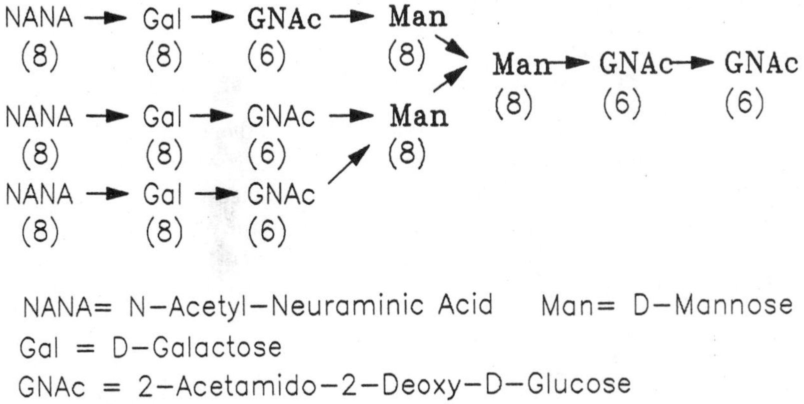

NANA= N—Acetyl—Neuraminic Acid   Man= D—Mannose
Gal = D—Galactose
GNAc = 2—Acetamido—2—Deoxy—D—Glucose

Fig. 1. Approximate number of possible structures in a tetradecasaccharide composed of four sugars in a ratio of $3:3:3:5$ is 3.51×10^{18}. The number is derived by: (1) The number of ways each sugar can be linked, given that it can be either α- or β-linked, is the product of $8 \times 8 \times 6 \times 8 \times 8 \times 8 \times 6 \times 8 \times 8 \times 8 \times 6 \times 8 \times 6 \times 6 = 1.0436771 \times 10^{12}$. Linkage informa-tion reduces this number to $2^{14} = 16,384$ and knowledge of the anomeric configuration would reduce the number of possibilities from 2^{14} to 1. (2) Number of sequence permutations of 14 units of 4 different sugars in a molar ratio of $3:3:5:3$ is $14!/3! \times 3! \times 3! \times 5!) = 3,363,360$. Knowledge of the biosynthetic pathway leading to the **core structure** eliminates all but $8!/(3! \times 3! \times 2!) = 560$ structures to be resolved.

4. ANALYTICAL STRATEGY

The determination of the structure of an oligosaccharide derived from a larger oligosaccharide can be accomplished by responding to the following four basic questions.

4.1. Which Sugars and in What Molar Ratio?

Sugar analysis is accomplished by hydrolyzing completely the glycosidic linkages in such a manner as to minimize degradation of the individual monomers, followed by quantitative and qualitative analyses of the sugars by GC and GC–MS, as their corresponding alditol acetates.

4.2. Mode of Attachment?

Linkage analysis is achieved by quantitative and qualitative permethylation followed by complete hydrolysis and identification by the free hydroxyl groups by GC and GC–MS. The hydroxyl groups identify the linkage points in the original carbohydrate component. Determining the ring form as pyran or furan is accomplished for most cases by this analysis, but may, in the case of 4-linked residues, require further analysis. The sum of the different sugar derivatives should be in agreement with the results of the sugar analysis. Discrepancies in stoichiometry between sugar and linkage analyses may indicate the presence of alkaline-labile or acid-stable groups.

4.3. Anomeric Configuration?

Anomeric configuration may be determined with the aid of high-resolution NMR when sufficient amounts of *pure* material are available. Alternatively, chromic acid oxidation of peracetylated carbohydrate components will specifically degrade the β-linked sugar residues. A sugar analysis of the oxidized material will, when compared with the analysis of the native component, reveal which residues are originally α-linked.

4.4. Monomer Sequence?

Sequence analysis can be achieved through a combination of chemical modifications and analysis of specifically derivatized compounds by FAB–MS or desorption-chemical-ionization-MS.

In all analytical procedures described herein it is understood that all solvents and reagents are of highest purity and that all liquids have been freshly distilled. Furthermore, it is understood that all glassware is acid washed, and has been stored wrapped in aluminum foil no more than one week. Deviating from these norms may result in decreased reliability and ambiguity during analysis by GC–MS or quantitative analysis by GC or both.

5. QUANTITATIVE AND QUALITATIVE SUGAR ANALYSES

5.1. Introduction

If the physical and chemical properties of the sample show that it contains acidic functions such as uronic acid residues, Conrad's procedures should be used to reduce the sample with carbodiimide and sodium borodeuteride (34). The cleavage of glycosidic linkages by acid hydrolysis occurs at rates that vary widely with the type of sugars present in the polymers (1, 5). The rate of hydrolysis depends on the electron density at the ring oxygen or glycosidic oxygen. Thus, 6-deoxy and 2-acetamido-2-deoxy-glycosides hydrolyze at approximately 10 times the rate of hydrolysis of glucosidic linkages. Nonreducing terminal residues hydrolyze at rates two to five times that of their internal counterparts. Sialic acid, 2-deoxy, and dideoxy sugars hydrolyze at about 100 times the rate of hydrolysis of glucosidic lingages. In addition, free sialic acid residues and 2-deoxy sugar residues are also susceptible to acid catalyzed degradation. Hydrolytic conditions are commonly used that will degrade and incompletely hydrolyze glycosidic linkages in complex oligo- and polysaccharides. Glucosaminidic linkages, for instance, are very resistant to acid hydrolysis because of the protonated amino groups. These structural features are not commonly found other than in proteoglycans. They are formed during hydrolysis from the commonly found 2-acetamido-2-deoxy glycosides, however, at a rate sufficiently high to prevent complete hydrolysis of the original N-acetyl glycosaminidic linkage, when strong inorganic acids are used ($> 1\,M$ HCl) (5).

To completely hydrolyze a polysaccharide, to protect the more rapidly released sugar residues, and to re-N-acetylate hydrolyzed acetamido groups, Hellerqvist and co-workers (16, 35) prescribe use of a mixture of glacial acetic acid and sulfuric acid as described subsequently. This mixture is proposed to generate an inorganic–organic anhydride capable of N-acetylation and acylation of the glycosidic hydroxyl group.

5.2. Procedure for Sugar Analysis by GC–MS

1. The sample ($1–10\,\mu g$) is dissolved in a glass ampul in $200\,\mu L$ of $2\,M$ sulfuric acid. $1.8\,mL$ of glacial acetic acid is added and the sealed ampul is heated at $100°C$ for 9 h.

2. Acetic acid is removed by repetitive codistillation with water in a rotary evaporator or under nitrogen in a waterbath. Temperature should be kept at less than $40°C$ to minimize losses of volatile components.

3. The sulfuric acid is neutralized by the addition of an *equimolar amount* of $BaCO_3$. Excess precipitate will lower the recovery.

4. The slurry is vacuum filtered through a sintered glass funnel (pore size F) into a 15 mL pear-shaped flask, and washed twice with 1 mL of water. Filtrate and washings are combined.

5. To the combined filtrate and washings (< 4 mL) is added a spatula tip (~ 5 mg) of sodium borodeuteride. The mixture is kept for 1 h at ambient temperature. If microbubbles cannot be seen forming after 30 min, add more borodeuteride.

6. To terminate the reaction, add a small chip of dry ice to consume excess borodeuteride and to precipitate remaining barium ions as $BaCO_3$.

7. The mixture is then filtered through a sintered glass funnel into a pear-shaped flask. The residue is washed with 2×1 mL water and the filtrate and washings are combined.

8. Add approximately 3 mL of glacial acetic acid and methanol (~ 15 mL) to the filtrate and washings from step 7. Rotary evaporation removes the volatiles including the methyl borate that is formed. Before the mixture evaporates to dryness, add further methanol. Repeat the procedure of addition of methanol and evaporation three more times. Transparent sodium acetate crystals should be seen inside the flask. White rather than transparent crystals are indicative of the presence of sodium borate, the presence of which hinders acetylation. If borate is present, it can be removed by dissolving the sample in 1 mL of water adding 1 mL glacial acetic acid and 5 mL of methanol. Repeat evaporations with methanol alone three times. When the sample is completely free of borate, add absolute ethanol (10 mL) and evaporate to dryness.

9. The residue is acetylated by the addition of a one-half filled pasteur pipette (0.5 mL) of freshly distilled pyridine and one pipette (1 mL) of acetic anhydride. Pasteur pipettes must have been acid-washed like all other glassware used in these procedures. The flask is stoppered and is heated in a sandbath at 100°C for 30 min.

10. The reaction mixture is removed from the bath, toluene (~ 5 mL) is added. Pyridine and acetic anhydride are codistilled with toluene to dryness at 40°C using a rotary evaporator. Fresh toluene is added as needed (two or three times) to maintain efflux of liquid from the sample. Use of the azeotrope minimizes loss of volatile derivatives from the sample.

11. Prepare a filter unit from a pasteur pipette fitted with a glass wool plug and 3–4 mm of active charcoal. Wash the filter unit using several milliliters of ethyl acetate and discard the washings. Add the residue from step 10 above dissolved in ethyl acetate to the damp filter. Wash the filter twice with ethyl acetate (0.5 mL) and combine the filtrate and washings, which are then evaporated to dryness under a stream of nitrogen. The filtrate and washings are best collected in a pasteur pipette sealed just below the tapered portion. The sample is dissolved in ethyl acetate prior to analysis by GC and/or GC–MS.

5.3. Identification of Alditol Acetates by GC–MS

In our laboratory, the samples are analyzed by GC and GC–MS using an OV-225 fused silica column of 5 m length (Quadrex Corp.). Incidently, the same column has been used daily in one of the authors' laboratories for 8 years with occasional injection of 100 μL chloroform for cleaning.

Quantitatively, the flame-ionization-detector (FID) response should be determined for each sugar derivative. In the author's laboratory the response of a Perkin Elmer Sigma 1 GC to the alditol acetates is almost exactly proportional to the total number of carbons in the molecule; for example, the FID response to one mole of peracetylated rhamnitol is 16/18th of that of the corresponding glucitol derivative. There may be some variation between individual gas chromatographs depending on their individual characteristics. In an analysis using a gradient from 190 to 230°C at 8°C/min and a carrier gas flow rate of 1 mL/min, deoxyhexoses will elute within 4 min, pentoses within 8 min, hexoses within 10 min, and amino sugars within 20 min.

The tentative identification of particular peaks as representing specific sugars is confirmed or rejected by GC–MS analysis using a similar column and conditions to that used for the GC analysis. In this way, variations in relative retention times are kept to a minimum in order to cross-correlate the quantitative GC and the qualitative GC–MS analyses.

Figure 2 illustrates the simple primary fragmentation pathways seen for a hexitol acetate and 6-deoxy-hexitol acetate. Introducing deuterium into carbon-1 during the reduction step provides a uniqueness in the spectrum that allows one to distinguish opposite ends of the molecule. As can be seen in Fig. 2, fragments that include carbon-1 (C-1) have an even mass and those retaining carbon-6 (C-6) in hexoses and C-5 in pentoses have an odd mass. Each acetylated carbon in the chain has a mass of 72 daltons. The fragment ions are formed through fission between any two carbons in the alditol chain with the charge retained on either carbon. The mass spectrum of the molecule therefore yields peaks at

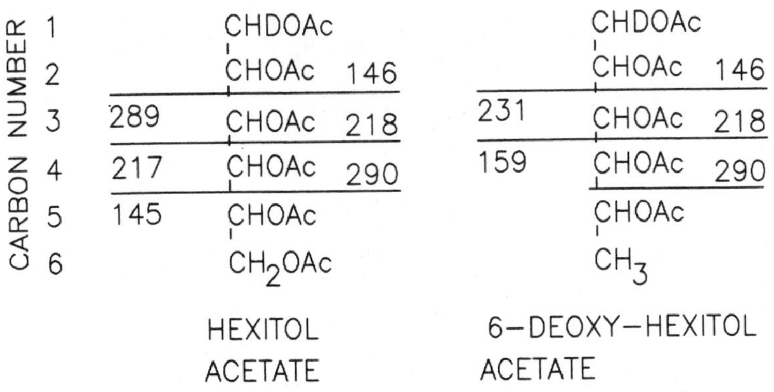

CARBON NUMBER		HEXITOL ACETATE				6–DEOXY–HEXITOL ACETATE	
1			CHDOAc			CHDOAc	
2			CHOAc	146		CHOAc	146
3	289		CHOAc	218	231	CHOAc	218
4	217		CHOAc	290	159	CHOAc	290
5	145		CHOAc			CHOAc	
6			CH$_2$OAc			CH$_3$	

Fig. 2. The primary fragment ions represented by peaks in the mass spectra are formed by fission between carbons in the acetylated chain. Charge is retained on either carbon at the cleavage site. A primary fragment ion containing the deuteride-reduced carbon-1 has a mass of $(n \times 72) + 2$ daltons, where n is the number of acetoxylated carbons in the alditol fragment ($+2$ is for the deuterium on carbon-1). Primary fragments containing acetoxylated carbons from C-6 and up are represented by fragment ion peaks at $m/z = (n \times 72) + 1$ in aldoses and by $(n \times 72) + 15$ for 6-deoxy-aldoses.

$m/z = (n \times 72) + 2$ (where n equals the number of acetylated carbons in the fragment) when the fragment includes C-1 with a deuteride and at $m/z = (n \times 72) + 1$ when the charged fragment contains C-6. In the event the original material contained uronic acid residues, which were reduced prior to the analysis, these would be qualitatively and quantitatively determined by the presence of fragment ion peaks at $m/z = (n \times 72) + 3$ as illustrated in Fig. 3. The 6-deoxy-hexose yields the usual even-mass fragments containing C-1. The deoxy function is evident by fragment ion peaks having $m/z = 15 + (n \times 72)$ from the C-6 end.

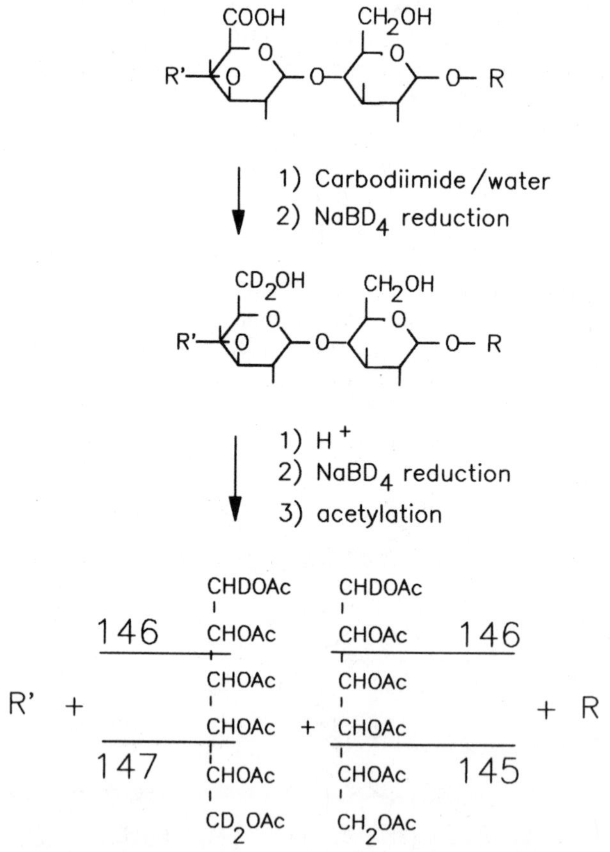

Fig. 3. The reaction scheme shows an oligosaccharide-containing uronic acid being deuteride-reduced by the carbodiimide–water method (34) prior to hydrolysis. The deuteride-reduced alditol, corresponding to the uronic acid residue in the native polysaccharide, yields fragment ions from C-6 and up with a mass of $(n \times 72) + 3$, where n is the number of acetylated carbons in the fragments. These primary fragments distinguish the carboxyl group from the primary alcohol in the neutral sugar shown to the right. Both derivatives yield fragment ion peaks at $m/z = (n \times 72) + 2$ from C-1 and down.

The advantage of and need for the deuteride-reduction step is best illustrated in Fig. 4. A naturally occurring 3-O-methyl- or 4-O-methyl-D-galactosyl residue would, upon reduction and subsequent acetylation, yield isomeric alditol acetates that are indistinguishable on the gas chromatograph. However, because fragmentation following EI favors charge retention on the methylated carbon (Fig. 4), the mass spectrum would unequivocally identify the compounds by the pairs of peaks at m/z 190, 261 and 262, 189, respectively.

Molecular ions from alditol acetates are normally not seen in an electron-impact spectrum using a quadrupole mass spectrometer (see Figs. 5a and 5b). However, the mass spectrum from an ion-trap mass spectrometer seen in Figs. 5c and 5d, will contain a peak for the protonated molecule (MH^+) or $(MH^+ - 60)$ (loss of acetic acid) or both (37), in addition to the preceding fragment ions. Figures 5a and 5b are the spectra of glucitol acetate (mol wt = 435) and glucosaminitol acetate (mol wt = 434), respectively, obtained using a Nermag R-10-10C quadrupole mass spectrometer in the electron-impact mode. The analogous spectra acquired with a Perkin-Elmer ion-trap mass spectrometer are shown for comparison in Figs. 5c and 5d. The amino-deoxy sugar can be positively identified by the fragments shown in Figs. 5b and 5d.

The mass spectra in Fig. 5 illustrate the advantage of the ion-trap mass spectrometer in providing key fragment ion peaks, as well as a peak for the intact protonated molecule or at least a peak representing loss of acetic acid (60 u) from the protonated molecule. The distribution of ion current for the MH^+-60 ion relative to that for other fragment ions can be controlled by altering the temperature in the ion source. Only a low abundance of the protonated molecule is needed to corroborate the identification given tentatively by the retention time and confirmed by the expected fragmentation pattern.

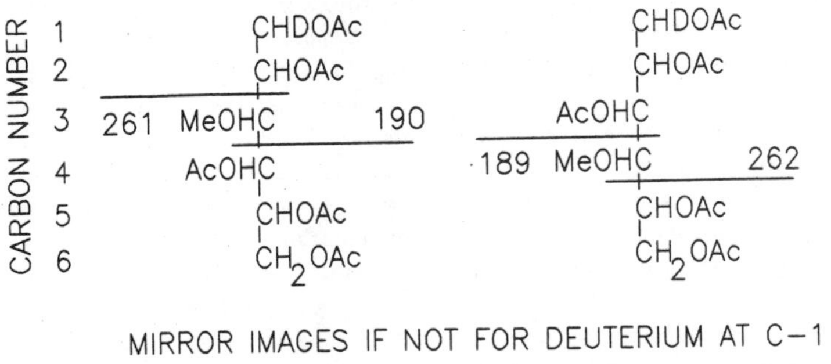

CARBON NUMBER			
1		CHDOAc	CHDOAc
2		CHOAc	CHOAc
3	261 MeOHC 190		AcOHC
4	AcOHC		·189 MeOHC 262
5	CHOAc		CHOAc
6	CH₂OAc		CH₂OAc

MIRROR IMAGES IF NOT FOR DEUTERIUM AT C—1

Fig. 4. These two structures, derived from 3-O-methyl and 4-O-methyl-O-galactosyl residues in the native material, are isomers that are indistinguishable by gas chromatography. The primary fragmentation occurs exclusively on either side of the methoxylated carbon (mass = 44). For the 3-O-methyl derivative, major fragmentations correspond to $(2 \times 72) + (1 \times 44) + 1 = 190$ daltons (C-1 and down) and $(3 \times 72) + (1 \times 44) + 1 = 261$ daltons from C-6 and up. The corresponding fragment ions for the 4-O-methyl derivative are 262 daltons for C-1 down to C-4 and 189 daltons for C-6 up to C-4.

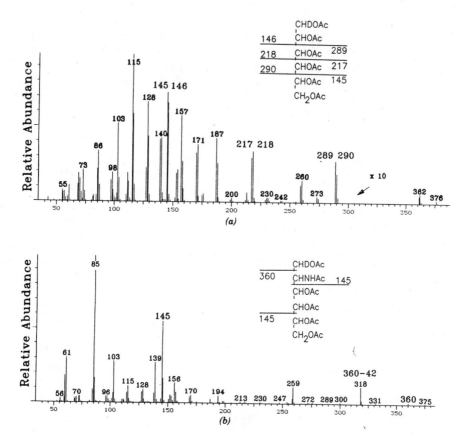

Fig. 5. (a) This mass spectrum of deuteride-reduced glucitol acetate (mol wt = 435) was recorded on a Nermag R 10-10 quadrupole instrument. The primary fragments illustrated in the structure (formed as discussed in Fig. 3) are all present as well as secondary fragments derived from loss of acetic acid residues (−60 daltons) or ketene groups (−42 daltons) or both from the primary fragments. The rarely seen minor peak at m/z 376 at × 10 magnification could represent $M^+ − 59$. (b) The EI mass spectrum of acetylated deuteride-reduced 2-amino-hexitol (mol wt = 434) was obtained with a Nermag R 10-10 quadrupole instrument. The primary fragmentation as illustrated in the structure, involves the acetamidylated carbon yielding 145 mass units, C-1 down, with loss of 42 u to form the ion represented by the significant peak at m/z-103. The C-6→C-2 fragment ion of mass 360 is of low abundance, but yields the secondary fragment ion peak at $m/z = 318$, formed by loss of ketene. The peak at $m/z = 259$ corresponds to the ion formed from m/z-318 by loss of acetamide (−59 daltons).

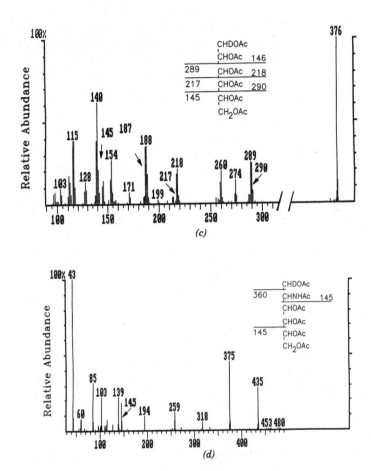

Fig. 5. (continued). (*c*) The mass spectrum of deuteride-reduced glucitol acetate (mol wt = 435) recorded with an ion-trap mass spectrometer yields the primary fragment ions formed by fission between the acetylated carbons in the alditol chains as illustrated in the structure: $m/z = (n \times 72) + 2$ for C-1→down and $m/z = (n \times 72) + 1$ for C-6→up. In addition, a significant peak at $m/z = 376$ is seen representing $MH^+ - 60$. (*d*) The mass spectrum of acetylated 2-amino hexitol (mol wt = 434) was obtained with an ion-trap detector. An amino sugar is readily identified with an ion-trap mass spectrometer as the corresponding deuteride-reduced alditol acetate by the presence of a peak corresponding to MH^+, here $m/z = 435$. This is corroborated by $MH^+ - 60$, $m/z = 375$. The 2-acetamido function is identified by the overlapping fragment ion peaks at $m/z = 145$ and $145 - 42 = 103$ from C-1→down and $m/z = 360 - 42 = 318$ and $m/z = 259 = 318 - 59$ from C-6→up.

6. LINKAGE ANALYSIS USING PERMETHYLATED DERIVATIVES

Linkage analysis by permethylation involves complete alkylation of all hydroxyl groups in the structure. Identifying the location of the free hydroxyl group within a monomer will reveal the mode of attachment in the native component. Data from the sugar analysis are added to the database for the compound under investigation. The presence of uronic acids, dideoxy hexoses, acetamido deoxy hexoses, and so forth, requires specific precautions to obtain quantitative as well as qualitative information.

If uronic acid residues are present, the reduction should be done prior to methylation to obtain maximum structural information from the analysis. As an alternative to the more preferable Conrad procedure (34) mentioned previously, the sample can be reduced with lithium aluminum deuteride after the methylation (17). This reduction converts N-acetyl functions to N-ethyl groups.

3,6-Dideoxy hexoses as well as 2-deoxy hexoses are extremely acid labile; in addition, they yield volatile derivatives so their quantitative determination may require precautions to avoid losses during sample preparation. Using a modified hydrolytic procedure that utilizes a two-step hydrolysis may circumvent this problem (4). The presence of amino sugars precludes use of cation exchange resins in the work up procedure following hydrolysis.

To determine the mode of attachment of the individual residues in the original compound, the quantitative conversion of *all free* hydroxyl groups is required. This is commonly and most efficiently accomplished by the Hakomori procedure (37), which utilizes methyl sulfinyl sodium as the proton extractor. The specifics of this procedure involve preparation of the base, proton extraction, and alkylation. As an alternative to the following procedure, sodium hydride may be added to the sample dissolved in DMSO (38). Finely powdered NaOH in DMSO has also been reported as an adequate proton extraction agent for alkylation (39).

6.1. Preparation of Methyl Sulfinyl Sodium

Methyl sulfinyl sodium (2 M) is prepared in small batches of 5 mL in serum vials. Finely powdered sodium hydroxide (39) or metallic sodium (40) can be used as an alternative to the sodium hydride in this procedure.

1. Into a high-walled container, place a small beaker of dry petroleum ether (drying agent, calcium hydride), a small beaker of ethanol, and three pasteur pipettes with latex bulbs.

2. Create an inert atmosphere in the container by rigging a funnel, connected to a nitrogen tank, over it.

3. Place a serum vial containing 500 mg NaH/oil 1 : 1 inside the high-walled container.

4. Add 5 mL of the petroleum ether to the NaH. Swirl to mix and allow to settle.

5. Transfer the petroleum ether to the beaker with the absolute ethanol. The purpose of this is to remove the oil from the NaH. Discarding the petroleum ether in the ethanol prevents an unintentional fire.

6. Repeat steps 4 and 5 and allow the NaH to dry, still under nitrogen.

7. Add 5 mL of freshly distilled DMSO and cap the vial. Remove and apply the metal seal.

8. Sonicate the reaction mixture in a waterbath for 2 h at 50°C. Occasionally, release the pressure by inserting a fine needle through the septum. If a dry vacuum is available from a small vacuum pump, it can be connected to the needle that is inserted through the septum for continuous evacuation.

9. The methyl sulfinyl anion should have a green color. Test it by withdrawing a few drops and slowly pushing out a drop and then placing it on a triphenylmethane crystal. The droplet should solidify from reaction with moisture and the crystal should become deep red as the triphenylmethyl carbanion is formed.

10. Titrate a small aliquot against a known amount of acid to confirm molarity of $> 2\,M$.

6.2. Procedure for Methylation

Permethylation of carbohydrates involves treatment with strong base. Therefore, special precautions are warranted when the carbohydrate component is an oligo- or polysaccharide with a reducing end. The carbonyl function at the reducing end makes any linkage to its β-carbon susceptible to base-catalyzed β-elimination. A polysaccharide composed of 3-linked glycosides would be completely degraded within minutes. A residue linked to C-4 of the reducing end will be eliminated at a slower rate because an alkaline-catalyzed migration of the carbonyl from C-1 to C-2 must precede the elimination reaction. Thus, the sample to be methylated should be reduced with sodium borodeuteride in order to prevent β-elimination or *alkaline peeling* from the reducing end. As a spin-off from this step, it follows that the reducing end will appear as a penta-O-methyl-hexitol or tetra-O-methyl-pentitol, and so forth, thereby yielding important sequential information. This is valuable with oligomers having a degree of polymerization under 50, since a fairly accurate molecular weight can be determined.

1. Transfer sample ($10–1000\,\mu g$) into a glass reacti-vial and add 0.3–1 mL dry distilled DMSO. Flush with nitrogen and seal the vial.

2. Sonicate the vial in a waterbath until the sample is dissolved. Solubility may increase at low temperatures ($10°C$) or elevated temperatures ($50°C$) depending on the sample.

When working with polysaccharides of very limited solubility, but available in large amounts, it may be feasible to sonicate the sample with a sonicator probe in order to partially dissolve the material. Sonicating in water is continued until the suspension is converted to a solution. The sample can then be reduced with borodeuteride, lyophilized, and dissolved in DMSO.

3. Add methyl sulfinyl sodium 2 M of equal volume to the DMSO. Sonicate for 30 min, let sit for 6 h to overnight at room temperature.

4. Withdraw a minute droplet of the reaction mixture and place it on a triphenyl methane crystal. The crystal will turn bright red if base is still present.

5. If base is present, add freshly distilled methyl iodide (equal volume to the base previously added). MeI is taken up in a dry syringe and added dropwise to the reaction mixture, which is kept chilled at less than 15°C in an ice water bath.

6. Sonicate the solution in the cold room in a sonicator bath until the solution becomes clear. After 60 min, if it will not clear, add half the volume of DMSO.

7. The methylated carbohydrate can be recovered by either (a) dialysis, (b) chloroform extraction, or (c) through adsorption on C_{18} Sep-Pak.

a. Add chloroform to the reaction mixture and transfer to a dialysis bag containing at least 10 mL of water. Wash the vial twice with chloroform and add to the bag. Chloroform will remain in the bag over a 48 hr dialysis period and prevent losses of even relatively low-molecular-weight components.

b. Countercurrent chloroform water extraction can be used with low-molecular-weight components.

c. Evaporate excess methyl iodide. Dilute the sample 1 : 1 with water and apply it with a syringe to a C_{18} Sep-Pak that has been washed sequentially with 10 mL each of chloroform, DMSO, methanol, acetonitrile, and water. After the sample has been applied, wash with 10 mL of water and 4 mL of acetonitrile : water 15 : 85. The sample is then eluted with 5 mL of chloroform. Save all phases just in case!

8. The chloroform phase is transferred to an ampul and dried under nitrogen; 1.8 mL glacial acetic acid is added and the sample is briefly sonicated; 0.20 mL of 2 M sulfuric acid is added and the ampul is sealed and heated at 100°C for 9 h.

9. Follow the procedures described in steps 2–1 for quantitative and qualitative sugar analysis.

6.3. Linkage Analysis

The samples are quantitatively analyzed by GC isothermally (e.g., on 25-m OV-225 fused Silica Column) in order to determine relative retention times. Relative retention times for a number of partially methylated alditol acetates are given in Table 1. These times were established using an early-eluting standard 1,5-di-O-acetyl-2,3,4,6-tetra-O-methyl-glucitol and a late-eluting standard, 1,4,5,6-tetra-O-acetyl, 2,3-di-O-methyl-glucitol. We use a software program written in BASIC to analyze automatically the chromatogram relative to those or any other two standards (41). The reproducibility of relative retention times is within ±2%, even as the column ages and samples elute faster.

Standards are readily prepared by subjecting methyl-glycosides to partial

TABLE 1

Isothermal Separation of Partially Methylated Alditol Acetates on an OV-225 Column

Location of Methyl Group	Relative Retention Times[a]					
	Xyl	Gal	Glc	Man	Fuc	Kha
2	2.15		6.6	5.65	1.43	1.37
3	2.15		7.6	6.8		1.67
4	2.15		8.4	6.8	1.71	1.57
6			5.0	4.1		
2,3	1.19	4.7	4.50[b]	3.69		0.92
2,4	1.06	5.1	4.21	4.51	1.02	0.94
2,5		4.65				
2,6		3.14	3.38	2.99		
3,4	1.19	5.5	4.26	4.06		0.87
3,5		5.1		4.51	0.96	
3,6			3.73	3.67		
4,6			3.49	2.92		
2,3,4	0.54	2.89	2.22	2.19	0.58	0.35
2,3,5		2.76			0.47	
2,3,6		2.22	2.32	2.03		
2,4,6		2.03	1.82	1.90		
2,5,6		1.95				
3,4,6		2.15	1.83	1.82		
2,3,4,6		1.19	1.00[b]	1.00		
2,3,5,6		1.10				

[a]Most of the relative retention times were established during Hellerqvist's tenure at the University of Stockholm.
[b]1.00 early std; 4.50 late std.

methylation by using equimolar rather than excess amounts of base or methyl-iodide or by using other methods for methylation (5). The partially methylated glycosides are converted to the corresponding deuteride-reduced alditol acetates and analyzed by GC to determine retention times relative to an early and late standard and by GC–MS to identify the individual peaks in the chromatogram. The procedure is illustrated in Fig. 6. In this manner standard retention times for all possible substitution patterns can be determined rapidly for any given sugar, and a retention time table can be created for any particular column.

Identifying partially methylated alditol acetates by GC requires the determination of relative retention times as listed in Table 1. In some cases, the GC method may lead to ambiguous solutions such as in the case of 2,4,6-glc or 3,4,6-man, which both have relative retention times of 1.82. GC–MS, however, provides unequivocal information for each component. Figure 7 illustrates the primary fragments formed by the fragmentation rules outlined below and which have been previously determined (5). Introducing a deuterium label by re-

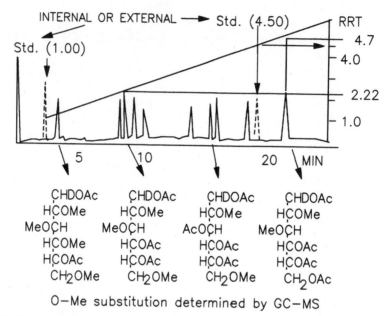

O–Me substitution determined by GC–MS

Fig. 6. This gas chromatogram represents a mixture of galactoside derivatives resulting from deliberate incomplete methylation (5) and conversion to the corresponding deuteride-reduced alditol acetates. The relative retention times (RRT) are recorded for each peak relative to an early standard (2,3,4,6-tetra-O-methyl-glucitol, RRT = 1.00) and a late-eluting standard (2,3-di-O-methyl-glucitol, RRT = 4.50) (see Table 1). The elution position of the standards can be determined by their inclusion in the sample or by pre- and postinjection to the mixture of interest. The fourth peak in this chromatogram is given an RRT of 2.22 and the last peak an RRT of 4.7. Subsequent analysis of this mixture by GC–MS will determine that the peak with an RRT of 2.22 is the 2,3,6-tri-O-methyl- and that the peak at RRT 4.7 is the 2,3-di-O-methyl-galactose derivative.

duction of carbonyl groups gives each compound a unique mass spectrum. Note that if hydride rather than deuteride had been used for reduction, the primary fragments indicated in Fig. 7 from the two compounds would have been identical in mass. Quantitatively, the sum of all partially methylated derivatives of each sugar should equal the amounts found in the sugar analysis.

6.4. Fragmentation Rules

In 1967 Björndal, Lindberg, and Svensson (3) observed that the methylated carbon, when present in an alditol acetate derivative, dominated the fragmentation pattern of the alditol chain in such a way that it would be the exclusive carrier of the charge generated by EI. The fragmentation rules for partially methylated alditol acetates, including aminosugars (5), predict formation of fragment ions of decreasing abundance formed by cleavage of the alditol chain

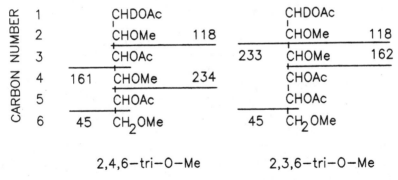

Fig. 7. Representative structures of partially methylated alditol acetates. Primary fragments are formed by fission between methylated, and between methylated and acetylated carbons. The charge is exclusively retained on a methylated carbon at the site of cleavage. These ions are prominent in the EI or ion-trap mass spectra of partially methylated alditol acetates. Fragment ions formed from C-1→down or C-6→up will always end at a methylated carbon, which retains the charge. The mass of a given fragment ion from C-1→down equals $(n \times 72) + (m \times 44) + 2$ and from C-6→up equals $(n \times 72) + (m \times 44) + 1$, where n is the number of acetylated carbons and m is the number of methylated carbons in the fragment ion.

C-1→Down			Fragment Ion
m/z 118	$n = 1$	$m = 1$	2^+-O-Me
m/z 162	$n = 1$	$m = 2$	$2,3^+$-di-O-Me
m/z 234	$n = 2$	$m = 2$	$2,4^+$-di-O-Me

C-6→Up			Fragment Ion
m/z 45	$n = 0$	$m = 1$	6^+-O-Me
m/z 161	$n = 1$	$m = 2$	$6,4^+$-di-O-Me
m/z 233	$n = 1$	$m = 2$	$6,3^+$-di-O-Me

between:

1. an (N-acetyl-N-methyl) aminated carbon and a methylated carbon with charge retention predominantly on the aminylated carbon, which proceeds to lose ketene;

2. two methylated carbons with charge retention on either carbon (the intensities of the signals due to mass discrimination are inversely proportional to the size of the resulting fragment);

3. a methoxylated and an acetylated carbon with charge retention exclusively on the methylated carbon.

One important exception, 1,2-di-O-methyl derivatives resulting from a 5,6-di-O-methylated hexitol, yield m/z 89 as a strong primary fragment (5).

6.5. Identification of Partially Methylated Alditol Acetates by GC–MS

The spectra obtained from neutral alditol derivatives are readily identifiable whether obtained using either a quadrupole or an ion-trap instrument. The accompanying figures exemplify the principles outlined above. Figures 8a–8d demonstrate how the substitution pattern of O-methyl groups is identified by the primary fragment ions in neutral sugars, while Figs. 9a–9e show the corresponding patterns from 2-amino-2-deoxy-hexose derivatives.

Applying the fragmentation rules noted earlier to the data shown in Fig. 8a, unequivocally identifies a 2,3,4,6-tetra-O- methyl substitution pattern on the hexitol. The ion-trap mass spectrometer produces the peaks at $m/z = 292$ for $MH^+ - 32$ (loss of methanol) and $m/z = 264$ for $MH^+ - 60$ (loss of acetic acid) normally not seen in a quadrupole generated EI spectrum. The peak at m/z 145 is derived from m/z 205 with loss of acetic acid from C-5.

Figure 8b represents the ion-trap-recorded mass spectrum of a 2,3,4,-tri-O-methyl-hexitol derived from a chain residue-linked at C-6 in the native compound. The peak at m/z 292 representing $MH^+ - 60$ is not normally seen in the EI spectra. The primary fragment ions at m/z 118, 162, 189, and 233

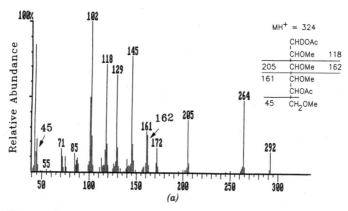

Fig. 8. (a) The mass spectrum of a 2,3,4,6-tetra-O-methyl-hexitol of mol wt 323 daltons, representing a nonreducing terminal residue, recorded with an ion-trap mass spectrometer. The primary fragments identify the 2,3,4,6-tetra-O-methyl substitution pattern.

C-1→Down			Fragment Ion
m/z 118	$m = 1,$	$n = 2$	2^+-O-Me
m/z 162	$m = 1,$	$n = 2$	$2,3^+$-di-O-Me

C-1→Up			Fragment Ion
m/z 45	$m = 0,$	$n = 1$	6^+-O-Me
m/z 161	$m = 1,$	$n = 2$	$6,4^+$-di-O-Me
m/z 205	$m = 1,$	$n = 3$	$6,4,3^+$-tri-O-Me

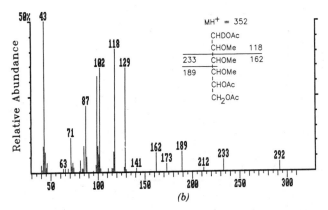

Fig. 8. (*b*) EI mass spectrum of a 2,3,4-tri-*O*-methyl-glucitol derivative representing a 6-linked internal glycoside, or chain residue, recorded on an ion-trap instrument. Background subtracting appears to have eliminated isotope peaks above *m/z* 162.

C-1→Down			Fragment Ion
m/z 118	$m = 1$,	$n = 1$	2^+-*O*-Me
m/z 162	$m = 1$,	$n = 2$	$2,3^+$-di-*O*-Me

C-1→Up			Fragment Ion
m/z 189	$m = 2$,	$n = 1$	4^+-*O*-Me
m/z 233	$m = 2$,	$n = 2$	$4,3^+$-di-*O*-Me

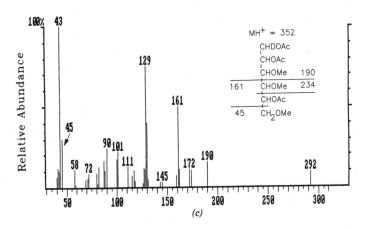

Fig. 8. (*c*) Ion-trap-recorded mass spectrum of a 3,4,6-tri-*O*-methyl-hexitol of (mol wt 352 daltons). The residue would be derived from a 2-linked hexosyl residue. The spectrum is described in detail in the text.

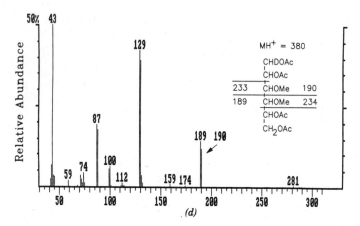

Fig. 8. (*d*) Ion-trap mass spectrum of 3,4-di-*O*-methyl hexitol acetate (mol wt 379 daltons) originating from a 3,6-di-substituted hexosyl residue. Details of this spectrum are discussed in the text.

positively identify the substitution, obviating the need for any of the secondary fragments at m/z 173, 129, and 102 for identification. All secondary fragments are formed by loss of acetic acid (-60 daltons) from primary fragments.

A C-2 linked hexosyl residue would give rise to the derivative 1,2,5-tri-*O*-acetyl-3,4,6-tri-*O*-methyl-hexitol shown in Fig. 8*c*. The substitution pattern is derived from finding the primary fragments that correspond to $m/z = (m + 72) + (n \times 44) + 2$ if C-1 is included as follows:

C-1 → down			Fragment Ion
m/z 190	$m = 2,$	$n = 1$	3^+-*O*-Me
m/z 234	$m = 2,$	$n = 2$	$3,4^+$-*O*-Me

or fragment ion peaks at $m/z = (m \times 72) + (n \times 44) + 1$ if C-6 is included as follows:

C-6 → Up			Fragment Ion
m/z 45	$m = 0,$	$n = 1$	6^+-*O*-Me
m/z 161	$m = 1,$	$n = 2$	$6,4^+$-di-*O*-Me
m/z 233	$m = 2,$	$n = 2$	$6,4,3^+$-tri-*O*-Me

(n is the number of methoxylated carbons, m is the number of acetylated carbons, and "$+$" indicates the carbon on which the charge is localized in the alditol chain). The fragment ion peaks at m/z 234 and 233 will appear depending on amounts of material analyzed and conditions used for MS analysis. Their absence demonstrates the extent to which cleavage is preferred between two methylated carbons over that between an acetylated and methylated carbon. The ion of mass 190 loses acetic acid $(60\,\mu)$ from C-1 to form an ion of mass 130. The ion of mass 161 loses methanol $(32\,\mu)$ from C-6 to form an ion of mass 129.

A 2,6-di-substituted hexosyl (Fig. 8d) would yield a 3,4-di-O-methyl-hexitol acetate with fragments formed as follows:

C-1 → Down		Fragment Ion
m/z 190	$m = 2$, $n = 1$	3^+-O-Me

C-6 → Up		
m/z 189	$m = 2$, $n = 1$	4^+-O-Me

Peaks at m/z 233 and 234 are weak (described in the previous paragraph) in this case because of the much more favorable cleavage between two adjacent methylated carbons (C-3 and C-4). In these cases, cleavage between C-2 and C-3 with charge retention on the methylated C-3 carbon (m/z 233) may or may not be observed; in the example illustrated in Fig. 8d, such cleavage is not significant. Similarly, cleavage between C-4 and C-5 could occur (m/z 234), but in the case presented in Fig. 8d, it is not observed.

6.6. Identification of Partially Methylated Amino-Deoxy Alditol Acetates by GC–MS

The fragmentation patterns obtained with the partially methylated derivatives of 2-amino-2-deoxy sugars in EI mass spectrometry are dominated by the N-methyl acetamido fragment ion of mass 159 and its daughter fragment ion (159–42) of mass 117. The low abundance of other fragment ions causes some difficulty for the determination of the number of methylated carbons. This difficulty plus the generally poor recovery observed with aminosugar derivatives in the linkage analysis using the quadrupole instrument is eliminated with the ion-trap instrument in the configuration provided by Perkin Elmer (Fig. 9a–9e).

The mass spectrum in Fig. 9a and primary fragmentation rules depicted with the structure identify the N-methyl-3,4,6-tri-O-methyl substitution of the native nonreducing terminal 2-acetamido-2-deoxy-hexoside. The base peak at m/z 117 represents loss of 42 u from the primary fragment ion of mass 159 (formed by cleavage between C-2 and C-3 with charge retention on the aminated carbon). Diagnostic peaks at m/z 45, 161, 203, and 205 represent key fragment ions formed on the methylated carbon as predicted from the fragmentation rules. As with the unmethylated derivative, the peaks representing MH$^+$ and MH$^+$ − 60 in Fig. 9a give an undisputable identification of the sugar derivative.

C-1 → Down				Fragment Ion
m/z 159	$m = 1,$	$m^N = 1,$	$n^N = 1$	$^2N^+$-Me
m/z 203	$m = 1,$	$m^n = 1,$	$n^n = 1,$	$^2N,3^+$-di-Me
	$n = 1$			

m^N and n^N refer to N-acetyl and N-methyl, respectively. ^2N refers to a 2-amino-2-deoxy function and " + " refers to site of charge in the alditol chain.

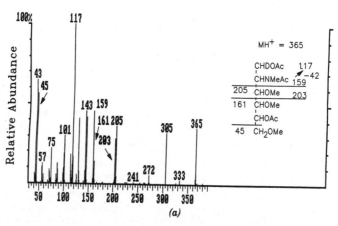

Fig. 9. (a) The mass spectrum of a 2-amino-2-deoxy-N-methyl-3,4,6-tri-O-methyl-hexitol acetate (mol wt 364 daltons) representing a nonreducing terminal 2-acetamido-2-deoxy-glycosyl residue recorded with an ion trap mass spectrometer.

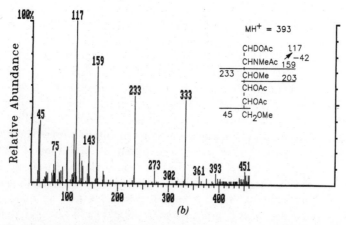

Fig. 9. (b) The ion-trap-recorded mass spectrum of an originally 4-substituted 2-acetamido-2-deoxy-glycoside. The substitution pattern N-methyl-3,6-di-O-methyl is readily identified. Peak at m/z 393 represents MH$^+$.

C-6 → Up			Fragment Ions
m/z 45	$m = 0,$	$n = 1$	6^{+}-O-Me
m/z 161	$m = 1,$	$n = 2$	$6,4^{+}$-di-O-Me
m/z 205	$m = 1,$	$n = 3$	$6,4,3^{+}$-tri-O-Me

An originally 4-linked 2-acetamido-2-deoxy-hexoside would yield the derivative shown in Fig. 9b. The ion-trap mass spectrum contains peaks correspond-

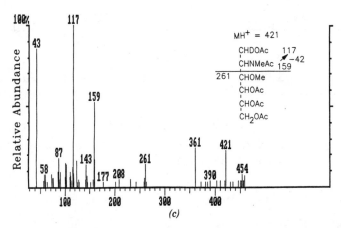

Fig. 9. (c) Mass spectrum of a $\mathcal{N}$-methyl-2-acetamido-3-O-methyl-hexitol acetate as recorded with an ion trap mass spectrometer; mol wt 420 daltons. The peaks at m/z 421 and 361 represent MH^{+} and MH^{+} − 60, respectively.

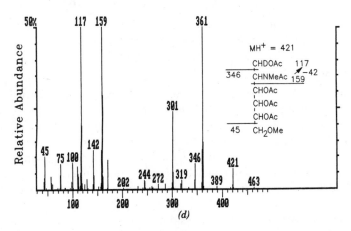

Fig. 9. (d) Mass spectrum of a 2-acetamido-2-deoxy-$\mathcal{N}$-methyl-6-O-methyl-hexosyl derivative. The molecular weight of 420 daltons is deduced from the peak at 421 for MH^{+} seen in this ion-trap-recorded spectrum.

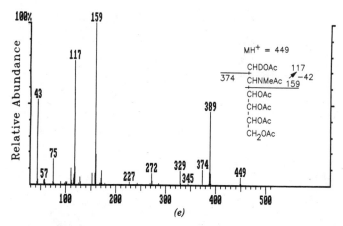

Fig. 9. (*e*) The mass spectrum of a 2-acetamido-2-deoxy-*N*-methyl-hexose derivative originating from a 3,4,6-tri-substituted residue recorded on an ion-trap mass spectrometer.

ing to fragments from the *N*-methyl-3,6-di-*O*-methyl-substituted structure as depicted in Fig. 9*b*. The fragment ions formed are:

	C-1 → Down			**Fragment Ion**
m/z 159	$m = 1$,	$m^N = 1$,	$n^N = 1$	$^2N^+$-Me
m/z 203	$m = 2$,	$m^N = 1$,	$n^N = 1$,	$^2N,3^+$-di-Me
	$n = 1$			

	C-6 → Up		**Fragment Ion**
m/z 45	$m = 0$,	$n = 1$	6^+-*O*-Me
m/z 233	$m = 2$,	$n = 2$	$6,3^+$-di-*O*-Me

The ion of mass 203, which is not observed, would represent a fragment predicted by the fragmentation rules; that this ion is produced is corroborated by the secondary fragment peak at *m/z* 143 [which corresponds to loss of the elements of acetic acid (60 u) from the ion of mass 203]. The ion of mass 233 verifies the 3-*O*-methyl group and *m/z* 45 the 6-*O*-methyl group. Also very important for assigning weak signals is the presence of the peak at *m/z* 393 representing MH$^+$ and at *m/z* 333 (for MH$^+$ − 60), which defines the derivative as an *N*-methyl-di-*O*-methyl derivative of a 2-acetamido-2-deoxy-hexosyl residue in the native compound.

A 2-amino-2-deoxy-hexosyl residue substituted at C-4 and C-6 would, upon linkage analysis, yield the 3-*O*-methyl derivative shown in Fig. 9*c*. The peaks at *m/z* 421 and 361 represent MH$^+$ and MH$^+$ − 60, respectively, of a *N*-methyl-mono-*O*-methyl hexosamine derivative. The fragment ions depicted in the structure give:

C-1 → Down				Fragment Ion
m/z 159	$m = 1$,	$m^N = 1$,	$n^N = 1$	$^2N^+$-Me
m/z 203	$m = 1$,	$m^N = 1$,	$n^N = 1$, $n = 1$	$^2N,3^+$-O-Me

C-6 → Up		Fragment Ion
m/z 261	$m = 3$, $n = 1$	3^+-O-Me

The peak at m/z 159 defines the 2-acetamido function in the native molecule. The position of O-methyl at C-3 is indicated by the fragment ion peak at m/z 261, which is corroborated by the peak at m/z 143 (corresponding to ion of mass 203 losing 60 u).

The branched aminosugar linked through C-3 and C-4 yields on linkage analysis the spectrum shown in Fig. 9d. The peak at m/z 421 corresponds to MH$^+$ for the mono-O-methyl-N-methyl substitution. The peaks at m/z 159 and 346 identify the 2-acetamido-N-methyl function on a six-carbon chain. The O-methyl is located at C-6 as indicated by the peak at m/z 45.

The presence of cyclic acetal on an internal 2-acetamido-2-deoxy-hexosyl residue would yield an N-methyl derivative with no O-methyl groups. The mass spectrum shown in Fig. 9e characterizes such a derivative. The peak at m/z 449 represents MH$^+$. The 2-acetamido-2-deoxy-N-methyl function is identified by the fragment ion peaks at m/z 159 and 374.

The mass spectrum in Fig. 10 characterizes a 3,4,6-tri-O-methylated 2-acetamido-2-deoxy-hexose derivative originating from a nonreducing terminal residue in the native component. Unsuccessful N-methylation may be indicative of an alkaline stabile N-substitution or an imcomplete methylation.

The substitution is readily identified from:

C-1 → Down				Fragment Ion
m/z 145	$m = 1$,	$m^N = 1$,	$n^N = 0$	N^+-AC
m/z 189	$m = 1$,	$m^N = 1$,	$n = 1$	$N,3^+$-O-Me

C-6 → Up		Fragment Ion
m/z 45	$m = 0$, $n = 1$	6^+-O-Me
m/z 161	$m = 1$, $m = 2$,	$6,4^+$-di-O-Me
m/z 205	$m = 1$, $m = 3$	$6,4,3^+$-tri-O-Me

The identity of the molecule is corroborated by the peak at m/z 351, which represents MH$^+$.

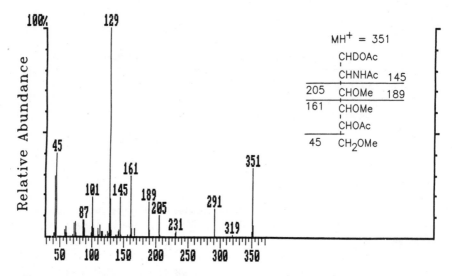

Fig. 10. Mass spectrum of a 2-acetamido-2-deoxy-3,4,6-tri-O-methyl-hexose derivative prepared from a nonreducing amino sugar which was not N-methylated, possibly due to an alkaline stabile N-substitution.

6.7. Quantitation by Selected Ion Monitoring

The FID is one of the least sensitive detectors used in analyses by GC and GC–MS. The FID response, however, is quantitative in that response is proportional to the number of carbons in the molecule. Figure 11a illustrates the problem and Fig. 11b illustrates the solution to the problem of having less than sufficient amounts of material for a quantitative analysis by GC.

Methylating 0.1 μg of a polysaccharide mannan and analyzing the corresponding partially methylated alditol acetate by GC yields a chromatogram and reconstructed total ion chromatogram with no interpretable peaks (Fig. 11a). The fragmentation rules described previously, indicate that most partially methylated derivatives are characterized by the presence of four primary fragments of variable abundance. For instance, Fig. 7 illustrates that 2,3,6- and 2,4,6-tri-O-methyl substitutions are characterized by peaks at m/z 45, 118, 162, 233 and at m/z 45, 118, 161, 234, respectively. Similarly, as shown in Fig. 8d, the mass spectrum of the 3,4-di-O-methyl substitution is characterized by peaks at m/z 189, 190, (233), and (234). However, selectively monitoring a set of primary fragment ion currents at m/z 45, 118, 161, 162, 233, 234, 189, and 190, the analytical results change dramatically as shown in Fig. 11b. The compounds represented by peaks at 5.21, 6.27, 6.36, and 7.57 min are identified by their mass spectra, recorded as selected ion chromatograms (Fig. 12) as the, 2,3,4,6-tetra-, 3,4,6-tri-, 2,4,6-tri-, and 3,4-di-O-methyl derivatives, respectively.

The selected ion current chromatogram (Fig. 11b), however, cannot be used

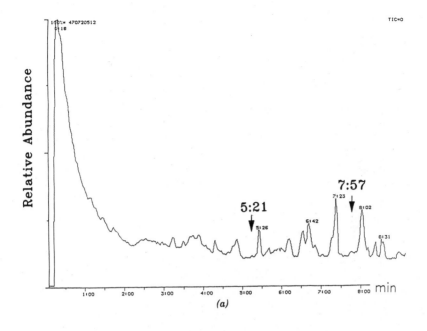

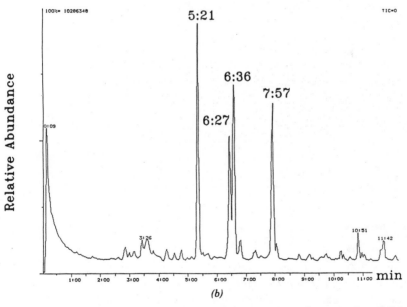

Fig. 11. (*a*) Reconstructed total ion current chromatogram from results of linkage analysis of a polysaccharide mannan by GC–MS on a quadrupole mass spectrometer equipped with an OV-225 fused silica capillary (25 m × 0.24 mm) column. Analysis by on-column injection at 90°C followed by a gradient of 10°C/min to 240°C. (*b*) Reconstructed selected ion chromatogram from the analysis described in Fig. 11a. The "total ion current" represents the combined intensities of the fragment ions *m/z* 45, 118, 161, 162, 233, 234, 189, and 190.

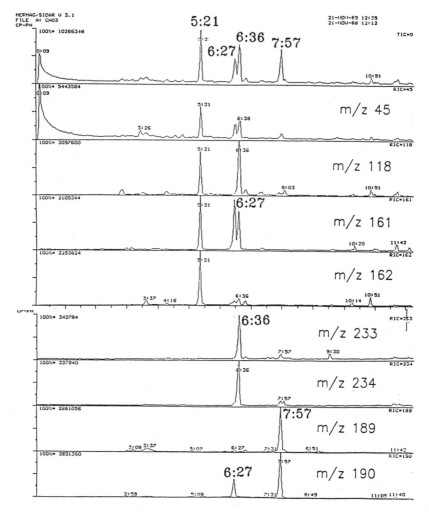

Fig. 12. Reconstructed mass chromatograms for each of the selected primary fragments formed from partially methylated alditol acetates. Reading from top to bottom gives:

Peak at 5:21 min; m/z 45, 118, 161, 162 (Fig. 8a)
Peak at 6:27 min; m/z 45, 161, 190, (234) (Fig. 8c)
Peak at 6:36 min; m/z 45, 118, 161, 233, 234 (Fig. 7)
Peak at 7:57 min; m/z 45, 189, 190, (233), (234) (Fig. 8d)

The depicted figure references show the origin of the primary fragment ions listed for each peak. Peaks in parentheses are not always present.

TABLE 2

Methyl Ethers Obtained upon Methylation Analysis of
Native and CrO_3-Oxidized Polysaccharides

Methyl Ethers	Native (mol%)	Oxidized (mol%)
2,3,4,6 Man	33	33[a]
3,4,6 Man	15	15
2,4,6 Man	13	14
3,4 Man	32	3

[a]Normalized to residue in native polysaccharide.

for quantitative purposes because the individual responses depend on the relative stability of ions formed, rather than on the number of carbons in the residue. Relative quantitation can be achieved, however, by analysis (by both GC and GC–MS) of a standard sample of mixed, partially methylated alditol acetates, obtained by partial methylation of a methyl glycoside (Fig. 6). The selected ion current chromatogram can then be quantitatively compared to the FID response of the individual components in the standard mixture. Correction factors can thus be established and applied to obtain a quantitative estimate of components in the unknown sample as analyzed only by GC–MS. The results of quantitative linkage analysis of the mannan are given in Table 2.

7.   ANOMERIC CONFIGURATION

7.1.   Introduction

NMR analysis, when sufficient pure material is available, gives significant information about the anomeric configuration and linkages of individual residues in small oligosaccharides. However, some investigators tend to use NMR as their only tool and go far beyond its capabilities. Theoretically, an unknown hexasaccharide can have several million isomeric structures, which is far beyond the resolving power of any modern instrument. The N-linked oligosaccharide in Fig. 1 with 10^{18} possibilities illustrates the degree of complexity that must be addressed.

Determining the anomeric configuration by GC–MS involves identification of sugar residues in the peracetylated carbohydrate component that are resistant to chromic acid oxidation. The point of attachment of β- or α-linked residues can be determined by subjecting the oxidized material to linkage analysis as described above. The method is based on the observation of Angyal and James (42) that axial-linked peracetylated alkyl glycosides are resistant to chromic acid oxidation in glacial acetic acid, whereas the equatorially linked are oxidized to the corresponding 5-keto-hexulosonates. Using chromic acid oxidation to analyze anomeric configurations in complex polysaccharides (43) was developed during an extensive study of model oligosaccharides (44).

7.2. Procedure for Determination of Anomeric Configuration by GC–MS

The anomeric configuration of individual residues in a polymer or oligomer, available in minute quantities, can be obtained by the following procedure, which is adapted from that described by Hellerqvist et al. (45).

1. The polysaccharide ($< 200\ \mu g$) in formamide ($200\ \mu L$) is acetylated by the addition of acetic anhydride and pyridine (1 mL, 1 : 1). (For oligosaccharides, omit the formamide.) The mixture is left at ambient temperature overnight.

2. Pyridine and acetic anhydride are removed by codistillation with toluene. The oligosaccharide sample is dissolved in acetonitrile ($200\ \mu L$) and $800\ \mu L$ of water is added. The mixture is applied to a C_{18} Sep-Pak cartridge, as described previously for purification of permethylated samples. Polysaccharides in $200\ \mu L$ of formamide are diluted with $800\ \mu L$ of water before application to the C_{18} Sep-Pak cartridge. The samples are eluted with chloroform.

3. The chloroform phase is dried with $MgSO_4(s)$ and transferred to a reactivial and dried under nitrogen. Add approximately 2 mg of crystallized chromic acid, $200\ \mu L$ of glacial acetic acid, and sonicate the reaction mixture at $50°C$ in an ultrasonic waterbath for 1 h.

The β-linked residues in the peracetylated sample are oxidized in this step to the corresponding 5-keto-hexulosonate derivatives. As a consequence, the alkaline-stable β-glycosidic linkages are converted to alkaline-labile ester linkages, but the polysaccharide retains the same degree of polymerization.

4. The oxidized sample is filtered through a glass wool plug in a pasteur pipette, applied to a C_{18} Sep-Pak after 1 : 5 dilution with water, eluted with chloroform, and transferred to a reactivial. Ten percent of the sample is removed and subjected to sugar analysis. The remainder is dried and subjected to methylation analysis.

The data in Table 2 are obtained from the application of this methodology to the polysaccharide to give the results of the linkage analysis shown in Figs. 11 and 12. Comparing the methyl ethers obtained from native and oxidized polysaccharides shows that the 2,6-di-substituted residues in the original polysaccharide are absent in the CrO_3-oxidized material. Therefore, these residues, represented originally by the 3,4-di-O-methyl derivatives, are β-linked in the original polysaccharide. The absence of derivatives containing methylated hydroxyl groups which would be generated upon cleavage of the ester bond, indicates that the β-linked residues are linked together in glycosidic bonds in the native polysaccharide. It follows that when β-linked residues alternate among α-linked residues and the oxidized material is subjected to methylation analysis, "new" derivatives will appear which are indicative of the linkage position for the β-linked residues. For an example of such a study, the reader is referred to the results of a sequence analysis of a lipopolysaccharide (45).

The partial sequence information obtained by this technique is no longer cost effective with respect to material needed in light of current available methodology discussed in Section 8. However, chromic acid oxidation is cost effective as a means of determining the presence of oxidizable β-linked residues. Internal standards are required for this analysis particularly if all residues in the unknown sample are β-linked. The original sugar analysis determines which internal nonoxidizable standard component should be used in the analysis. Hoffman et al.'s study (44) suggests several oligosaccharides that can be used as standards.

8. SEQUENCE ANALYSIS

8.1. Introduction

Prior to 1980, mass-spectrometric sequence analysis of oligosaccharides was limited to relatively low-molecular-weight compounds (7) because of instrumental limitations such as usable mass range and limitations in ion transmission. Additionally, available ionization modes such as electron-impact ionization, chemical ionization, and field desorption were limited in their applicability to oligosaccharide sequence determination. Chemical ionization mass spectrometry using ammonia or isobutane as reagent gases, for example, provided data to only partially sequence permethylated tri- and tetrasaccharides (46).

Fortunately, recent significant technological advances in mass spectrometry have narrowed the gap between biological complexity and analytical capability. The development of high-resolution, high-field, multisector magnetic mass spectrometers capable of analyzing high-mass ions at high ion transmissions, with high-performance data systems and ionization techniques such as fast-atom bombardment (FAB), direct chemical ionization (DCI), laser desorption (LD), and plasma desorption (PD) which allow "soft" ionization of large polar molecules have dramatically expanded the usefulness of mass spectrometry. Collisional activation using neutral gas also enhances the structural information available from FAB ionization of oligosaccharides (47). Newer techniques for sample introduction, such as HPLC–MS and continuous flow FAB–MS, will surely play an important role in future elucidation of oligosaccharide structures.

The key to effective sequence analysis of oligosaccharides, therefore, lies in the use of these modern instrument types and techniques in combination with appropriate techniques of sample isolation and chemical modification. A few examples are described in this section to illustrate some of the general principles of oligosaccharide sequencing. Most of the example spectra were obtained with a high-field (mass range of ∼2600 daltons at a full accelerating voltage of 6 kV) VG 70-250 instrument equipped for FAB ionization. Larger instruments having higher full accelerating voltages are capable of detecting ions arising from carbohydrates with molecular weight heavier than 5000 daltons. The reader is referred to the elegant work of Dell and co-workers (10, 48) and Egge et al. (49) for examples. ^{252}Cf-PD mass spectrometry shows great promise for obtaining molecular weight information for underivatized, complex lipooligosaccharides (50), but this technique is considered beyond the scope of this chapter.

8.2. Ionization Methods

8.2.1. DIRECT CHEMICAL IONIZATION

Direct (or desorption) chemical ionization (DCI) is useful for analyzing the sequence of oligosaccharides. A sample is placed on an electrically resistant wire or emitter that is coated with a protective surface such as polyamide to assist the process of desorption. A programmed heating current is passed through the emitter to promote thermal desorption (51–54). Spectra acquired early in the run typically show a high abundance of ions related to the intact structure, while spectra acquired later in the run show an increasing abundance of low-mass fragments associated with the increasing extent of pyrolysis of the sample. These two sets of spectra often provide complementary information about molecular weight and structure. DCI also can be applied to the sequence analysis of oligosaccharides. It appears to be most successful when applied to oligosaccharides that have been permethylated using the Hakomori procedure (37) (as detailed previously) and using ammonia as reagent gas.

The advantages of using DCI are that abundant structural information can usually be obtained using considerably less sample than that obtained using FAB–MS. The disadvantages of the technique are that permethylation of an oligosaccharide substantially increases its molecular weight. Above a molecular weight of ~2500–3000 daltons, pyrolytic decomposition rather than desorption appears to be the predominant process.

8.2.2. FAST-ATOM-BOMBARDMENT MASS SPECTROMETRY

FAB–MS, first introduced in 1981 by Barber and co-workers (55), had an immediate and profound impact on the ability of scientists to obtain structural information about carbohydrates. To conduct a typical FAB–MS experiment, a thin layer of viscous liquid (termed matrix) having low volatility is applied to a small metallic target and a solution ($1-2\,\mu L$) of the analyte of interest (in an appropriate solvent) is added via a syringe to the center of the target. The surface of the matrix plus the analyte on the target is then bombarded with a beam of accelerated xenon or argon atoms (or sometimes ions such as cesium). The resultant transfer of kinetic energy causes surface molecules of both analyte and matrix to be converted into both positive and negative ions and sputtered into the vapor phase where they are extracted and mass analyzed using the ion source and optical system of the particular mass spectrometer.

8.2.3 INSTRUMENTAL PARAMETERS

The examples presented here were obtained with the VG FAB probe and associated Ion Tech B 11N saddle-field gun. In this system, the target (a rectangular stainless-steel plate ~ 1.5 mm $\times$ 6 mm) is bombarded with xenon atoms having an energy of 8 keV. Sufficient xenon is leaked into the system to raise the pressure of the ion source region to 10^{-6} Torr and the analyzer region to 10^{-8} Torr. The mass spectrometer is adjusted to a static resolving power of about 2500 for low-resolution acquisition and scanned at 10 sec/decade using an accelerating voltage of 6 kV (mass range of about 2600 daltons), 5 kV (3120 daltons), or 4 kV (3900 daltons). Reducing the accelerating voltage causes a progressive decrease in available sensitivity (ion transmission). There is no particular problem from catalytic effects associated with the use of a stainless-steel target. Gold targets also provide good results, although when using thiol matrices, gold–thiol ion complexes tend to dominate the spectrum.

The characteristics of different matrices for FAB–MS have been reviewed recently by Gower (56). For the analysis of underivatized oligosaccharides by FAB–MS, the authors prefer to use glycerol or 1-thioglycerol as matrices. Dell and co-workers (10) suggest the use of a 1 : 1 mixture of glycerol and thioglycerol. Thioglycerol, while often yielding excellent results, is considerably more volatile than glycerol in the mass spectrometer and its use can lead to transient spectra due to matrix depletion. These same matrices have also been used for derivatized oligosaccharides (10).

We have obtained excellent results (12, 13) using 3-nitrobenzyl alcohol (3-NBA) as a matrix for positive ion FAB–MS analysis of peracetylated or periodate-oxidized, reduced, and peracetylated oligosaccharides; using 3-NBA leads to long-lasting spectra. Triethanolamine may be used to obtain negative ion spectra.

8.2.4. SAMPLE HANDLING

Because FAB–MS is both an operator- and sample-sensitive technique, the guidelines given previously for loading the target and obtaining the FAB spectrum should be rigidly adhered to. Analyte in solution should be added to the matrix. Analyte dried on the target before the addition of matrix will rarely yield good results, presumably because the matrix surface contains a low concentration of analyte and hence generates a greatly reduced yield of sputtered ions. The probe with a mixture of matrix and analyte in an appropriate solvent is inserted into the vacuum lock and most of the solvent is pumped away with the mechanical pump. Once initialized, the data system controls the scan functions of the mass spectrometer. The probe tip is then moved toward the ion source but not into the line of the atom beam. The atom gun is turned on and left to stabilize for one or two scan cycles before the probe is fully inserted to the operating position for the acquisition of consecutive spectra. The data system may then be used to average selected spectra or to subtract matrix contributions, and so forth. As a matter of practical operating procedure, the initial instrument tuning should be performed using matrix only on the target. This initial tuning simulates the analytical situation of the matrix plus analyte. The instrument can then be calibrated in the usual way by use of an alkali metal halide such as cesium iodide. It is important to note that tuning parameters can differ greatly between positive or negative ion extraction. Even though data systems can be used to alternate between positive and negative ion spectra on consecutive scans, it is likely that neither will be optimal. Thus, separate acquisition of positive or negative ion spectra is recommended if both are desired for a particular compound.

Oligosaccharides to be analyzed by FAB–MS must be dissolved in an appropriate solvent. Underivatized oligosaccharides should be dissolved in water or 2–10% aqueous acetic acid, while permethylated or peracetylated derivatives are best dissolved in methanol, chloroform, or other appropriate solvents.

The FAB–MS of underivatized carbohydrates are rarely useful in providing structural details other than confirmation of the molecular weight, which is normally calculated from the composition analysis. It is, however, of value to establish the presence or absence of chemically labile functional groups such as sulfates, phosphates, or acyls. Sample purity is of utmost importance because fragment ions in the spectra can lead to erroneous structural conclusions. For this reason, carbohydrates are usually derivatized prior to obtaining their FAB spectra.

Procedures for converting carbohydrates to their corresponding peracetyl or permethyl derivatives are well established in carbohydrate chemistry and details are given in previous sections of this chapter. Spectral details have been reviewed by Dell (10). The quality of FAB spectra of peracetyl and permethyl derivatives are superior to those of their nonderivatized forms, when using orders of magnitude less material. In general, derivatization leads to little fragmentation and molecular weight information. Adding trace amounts of a sodium salt allows one to confirm MH^+ as MNa^+. It should be stressed, however, that the improved quality affects only the spectrum and not the structural information that can be extracted. The spectrum does not distinguish between linkages nor can it distinguish between homologous types of sugar residues.

8.3. Periodate Oxidation in Sequence Analysis

To address sequence problems, Angel, Lindh, and Nilsson (11) reintroduced periodate oxidation. Oligosaccharides are sequentially oxidized with periodate and reduced with sodium borodeuteride, and the resulting product is permethylated. The FAB spectrum of the permethylated product is obtained using 1-thioglycerol as matrix. This procedure leads to product residues that vary in mass depending on the substitution of the individual residues (11). Figure 13 illustrates that hexosyl residues substituted at C-2 or C-4 give product residues of 208 daltons, those substituted at C-3 yield 204 daltons, and the C-6-substituted derivative contributes 164 daltons to the m/z value. The C-2 and C-4 substitution can be distinguished by the fact that the fragmentation pathway of the C-2-substituted moiety involves elimination of methanol, while that of the C-4-substituted moiety does not.

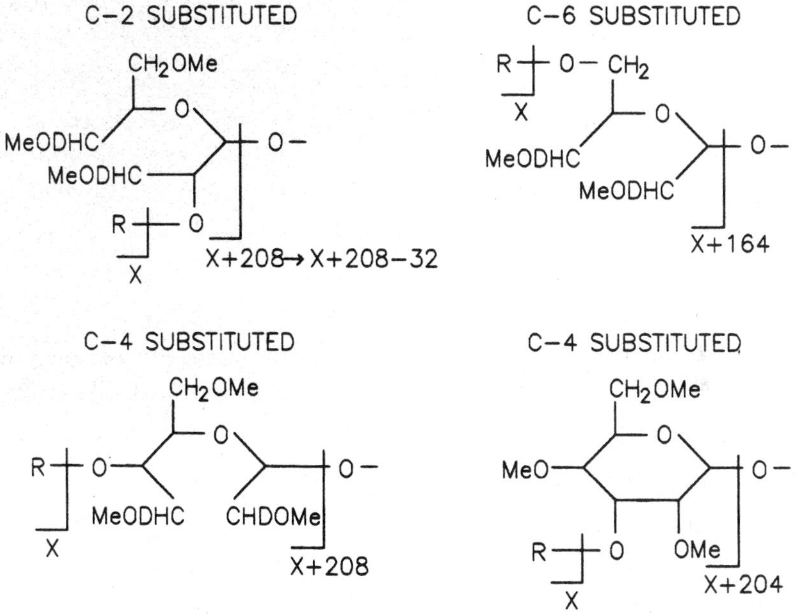

Fig. 13. Products formed after periodate oxidation, borodeuteride reduction, and methylation of internal hexosyl residues substituted at C-2, C-6, C-4, and C-3, respectively. Fragments formed by a primary cleavage are indicated.

The authors have extended the periodate oxidation technique for sequencing polysaccharides and oligosaccharides, and obtained improved results by adapting the consequences of the fragmentation rules given previously which suggest that cleavage with charge retention at either side of the oxidized ring oxygen or glycosidic oxygen will be preferred over cleavage at the acetoxylated carbons. In addition, analyzing the derivatives by FAB–MS after purification on HPLC in a 3-nitrobenzyl alcohol rather than in a 1-thioglycerol matrix gives an improved signal to noise ratio.

Periodate oxidation of nonreducing terminal hexoses, and 6-deoxy hexoses, and internal hexoses substituted at C-6 in poly- and oligosaccharides results in loss of C-3 as formic acid. Periodate oxidation of internal hexoses that are linked at C-2 or C-4 produces oxidatively opened rings without the loss of carbons (Figs. 14 and 15). Hexoses that are 3-substituted, with or without additional linkages, are also not oxidized. 3,6-Di-deoxy-hexoses and branched hexoses substituted at C-2 and C-4 are also not oxidized. The reducing sugar is oxidized with participation of the hemiacetal at C-1. Figure 14 illustrates the chemical modification required for sequencing oligosaccharides; the reactions required for sequencing polysaccharides are illustrated in Figs. 15 and 16. The arrows in Fig. 16 illustrate possible sites of hydrolysis. FAB–MS spectra show fragmentation on both sides of the glycosidic oxygen (type B and C fragments) and in the oxidized

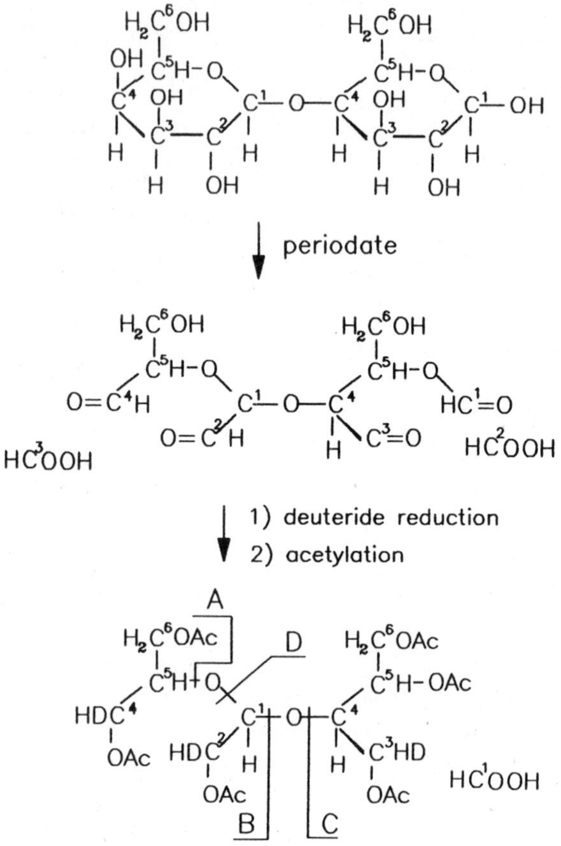

Fig. 14. Periodate oxidation, deuteride reduction, and acetylation of oligosaccharides for FAB–MS sequence analysis.

residues on both sides of the ring oxygen (type A and D fragments) as illustrated in Figs. 14 and 16. The charge, however, is retained on the carbon side of the cleavage point. This then yields overlapping fragments from *both* the reducing and nonreducing end of the molecule. The technique is currently applicable at the low nanomole level for sequencing of linear and branched oligosaccharides, native or derived from polysaccharides by intentional Smith degradation. Oligosaccharides containing a sialic acid residue after periodate oxidation yield an interresidue lactone linked to galactose (57).

The very simple fragmentation patterns, illustrated in Figs. 17–22, obtained through cleavage predominantly on either side of the glycosidic oxygen and ring oxygen in oxidized ring structures were used to generate the computer program, GLYCOSPEC, written in Turbo Pascal (Borland). The current database can be used to analyze spectra resulting from the periodate oxidized, borodeuteride-reduced, and peracetylated carbohydrate derivatives. However, it can be modified easily to accommodate other periodate oxidized derivatives.

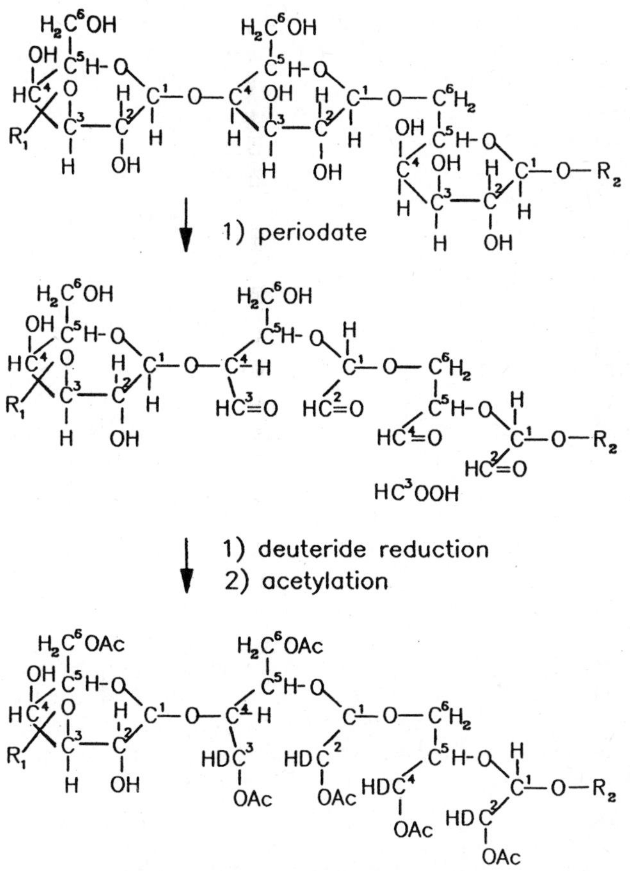

Fig. 15. Periodate oxidation, deuteride reduction, and acetylation of polysaccharides.

8.4. Procedures for Periodate Oxidation

As always, analytical procedures are conducted using acid-washed glassware and glass-distilled highest-purity solvents.

1. Periodate oxidation is effected by dissolving the sample (0.5–2 mg) at a concentration of 1 mg/mL in an aqueous solution of sodium periodate (0.12 M). The mixture is kept in the dark for 48 h at 4°C.

2. The reaction mixture is applied to a Dowex-1 x 4 anion exchange column (1 × 5 cm, chloride form) which has been thoroughly prewashed with glass-distilled water. Ten milliliters of water are used to elute the sample from the bed. The procedure removes excess periodate and iodate from the reaction mixture. Sep-Pak ion exchange cartridges should be a convenient alternative.

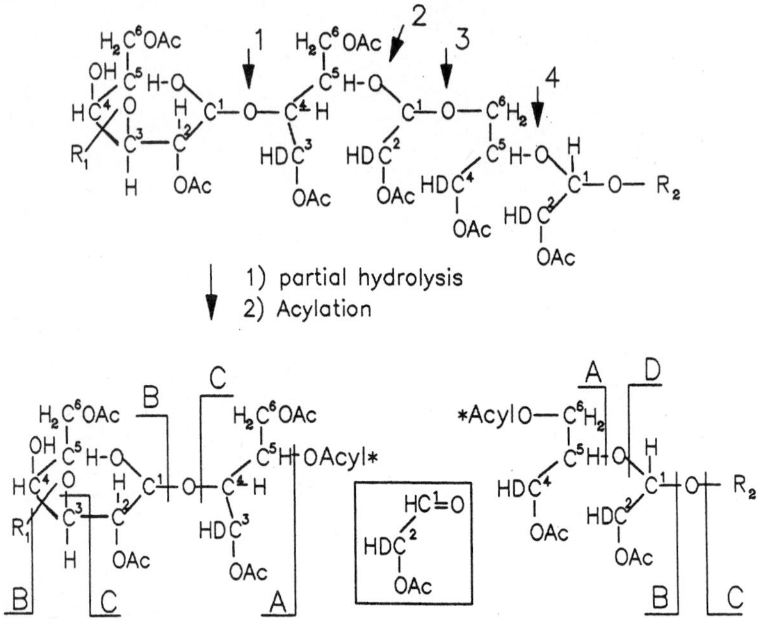

Fig. 16. Partial hydrolysis and acylation of hydroxyl groups, liberated as a result of acid degradation. The mixture of oligosaccharides is separated on HPLC and subjected to FAB–MS analysis. The arrows numbered 1 through 4 indicate four possible sites of hydrolysis; in this scheme hydrolysis occurs at sites 2 and 3. Asterisks denote acyl groups introduced after hydrolysis.

3. Excess (10 mg) sodium borodeuteride is added to the eluate and kept 2 h at ambient temperature. Excess borodeuteride is destroyed and sodium is removed by the addition of a slight excess Rexyyn-101 cation exchange resin (Fisher) H^+ form. The resin has to be prewashed with 20 bed volumes of acetic acid followed by methanol and water.

4. The mixture is filtered through a small acid washed and thoroughly rinsed sintered glass funnel to a 15-mL pear-shaped flask. Boric acid is removed as methyl borate by twice repeated codistillation with methanol. The residual moisture is removed by codistillation with absolute ethanol.

5. The sample is acetylated with acetic anhydride pyridine 1:1 (1 mL) at 100°C for 30 min. After pyridine and acetic anhydride are removed as azeotropes with toluene, the residue is dissolved in chloroform with brief sonication and transferred to a reactivial and evaporated to about 20 µL under nitrogen. The positive ion FAB spectrum is obtained, as described previously, by using 2 nmol of sample.

6. After polysaccharides are subjected to steps 1–5, the fully acetylated sample is hydrolyzed with 1 mL trifluoro acetic acid for 45 sec at room temperature before adding 4 mL of acetic anhydride. After 10 min at ambient temperature

acetic anhydride and trifluoro acetic acid are removed as azeotropes with toluene. As an alternative, deuterated acetic anhydride or an analog, propionic anhydride, can be used to tag the site of hydrolysis in the polymer.

The degree of desired degradation is determined by the duration of the hydrolysis step. The more oxidation sites in the molecule, the shorter the hydrolysis time. The number of oxidation sites in the polymer is assessed by the linkage analysis described earlier. If a limited amount of sample is available, the exact hydrolysis conditions should be worked out first, using commercial polysaccharides with similar type linkages. The conditions described for periodate oxidation yield complete oxidation with minimum overoxidation.

7. The acetylated polysaccharide derivative is dissolved in chloroform and extracted with water. The chloroform phase is dried and the sample is dissolved in acetonitrile:water, 17:7, and applied to a reverse phase HPLC column (Bio-Rad ODS-10 150X4mm). The column is developed in acetonitrile:water 17:7 on a Waters Model 440 liquid chromatograph equipped with a differential refractometer and UV detector. The individual fractions are collected, dried under nitrogen, redissolved in chloroform, and analyzed by FAB–MS as described previously.

8.5. Sample Analysis by FAB–MS

The successful application of this sequence methodology requires substantial information regarding the mode of attachment of the individual residues, preferably by having subjected the original material to a linkage analysis, as described previously. When only limited amounts of material are available, linkage information necessary for a successful structural determination might be obtained in the analytical and biochemical literature dealing with related compounds.

The FAB–MS spectra of small oxidized, reduced, and acetylated oligosaccharides show simple, readily interpretable cleavage patterns. The FAB mass spectrum of the compound derived from lactose (Fig. 17) illustrates the four simple and predominant types of cleavage observed. Figure 17 contains an abbreviated version of the structure shown in Figure 14, which shows all the deuterium atoms that were installed during the deuteride reductions. The FAB–MS spectrum in Fig. 17 indicates that A, B, C, and D fragments are represented by significant peaks.

Fragmentation of the molecule with charge retention on the *nonreducing* end results in ions with m/z 160 and 263. The ion with m/z 160 arises by cleavage between C-5 and the ring oxygen of the original nonreducing terminal residue (Fig. 17). The ion with m/z 263 results from cleavage between the glycosidic carbon and oxygen.

Fragmentation of the molecule with charge retention on the *reducing* end results in ions having m/z 232 and 335. The ion having m/z 232 represents cleavage between the glycosidic oxygen and aglycone carbon (type C). The ion

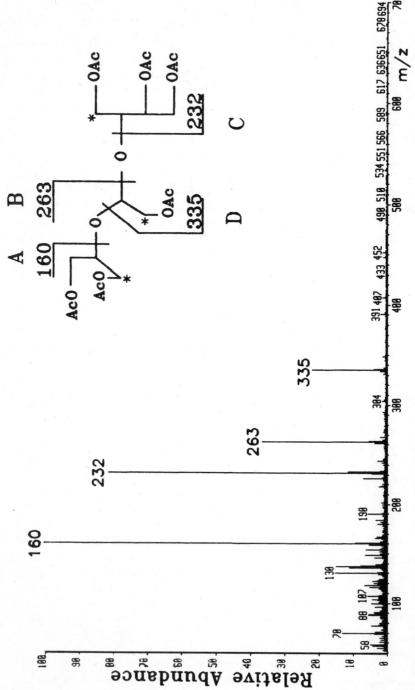

Fig. 17. FAB–mass spectrum of periodate-oxidized, deuteride-reduced, and acetylated lactose (mol wt 511). Asterisks denote those carbons to which a deuterium atom is attached as a result of the deuteride reduction; see Fig. 14 for a more complete structure.

having m/z 335 represents cleavage between the glycosidic carbon and ring oxygen (type D). The FAB–MS spectrum, although simple, does not by itself exclude a reducing terminal pentose. Sugar and linkage analysis are needed for a complete structural analysis even of such a simple compound as that illustrated in Fig. 17.

In the absence of the periodate oxidation step, an acetylated disaccharide shown in Fig. 18 gives a fragmentation pattern common to 16 different possible disaccharides. All of these would have the identical primary fragment peaks at m/z 331 and 619 with a peak for MH$^+$ at m/z 701. In fact, more than 150,000,000 hexasaccharides can be constructed, all of which would yield the same MH$^+$ and the primary fragment ions would be mostly the same. These considerations indicate that FAB–MS of acetylated or methylated native oligosaccharides yield limited, if any, sequence information.

Fucosyllactose, comprised of nonreducing terminal L-fucose, 2-linked galactose, and 4-linked glucose residues, is used as a model to evaluate the applicability of the above procedure to the analysis of small amounts of compound. Approximately 2 nmol (1 μg) of starting material, subjected to the derivatization procedure, gave the spectrum shown in Fig. 19. This spectrum demonstrates clearly that the compound can be sequenced readily in a manner similar to that described for lactose (Fig. 17). For this quantity of sample, the matrix peaks m/z 136, 154, 289, 307, and 460 are evident as are the peaks derived from the modified fucosyl lactose. Use of larger sample quantities leads to the total suppression of these matrix peaks. Type A fragments having m/z 102 and 160 characterize the oxidized ring structures of the nonreducing terminal fucose and the 2-linked galactosyl residues, respectively. The sequence fuc-(1-2)-gal follows from the two sequential type B fragments m/z 205 and 497. From the linkage information and the ascending type C fragments at m/z 232 and 524, it follows that the 4-linked glucose is the reducing end. The type D fragments at m/z 569 and 627 corroborate the conclusions regarding the sequence. The peak at m/z 768 is probably due to the presence of MNa$^+$. The data suggest that the above methodology can be used to generate sequence information on low nanomole amounts of oligosaccharides.

Periodate oxidation and partial hydrolysis (Smith degradation) of carbohydrates often yields mixtures of oligosaccharides that can be completely separated only with difficulty and with subsequent loss of material. The FAB–MS mass spectrum of nigeran tetrasaccharide (Fig. 20) illustrates this problem and the capacity of the sequencing strategy described here to resolve mixtures of oligosaccharides. The peaks at m/z 1186 and 822 represent the natriated molecules (M + Na$^+$) of nigeran-derived tetra- and trisaccharides, respectively. Based on available linkage information, the oligosaccharide is composed of glucose residues substituted at C-3 and C-4. The fragment ion peaks at m/z 160, 263, 551, 740, and 843 represent types A, B, B, A, and B fragmentation from the nonreducing end, respectively. Peaks at m/z 160 and 263 represent ions derived from the nonreducing terminal residue. The fragment having m/z 551 demonstrates that the nonreducing terminal residue *(m/z* fragment 263) is linked to C-3

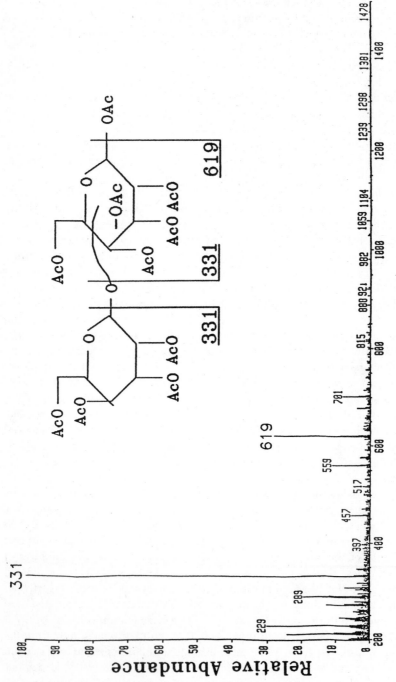

Fig. 18. FAB–mass spectrum of unoxidized peracetylated lactose (mol wt 678 common to 16 possible pyranose structures).

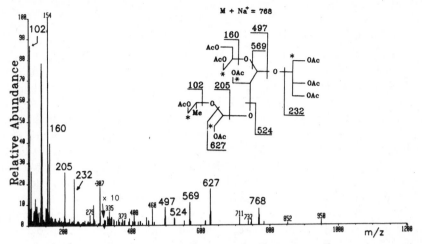

Fig. 19. FAB–mass spectrum of periodate-oxidized, deuteride-reduced, and acetylated fucosyllactose (mol wt 745). The identity of the molecule is given by the mass spectrum that distinguishes it from 2304 other possible trisaccharides with the same sugar composition. In the absence of periodate oxidation, there would be 64 different oligosaccharides fuc → gal → glc with the identical spectrum. Asterisks on the structure indicate which carbons have a deuterium atom as a result of deuteride reduction of the original molecule.

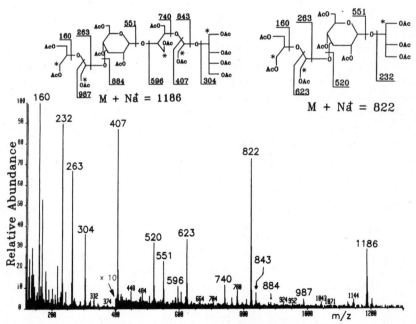

Fig. 20. FAB–mass spectrum of derivatives of periodate oxidized, deuteride reduced and acetylated nigeran tetrasaccharide (mol wt 1085). Asterisks on the structure indicate which carbons have a deuterium atom as a result of deuteride reduction of the original molecule.

135

of the aglycon. If the second residue had been linked at C-4, the expected type B cleavage would have shown a peak at m/z 555. Linkages to either C-2 or C-6 would be unexpected. If present, a C-2 linkage would yield a peak at m/z 555 that would lose acetic acid (60 daltons). A C-6 linkage would result in a peak at m/z 483.

The peak at m/z 740 could be derived by the addition of an 189 dalton moiety to m/z 551. This shows that the 3-linked residue is linked to the 4-position of an oxidized ring structure. The fragment m/z 843 represents an oxidized 4-linked residue added to the disaccharide derivative represented by m/z 551. The sequence from the nonreducing end based on these data is, therefore, Glc-(1-3)-Glc-(1-4)-Glc-X, where X is an oxidized reducing terminus.

Oxidized hexoses at the reducing end yield type C fragments that are unique to the mode of attachment. Hexoses at the reducing terminus substituted at C-2, C-3, C-4, and C-6 would yield m/z 161, 304, 232, and 160, respectively. The spectrum shows both m/z 304 and 232, demonstrating the presence of both 3-linked and 4-linked hexose residues at the reducing end. Given the available linkage information, the next type C fragment would be the addition to the reducing end, of 288 daltons for a 3-linked or 292 daltons for a 4-linked residue. The spectrum contains peaks at m/z 520 and 596 that suggest the presence of a 3-linked residue penultimate to the 4-linked reducing terminus (m/z 520), and a 4-linked residue penultimate to the 3-linked reducing terminus (m/z 596). The peak at m/z 884 is derived from the addition of 288 daltons to m/z 596, demonstrating that a 3-linked residue is linked to the 4-linked penultimate residue from the reducing end. In addition, type D fragments are seen 103 daltons higher at m/z 407, 623, and 987. The moiety of 103 daltons, represents C-1 and C-2 of a residue oxidized at C-3 and beyond. The presence of the peak having m/z 407 confirms the presence of a 4-linked hexose as the residue penultimate to the 3-linked reducing end. The peak at m/z 623 demonstrates that a nonreducing terminal residue is linked to C-3 of the residue linked 1-4 to the reducing end, thereby revealing the presence of a trisaccharide. The peak at m/z 987 is accounted for by the addition of 103 daltons to m/z 884 and demonstrates that an oxidized residue is linked also to the 3-linked derivative, which was linked 1-4 to the residue linked 1-3 to the reducing end.

From the preceding analysis it is apparent that the mass spectrum shown in Fig. 20 can only be derived from a mixture of a tri- and tetrasaccharides. This example shows the resolving power of the sequence method that gives structural information from both the reducing and nonreducing ends of the oligosaccharide derivatives. Thus, suspected sample degradation or a limited mixture of structures may be resolved without complete purification of each component. The redundancy of the overlapping information provides confidence in low-abundance, higher-mass ions. Note that ions arising from cleavages on either side of any of the ring or glycosidic oxygens are present in the spectrum. The sum of the m/z values of each of these pairs of complementary fragment ions plus sodium plus oxygen gives the expected natriated molecule for the tri- or tetrasaccharide at m/z 822 or 1186, respectively, as shown in Fig. 20.

TABLE 3

GLYCOSPEC printout of its Solutions to the Spectrum Shown in Fig. 20[a]

Proposed peak sources

m/z	Symbolic Representation	Corresponding Fragment of Intact Structure
232	(R4LHEX)	-4)-Glc
304	(R3LHEX)	-3)-Glc
263	(NRHEX)	Glc-(1-
520	(R4LHEX=232) + (3LHEX=288)	-3)-Glc-(1-4)-Glc
551	(NRHEX=263) + (3LHEX=288)	Glc-(1-3)-Glc-(1-
596	(R3LHEX=304) + (4LHEX=292)	-4)-Glc-(1-3)-Glc
623	(520) + (NRHEX E 103)	-Glc[C,1-2]-(1-3)-Glc-(1-4)-Glc
740	(551) + (4LHEX E 189)	Glc-(1-3)-Glc-(1-4)-Glc[C,3-6]
822	(740) + (OAc) + Na⁺	Glc-(1-3)-Glc-(1-4)-Glc + Na⁺
843	(551) + (4LHEX=292)	Glc-(1-3)-Glc-(1-4)-Glc-(1-
884	(596) + (3LHEX=288)	-3)-Glc-(1-4)-Glc-(1-3)-Glc
987	(884) + (NRHEX=103)	-Glc[C,1-2]-(1-3)-Glc-(1-4)-Glc-(1-3)-Glc
1186	(843) + (R3LHEX=304) + Na⁺	Glc-(1-3)-Glc-(1-4)-Glc-(1-3)-Glc + Na⁺

R4LHEX = Reducing 4-linked hexose
NRHEX = Non-reducing hexose
3LHEX = 3-linked hexose

[a]The database contained, in addition to FAB–MS data, information about the type of sugars and linkages present in the oligosaccharide.

Analysis from reducing end:
Hex 1 → 3 Hex 1 → 4 Hex
Hex 1 → 3 Hex 1 → 4 Hex 1 → 3 Hex

Analysis from nonreducing end:
Hex 1 → 3 Hex 1 → 4 Hex 1 → 3 Hex
Hex 1 → 3 Hex 1 → 4 Hex

The combined data from linkage, sugar, and FAB–MS analysis yields, when applied to the expert system GLYCOSPEC, the structural solutions shown in Table 3. Note that the information being processed by GLYCOSPEC represents sets of data, which when processed yields the two solutions.

8.6. Application to Polysaccharides

The applicability of the methodology for sequence analysis of complex branched polysaccharide structures is illustrated with the *Salmonella* polysaccharides *S. typhimurium LT2* (58) and *S. strasburg* (59). The lipopolysaccharides from these bacteria were subjected to oxidation, borodeuteride reduction, acetylation, partial acid hydrolysis, and reacetylation. The oligosaccharide derivatives were fractionated on HPLC into fractions containing tetra- and pentasaccharides and octa- through decasaccharides; these were analyzed by FAB–MS as described (Fig. 21).

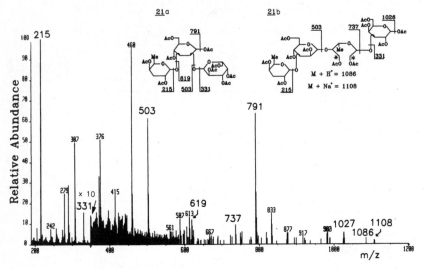

Fig. 21. FAB–mass spectrum of periodate-oxidized deuteride-reduced, acetylated, partially hydrolyzed, and reacetylated derivatives of lipopolysaccharide from *Salmonella typhimurium*. Asterisks on the structure indicate which carbons have a deuterium atom as a result of deuteride reduction of the original molecule.

Sugar and linkage analysis of the *LT2* lipopolysaccharide (58) shows that it contains equimolar amounts of nonreducing terminal abequosyl- (3,6-dideoxy-D-ribo-hexose = Abe), 4-linked L-rhamnosyl-, 3-linked D-galactosyl-, and 2,3-disubstituted D-mannosyl residues.

Theoretically, a nonreducing abequosyl residue should give a peak at m/z 215, while the other three residues, being internal, should give peaks at m/z 234, 288, and 245, respectively. The corresponding peaks of terminal residues are 43 daltons higher. The fragment ion of mass 331 arises from a type B or C cleavage and represents an unoxidized, nonreducing (B) or reducing (C) terminus. Owing to the partial hydrolysis employed (Figs. 15 and 16), an originally internal 3-linked hexosyl residue could be present at either end of an isolated oligosaccharide derivative. Either residue would give rise to a fragment ion as m/z 331. Originally branched residues may appear as chain residues (m/z 288) in the final derivative. A reducing-terminal rhamnosyl residue would give a peak at m/z 174 and a 3-linked hexose gives a peak at m/z 331 arising from the reducing end.

The actual mass spectrum derived from the partially degraded and purified *S. typhimurium* LT2 lipopolysaccharide is shown in Fig. 21. The nonreducing ends are Abe (NR36DDH) and nonreducing hydrolyzed 3-linked hexoses (NRH3LHEX), resulting from Smith degradation of the oxidized polysaccharide. Fragmentation from the nonreducing end yields type B fragments indicative of the linear structure (21*b*) and B and C fragments expected for the branched structure (21*a*).

Based on the fragmentation principles shown in the previous spectra, all of the fragments derived from the reducing end should also be found, although with decreasing intensities with increasing mass. The major fragment ion of mass m/z 503 and the minor fragment of mass m/z 619 would arise from the reducing end of the trisaccharide derivative gal-(1-2)-[abe-(1-3)]-man (21a) with a mass of 850 dalton by cleavage at the gal and abe linkage, respectively. Table 4 lists the possible solutions according to GLYCOSPEC to the m/z values in ascending order from the nonreducing end. The database processed by GLYCOSPEC contained the linkage analysis and the FAB–MS data, which to GLYCOSPEC again constitutes an unknown polysaccharide.

The spectrum obtained from an approximate decasaccharide HPLC fraction of partially degraded derivatives of *S. strasbourg* lipopolysaccharide are shown in Fig. 22. The polysaccharide differs from the previously described (Fig. 21) only in that the mannose residues are substituted at C-3 and C-6. Rhamnose is 4-linked and galactose is substituted at C-3, with tyvelose (3,6-dideoxy-D-arabino-hexose = Tyv) as a nonreducing terminal.

The type B fragments suggest the presence of both linear (m/z 737) and branched (m/z 791) nonreducing ends (Fig. 22). These could be combined with the two primary reducing ends, indicated by the type D fragments [m/z 1314 (upper structure) and m/z 923 (lower structure)], and depicted in Fig. 22. There are a total of four possible major structures, each of which reveal the sequence of all the individual residues identified in the linkage analysis.

TABLE 4

GLYCOSPEC Solutions to FAB–MS Data

m/z	*Symbolic Representation*	*Corresponding Fragment of Intact Structure*
Structure 21a		
215	(NR36DDHEX=215)	Abe-(1-
331	(NRH3LHEX=331)	Gal-(1-
791	(331) + [NR36DDH B 215]	Gal-(1-2)-Man-
	+ (B23LHEX=245)	Abe-(1-3)/
Structure 21b		
215	(NR36DDHEX=215)	Abe-(1-
503	(215) + (3LHEX=288)	Abe-(1-3)-Man-(1-
737	(503) + (4L6DHEX=234)	Abe-(1-3)-Man-(1-4)-Rha-(1-
1026	(737) + (3LHEX=288)	Abe-(1-3)-Man-(1-4)-Rha-(1-3)-Gal-(1-
1086	(1026) + (OAc) + 1 = M + H$^+$	Abe-(1-3)-Man-(1-4)-Rha-(1-3)-Gal-OAc + H$^+$

NR36DDHEX = Nonreducing 3,6-dideoxy hexose
NRH3LHEX = Nonreducing hydrolyzed 3-linked hexose
B23LHEX = Branched 2,3-linked hexose
3LHEX = 3-linked hexose
4L6DHEX = 4-linked 6-deoxy hexose

[a]Given a data base that contained all expected linkages from the linkage analysis and anticipated results from the partial acid hydrolysis step involved in the sample preparation.

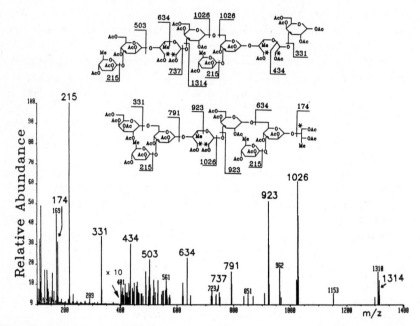

Fig. 22. FAB–mass spectrum of approximate decasaccharide HPLC fraction of periodate-oxidized, deuteride-reduced, acetylated, partially hydrolyzed, and reacetylated derivatives of lipopolysaccharide from *Salmonella strasbourg*. Asterisks on the structure indicate which carbons have a deuterium atom as a result of deuteride reduction of the original molecule.

The type B fragments m/z 215 and 331 demonstrate the presence of the nonreducing terminal tyvelosidic and hydrolyzed 3-linked galactosidic residues. The peaks m/z 503 and 791 represent the two different nonreducing ends both of which have tyvelosidic residues (m/z 215) as part of their structure. The absence of a peak at m/z 443 of (503 − 60) demonstrates that the tyvelosidic residue is linked to the 3-position of the 3,6-disubstituted mannose residue.

The spectrum clearly demonstrates that the fragmentation pattern obtained, owing to the redundancy of overlapping fragments, allows for the safe assignment of sequence for a hexasaccharide SFSU and for reasonable assessment of larger structures. Furthermore, the repetitive nature of the polysaccharide can be readily determined.

9. CONCLUSIONS AND FUTURE DIRECTIONS

The combined methodologies of sugar analysis, linkage analysis, anomeric configuration determination, and sequence analysis described herein constitute, in our experience, the most sample-conserving approaches, based on mass spectrometry, for deriving precise oligosaccharide structures. Current efforts are directed toward improving methods and developing computer programs, such as the expert system GLYCOSPEC, in order to deduce precise structures from analytical results obtained with ever smaller amounts of material. With biological systems communicating by means of only 10^5 specific carbohydrate protein interactions (28, 29), we will need to arrive at a state of the art where 10^{12} molecules will suffice for a *complete* structural analysis of a complex oligosaccharide epitope.

Subjecting a periodate-oxidized derivative, as described herein, to the high-transmission four-sector instruments with diode array detectors available today (60), would yield significant structural information from 10^{12} molecules. The simple principal fragmentations, seen with these derivatives, lend themselves to the analysis of parent and daughter ions for further sequential information. From the overall strategies discussed herein, it follows that existing partial information on biosynthesis in specific tissues and species as well as partially elucidated structures for common core elements in different types of complex carbohydrates, can give the investigator significant structural information in one analysis.

References

1. C. Croon, G. Herrström, G. Kull, and B. Lindberg, *Acta Chem. Scand.* **14**, 1338 (1960).

2. H. Björndal, B. Lindberg, and S. Svensson, *Acta Chem. Scand.* **21**, 1801 (1967).

3. H. Björndal, B. Lindberg, and S. Svensson, *Carbohyd. Res.* **5**, 433 (1967).

4. C. G. Hellerqvist, B. Lindberg, S. Svensson, T. Holme, and A. A. Lindberg, *Carbohyd. Res.* **8**, 43 (1968) (Citation Classic).

5. H. Björndal, C. G. Hellerqvist, B. Lindberg, and S. Svensson, *Angew. Chem.* **82**, 643 (1979) (Citation Classic).

6. K.-A. Karlsson, *FEBS Lett.* **32**, 317 (1973).

7. K.-A. Karlsson, I. Pascher, W. Pimlott, and B. E. Samuelsson, Biomed. *Mass Spectrom.* **1**, 49 (1974).

8. H. Egge, J. Peter-Katalinic, G. Reuter, R. Schauer, R. Ghidoni, S. Sonnino, and G. TeHamanti, *Chem. Phys. Lipids* **37**, 127 (1985).

9. V. N. Reinhold, *Mass Spectrometry in Biomedical Research*, 1986, Chap. 11, p. 181.

10. A. Dell, *Adv. Carbohyd. Chem. Biochem.* **45**, 19 (1987).

11. A.-S. Angel, F. Lindh, and B. Nilsson, *Carbohyd. Res.* **168**, 15 (1987).

12. R. S. Pappas, B. Sweetman, S. Ray, and C. G. Hellerqvist, *Glycoconj. J.* **5**, 293 (1988).

13. R. S. Pappas, B. Sweetman, S. Ray, and C. G. Hellerqvist, *Carbohyd. Res.* (in press) (1990).

14. V. N. Shibaer, *Adv. Carbohyd. Chem. Biochem.* **44**, 277 (1986).

15. C. G. Hellerqvist, B. Lindberg, S. Svensson, T. Holme, and A. A. Lindberg, *Carbohyd. Res.* **9**, 237 (1969).

16. C. G. Hellerqvist, U. Ryden, and P. H. Makela, *Eur. J. Biochem.* **25**, 96 (1972).

17. P. J. Garegg, B. Lindberg, T. Onn, and T. Holme, *Acta Chem. Scand.* **25**, 1185 (1971).

18. C. G. Hellerqvist, H. Sundell, and P. Gettins, *Proc. Natl. Acad. Sci. U.S.A.* **84**, 51 (1987).

19. Y. Nakanishi, M. Shimizu, K. Otsu, S. Kato, M. Tsuji, and S. Suzuki, *J. Biol. Chem.* **256**, 5443 (1981).

20. S. V. K. N. Murthy, M. A. Melly, T. M. Harris, C. G. Hellerqvist, and J. H. Hash, *Carbohyd. Res.* **117**, 113 (1983).

21. M. Hook, L. Kjellén, and S. Johansson, *Ann. Rev. Biochem.* **53**, 847 (1984).

22. A. Malmström, *J. Biol. Chem.* **259**, 161 (1984).

23. U. Lindahl and G. Pejler, *Acta Med. Scand., Suppl.* **715**, 139 (1987).

24. M.-C. Bourin, A.-K. Öhlin, D. A. Lane, J. Stenflo, and U. Lindahl, *J. Biol. Chem.* **17**, 8044 (1988).

25. Y.-T. Li and S.-C. Li, *Adv. Carbohyd. Chem. Biochem.* **40**, 235 (1982).

26. F. W. Hemming, in T. W. Goodwin (Ed.) *Biochemistry of Lipids, MTP Int. Rev. Sci. Biochem. Ser. One* **4**, 39–98 (1974).

27. R. T. Schwarz and R. Datema, *Adv. Carbohyd. Chem. Biochem.* **40**, 287 (1982).

28. P. H. Weingel, R. L. Schnaar, M. S. Kuhlenschmidt, E. Schmell, R. T. Lee, Y. C. Lee, and S. Roseman, *J. Biol. Chem.* **254**, 10830 (1979).

29. K. Krueger and C. G. Hellerqvist, *J. Biol Chem.* **256**, 8553 (1981).

30. E. A. Kabat, *J. Immunol.* **84**, 82 (1964).

31. V. N. Shibaev, *Adv. Carbohyd. Chem. Biochem.* **44**, 277 (1986).

32. B. Lindberg, J. Lonngren, and S. Svensson, *Adv. Carbohyd. Chem. Biochem.* **31**, 181 (1975).

33. B. V. McCleary and K. Matheson, *Adv. Carbohyd. Chem. Biochem.* **44**, 147 (1986).

34. R. L. Taylor and H. E. Conrad, *Biochemistry* **11**, 1383 (1972).

35. C. G. Hellerqvist and A. A. Lindberg, *Carbohyd. Res.* **16**, 39 (1971).

36. D. A. Cumming, C. G. Hellerqvist, M. Harris-Braedts, S. W. Michnick, J. P. Carver, and B. Bendiak, *Biochemistry* (submitted).

37. S. Hakomori, *J. Biochem. (Tokyo)* **55**, 205 (1964).

38. B. Lindberg, J. Lönngren, J. L. Thompson, and W. Nimmich, *Carbohyd. Res.* **25**, 49 (1972).

39. I. Ciucanu, and F. Kerek. *Carbohyd. Res.* **131**, 209 (1984).

40. C. G. Hellerqvist (unpublished).

41. J. Gailitt and C. G. Hellerqvist (unpublished).

42. S. J. Angyal and K. James, *Australian J. Chem.* **23**, 1209 (1970).

43. C. G. Hellerqvist, J. Hoffman, B. Lindberg, A. Pilotti, and A. A. Lindberg, *Acta Chem. Scand.* **25**, 1512 (1971).

44. J. Hoffman, B. Lindberg, and S. Svensson, *Acta Chem. Scand.* **26**, 661 (1972).

45. C. G. Hellerqvist, J. Hoffman, A. A. Lindberg, B. Lindberg, and S. Svensson, *Acta Chem. Scand.* **26**, 3282 (1972).

46. K. Harada, S. Ito, M. Suzuki, and A. Tatematsu, *Biomed. Mass Spect.* **10**, 5 (1983).

47. S. A. Carr, V. N. Reinhold, B. N. Green, and R. J. Hass, *Biomed. Mass Spect.* **12**, 288 (1985).

48. A. Dell and M. Pamico, in *Mass Spectrometry in Biomedical Research*, S. J. Gaskell, Ed., Wiley, New York, 1986, Chapter 10, p. 149.

49. H. Egge, J. Dabrowski, and P. Haffland, *Pure Appl. Chem.* **56**, 807 (1984).

50. I. Jardine, *Mass Spectrometry in Biomedical Research*, S. J. Gaskell, Ed., Wiley, New York, 1986, Chapter 16, p. 287.

51. A. G. Harrison, *Chemical Ionization Mass Spectrometry*, CRC Press, Boca Raton, FL, 1983.

52. V. N. Reinhold, *Mass Spectrometry in Biomedical Research*, S. J. Gaskell, Ed., Wiley, New York, 1986, Chapter 11, p. 181.

53. V. N. Reinhold and S. A. Carr, *Anal. Chem.* **54**, 499 (1982).

54. N. Takeda, K. Harada, M. Suzuki, A. Tatematsu, and I. Sakata, *Mass Spectroscopy* **33**, 59 (1985).

55. M. Barber, R. S. Bordoli, R. D. Sedgwick, and A. N. Tyler, *J. Chem. Soc. Commun.*, 325 (1981).

56. J. L. Gower, *Biomed. Mass Spectrom.* **12**, 191 (1985).

57. H. Krotkiewsky, E. Lisowska, A. S. Angel, B. Nilsson, *Carbohyd. Res.* **184**, 27 (1988).

58. C. G. Hellerqvist, B. Lindberg, S. Svensson, T. Holme, and A. A. Lindberg, *Carbohyd. Res.* **9**, 231 (1969).

59. C. G. Hellerqvist, B. Lindberg, A. Pilotti, and A. A. Lindberg, *Acta Chem. Scand.* **24**, 1168 (1970).

60. A. L. Burlingame, D. Maltby, D. H. Russell, and P. T. Holland, *Ann. Chem. Fund. Reviews* **60**, 294R (1988).

Peptide Sequencing by Mass Spectrometry

JOHN T. STULTS, *Protein Chemistry Department, Genentech, Inc., South San Francisco, California*

1. INTRODUCTION

The dramatic advances in molecular biology and recombinant DNA technology during the past 15 years have given scientists a new understanding of the molecular basis of life and have opened many new avenues of research. Contrary to earlier predictions, the growth of molecular biology has not meant the demise of protein chemistry, but rather it has elevated protein chemistry to new importance. Many of the advances in biochemistry and biotechnology can be traced to the combined efforts of molecular biologists and protein chemists. Determination of the amino acid sequences of peptides and proteins is one of the objectives of protein chemistry. The field of protein sequencing has, as a result, also seen advances in terms of efficiency and enhancements in sensitivity.

Mass spectrometry is part of that advancement. In the 1970s, the utility of mass spectrometry for sequencing was demonstrated in a few highly skilled laboratories. When fast atom bombardment (FAB) was introduced in 1981, explosive growth in new methods and applications began, because the requirements for volatility were eliminated. Advances in high-mass instrument development made mass spectrometry applicable to an ever-increasing number of peptides. Tandem mass spectrometry can now provide detailed structural information on many peptides.

Today mass spectrometry is used more and more by protein chemists as they strive to determine the primary structure of proteins. Mass spectrometry complements the traditional sequencing methods, giving protein chemists a greater variety of tools to solve structural problems. Likewise, mass spectrometrists are expending a great deal of effort toward understanding the fragmentations of peptides and toward improving the instrumentation and methodologies for studying peptides.

2. PEPTIDE AND PROTEIN STRUCTURE

The primary structure of a protein or peptide includes the amino acid sequence plus any covalently attached groups, for example, carbohydrate, phosphate, and lipid. The distinction between peptides and proteins is based on size; peptides are generally below 10 kDa in mass, proteins are larger. Table 1 lists the common amino acids, their single- and three-letter abbreviations, and their structures.

2.1. Posttranslational Modifications

The sequence of a protein is determined by the gene that encodes for it. Immediately following translation of the gene, the protein is composed of only the 20 "common" amino acids. Many proteins are subsequently acted on by a wide variety of enzymes that modify the protein in some manner. These posttranslational modifications include alterations to specific amino acid side chains, addition of carbohydrates, formation of disulfide bonds or other cross-links, and

TABLE 1

Common Amino Acids and Their Structures

Name	Abbreviations		Structure
Alanine	Ala	A	$CH_3-\overset{\overset{\displaystyle NH_2}{\mid}}{C}HCO_2H$
Arginine	Arg	R	$H_2N-\overset{\overset{\displaystyle NH}{\|\|}}{C}-NH-(CH_2)_3-\overset{\overset{\displaystyle NH_2}{\mid}}{C}HCO_2H$
Asparagine	Asn	N	$H_2N-\overset{\overset{\displaystyle O}{\|\|}}{C}-CH_2-\overset{\overset{\displaystyle NH_2}{\mid}}{C}HCO_2H$
Aspartic acid	Asp	D	$HO-\overset{\overset{\displaystyle O}{\|\|}}{C}-CH_2-\overset{\overset{\displaystyle NH_2}{\mid}}{C}HCO_2H$
Cysteine	Cys	C	$HS-CH_2-\overset{\overset{\displaystyle NH_2}{\mid}}{C}HCO_2H$
Glutamic acid	Glu	E	$HO-\overset{\overset{\displaystyle O}{\|\|}}{C}-(CH_2)_2-\overset{\overset{\displaystyle NH_2}{\mid}}{C}HCO_2H$
Glutamine	Gln	Q	$H_2N-\overset{\overset{\displaystyle O}{\|\|}}{C}-(CH_2)_2-\overset{\overset{\displaystyle NH_2}{\mid}}{C}HCO_2H$
Glycine	Gly	G	$H-\overset{\overset{\displaystyle NH_2}{\mid}}{C}HCO_2H$
Histidine	His	H	(imidazole ring)$-CH_2-\overset{\overset{\displaystyle NH_2}{\mid}}{C}HCO_2H$
Isoleucine	Ile	I	$CH_3CH_2-\overset{\overset{\displaystyle CH_3}{\mid}}{C}H-\overset{\overset{\displaystyle NH_2}{\mid}}{C}HCO_2H$
Leucine	Leu	L	$CH_3-\overset{\overset{\displaystyle CH_3}{\mid}}{C}H-CH_2-\overset{\overset{\displaystyle NH_2}{\mid}}{C}HCO_2H$
Lysine	Lys	K	$H_2N-(CH_2)_4-\overset{\overset{\displaystyle NH_2}{\mid}}{C}HCO_2H$
Methionine	Met	M	$CH_3-S-(CH_2)_2-\overset{\overset{\displaystyle NH_2}{\mid}}{C}HCO_2H$

Table 3.1 (*Continued*)

Name	Abbreviations		Structure
Phenylalanine	Phe	F	
Proline	Pro	P	
Serine	Ser	S	$HO-CH_2-CHCO_2H$ with NH_2
Threonine	Thr	T	$CH_3-CH-CHCO_2H$ with OH and NH_2
Tryptophan	Trp	W	
Tyrosine	Tyr	Y	
Valine	Val	V	$CH_3-CH-CHCO_2H$ with CH_3 and NH_2

cleavage or "processing" of amino acids from either end of the peptide chain. Processing at the C-terminal in particular may result in heterogeneity or "fuzzy ends." Many modifications have been discovered and more are being found as new proteins are isolated and characterized. Detailed listings can be found elsewhere (1–3).

Acetylation or formylation of the N-terminal amino group are among the most common modifications. Residues most often acetylated are Gly, Ala, Asp, Ser, and Met. The "blocked" N-terminus precludes traditional sequencing methods as described in the next section. Another blocking group is pyroglutamic acid (pGlu), which is formed by cyclization of an N-terminal Gln. Amidation is the most common modification of the carboxy-terminus.

Glycosylation is also observed fairly often. Carbohydrates may be attached to either Ser or Thr (O-linked) or Asn (N-linked). N-linked glycosylation requires the consensus sequence N-X-S/T (X can be any residue except proline, followed by either Ser or Thr). Identification of the glycosylation sites will be dealt with in a subsequent section. The carbohydrate portions of the molecule can be removed and analyzed using the procedures described in Chapter 2. Phosphorylation of hydroxyl groups (Ser, Thr, Tyr) may be observed as well, as it is an important aspect of many biological regulatory pathways.

Some of the modifications can be quite labile and are easily removed during isolation or characterization, especially when extremes in pH are employed. This factor should be considered when planning the purification steps. Likewise, steps in the isolation process can also introduce modifications that are not present in the native protein. For example, formic acid, a common solvent for peptides used extensively for cyanogen bromide digestions, can formylate free amino groups under certain conditions as described in greater detail in Section 3.2.

Disulfide bonds between cysteine residues are often found. These contribute greatly to the three-dimensional structure and stability of many proteins. Mapping the disulfide bonds is a necessary first step in determining the tertiary structure of a protein.

Mass spectrometry plays a very important role in identifying the posttranslational modifications of proteins. Based on the mass of a peptide and the predetermined amino acid sequence, it is often possible to identify the particular modification, a task that is considerably more difficult by other means. Furthermore, tandem mass spectrometry can be used to identify both the site and the identity of the modification.

2.2. Traditional Techniques for Sequence Determination

Several methods have been developed for determining the sequences of proteins and peptides. All involve sequential degradation of the molecule from one end or the other, removing and identifying the amino acids one at a time.

Sequencing peptides from the C-terminus is possible by a variety of chemical methods (4). All suffer from poor yields, which limit the number of residues that can be determined and most involve complex, multistep chemistry. Recent improvements in the thiohydantoin method (5) show promise for making C-terminal sequencing more practical.

More often, carboxypeptidases are used for C-terminal analysis (6–8). A number of carboxypeptidases are known which remove amino acids one at a time from the carboxy-terminus. The released amino acids are then identified. The enzymatic approach to C-terminal sequencing suffers from varying rates of hydrolysis for different amino acids, making its use less than ideal in practice. A slightly different approach using fast atom bombardment mass spectrometry measures the molecular weight of the remaining peptide at selected time intervals during the digestion (9). This method eliminates some of the drawbacks to the traditional approach, but limits the size of the peptide that can be sequenced.

N-terminal sequencing methods have more use. Several aminopeptidases cleave from the N-terminus inward, but suffer from the same drawbacks as the carboxypeptidases.

The most accepted N-terminal sequencing method is that first proposed by Edman (10). This approach involves reaction of the amino-terminus of the peptide with phenylisothiocyanate (PITC) to form the phenylthiocarbamoyl derivative (see Fig. 1). The N-terminal amino acid is then cleaved, converted to the more stable phenylthiohydantoin (PTH), identified, and quantitated. The remaining peptide is put through subsequent cycles of degradation. The manual approach to Edman degradation has been improved in recent years in terms of both efficiency and sensitivity (11).

The Edman procedure is also automated (12–15) and commercial units are available that can sequence at the low picomole level. The advances in this instrumentation have dramatically altered the field of protein chemistry by pushing the limits of sensitivity and providing tools that can be used in almost any laboratory.

Although amino terminal sequencing is sensitive and, as a result of automation, can be left unattended for long periods of time, the process is relatively slow, normally taking about 1 h per residue. It is of no use with N-terminally blocked peptides. Microsequencing (another term for automated Edman degradation) can yield uncertainty in certain residue assignments, especially when the quantity is small or mixtures contribute overlapping signals. As sequencing extends toward the C-terminus of a peptide, residue signals drop off gradually owing to imperfect repetitive yields. Furthermore, hydrophobic peptides can "wash out" as the C-terminus is approached owing to increased solubility of the residual peptide in the extraction solvents, resulting in less than complete sequence determination.

Undoubtedly, many posttranslational modifications are missed by Edman chemistry methods because of the relatively harsh conditions employed. The chromatographic identification of the PTH-amino acids is also prone to missing posttranslational modifications. Modified amino acids could be misassigned as another amino acid with identical retention time, or simply taken as an unassigned residue, especially when low levels are sequenced.

Owing to the advances in molecular biology, it is often possible to isolate, clone, and sequence the gene that encodes a protein with less effort than it would take to determine the complete amino acid sequence directly. This is especially true for large proteins and for proteins that are available in such small quantities that only limited amino acid sequence can be determined. The amino acid sequence can then be taken from the DNA sequence. Most often mRNA that codes for a particular protein is isolated. From it the complementary DNA (cDNA) is made and cloned. Methods for sequencing DNA can be found elsewhere (16–19). It should be kept in mind, however, that at least a partial amino acid sequence is usually required in order to isolate the DNA of interest.

The amino acid sequence deduced from the cDNA sequence is not the final answer, however. Error in reading the cDNA sequence from the gel is possible. The question of where translation of the mRNA begins and ends is not always trivial, nor is choosing the correct "reading frame" (three bases code for each amino acid, hence there are three reading frames for starting the DNA sequence

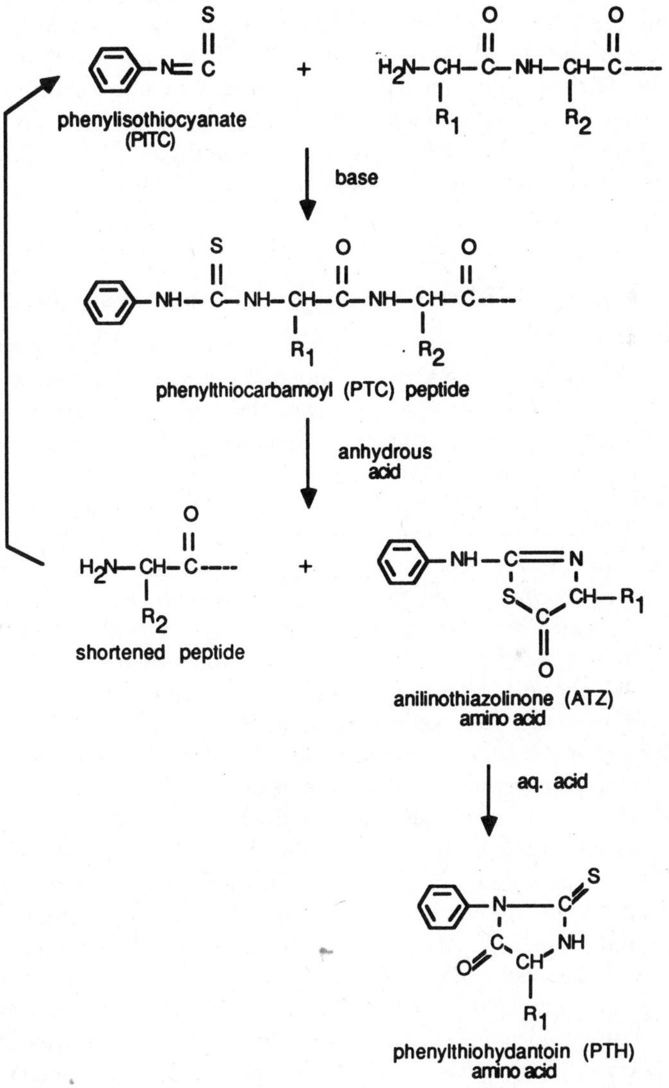

Fig. 1. Edman degradation chemistry. The peptide is coupled to PITC in base, then cleaved with acid to yield the shortened peptide plus the thiazolinone derivatives of the N-terminal amino acid. The shortened peptide is subjected to repeated cycles. The thiazolinone derivative is converted to the more stable PTH-amino acid, then identified and quantitated by HPLC.

interpretation). In mammalian genes, stretches of nontranscribed DNA, known as intervening regions or introns, are often found, which further complicate protein sequence deduction from genomic DNA. Following translation, amino acids may be enzymatically removed from either end and other modifications can be extensive, as already mentioned. A protein expressed by recombinant DNA techniques is not necessarily identical to the native molecule. The confirmation of the DNA-derived sequence is thus one of the areas where mass spectrometry is making a significant impact.

2.3. Integration of Mass Spectrometry and Microsequencing

Each of the traditional techniques for peptide sequencing has its advantages and also its drawbacks as described above. Many of the strengths of mass spectrometry for sequencing are in those areas where the other techniques have their weaknesses. Thus, mass spectrometry complements many of the traditional techniques for protein sequencing.

As an aid to microsequencing, mass spectrometry can improve both the efficiency and the accuracy of the operation. One of the most important contributions of FAB mass spectrometry to protein structure determination has been the ability to obtain precise, accurate molecular weights of peptides. Molecular weight measurements can usually be made on 10–50 pmole of sample, the same range as for automated Edman degradation and amino acid analysis. For an unknown peptide, the molecular weight is valuable to (a) confirm amino acid analysis accuracy, (b) determine how many cycles to program the automated microsequenator, (c) improve the confidence of residue assignment, (d) show whether the peptide was fully sequenced to the C-terminal, and (e) identify the presence of posttranslational modifications.

When a protein is to be sequenced, it is often first degraded under controlled conditions into several smaller peptides that are sequenced. After sequencing these smaller peptides, the intact protein is again cleaved but at different sites than the primary cleavage. Mass measurements of these secondary cleavage products provide the overlap data needed to piece together the entire sequence of the protein. A simple computer program can link all known sequences together in all possible combinations, identifying any molecular weight matches. Matches can be confirmed by molecular weight determination of the corresponding peptide after one or two cycles of manual Edman degradation, by one to two cycles on an automated microsequenator, or by amino acid analysis.

Confirmation of the sequence of synthetic peptides, or peptides and proteins produced by recombinant DNA technology, can be rapidly performed by mass measurement since the putative sequence is already known. Details of this process will be described subsequently. Considerable time can be saved in most cases because complete sequencing by Edman degradation is not required.

Mass spectrometry can be used directly to sequence an unknown protein. Such a task is not trivial, however. At present, mass spectrometry is usually used to sequence small peptides, or small proteins for which homologous sequences are already known. The general approach to sequencing by mass spectrometry is detailed in the last section of this chapter.

3. SAMPLE PREPARATION

Preparing a peptide sample for mass spectrometry involves two processes: isolation and purification of the original protein, then cleavage of the protein and separation of the smaller peptide fragments.

3.1. Protein Isolation and Purification

Protein purification is a broad field and any coverage of it is beyond the scope of this monograph. Most mass spectrometrists are likely not to be intimately involved with this aspect of the problem. However, it is useful to have some appreciation for the possible steps involved. More important, if one is involved at this stage and knows that mass spectrometry will ultimately be used in the analysis, there are some considerations that will increase the likelihood of success of the mass spectral analysis.

3.1.1. TRADITIONAL APPROACHES IN PROTEIN CHEMISTRY

A multitude of techniques is available for isolating and purifying a protein (20). The steps involved are dependent on the nature of the protein sought and the type of tissue or medium from which it is to be isolated. For example, cytosolic proteins are released by lysing the cells. Once the crude protein fraction of interest has been isolated, the tedious job of separating the protein of interest from many other proteins begins. Many chromatographic and electrophoretic techniques are employed. The goal is to recover the maximum quantity of active protein in the highest purity.

3.1.2. SPECIAL CONSIDERATIONS FOR MASS SPECTROMETRY

Many of the steps in protein purification involve chemicals that are incompatible with mass-spectrometric analysis. For derivatization, interferences in the chemistry can lead to undesirable by-products or poor reaction yields. In desorption ionization spectra, alkali metals readily attach to peptides. Many other compounds either compete for ionization or otherwise obscure the analyte of interest. This problem is particularly acute in fast atom bombardment; the ionization is based in part on the solubility and surface activity of the peptide in the matrix. Surfactants in even very low concentrations easily obscure peptide signals. Nonvolatile buffers often completely suppress the signals as well. Metals readily attach to the peptide, often resulting in addition of one, two, three, or more metal ions, spreading ion current over several peaks and sometimes making assignment of the molecular weight difficult or impossible. When peaks are poorly resolved, as is normally the case at high mass, alkali metal adduct peaks make accurate mass assignment difficult or impossible.

It is necessary to remove any complicating compounds as efficiently as possible before mass analysis. If possible, such compounds should be avoided altogether. For example, volatile buffers such as ammonium bicarbonate, pyridinium acetate, or *N*-ethyl morpholine can often be substituted for other nonvolatile buffers.

When use of potentially interfering compounds cannot be avoided, it is necessary to remove them from the sample before analysis by mass spectrometry. Fortunately, retention of biological activity is not necessary for mass spectral measurements. The most efficient, cleanest method of purification is reversed-phase HPLC using a water/acetonitrile/trifluoroacetic acid gradient. Care must be used in the chromatography. If salts, surfactants (e.g., SDS, Tween, Triton), or polyethylene glycol have previously been used in the HPLC system or column, there is the chance that these components may slowly elute along with the analyte. Other techniques may never give evidence of their existence. Should a sample not give the expected signal and contaminants appear likely (as evidenced in the low-mass region), one can check the final purification step using a standard of similar composition and quantity. All too often protein chemists write off mass spectrometry when their first sample fails to give a signal. Like all techniques, mass spectrometry has its own idiosyncratic requirements and learning these is part of the challenge of research.

3.2.   Cleavage into Smaller Peptides

Most proteins and peptides must be cleaved into smaller pieces to make their size compatible with mass spectrometry. Several monographs are especially recommended for more details on the cleavage and separation methodologies (21–23). The methods are divided into two categories, chemical and enzymatic.

3.2.1.   CHEMICAL METHODS

The most common chemical method uses cyanogen bromide (CNBr). CNBr specifically cleaves at the C-terminal side of methionine. Since methionine occurs relatively infrequently, CNBr fragments may be fairly large (up to 10 kDa or more). The reaction is straightforward (24):

> The protein is dissolved in 200 μL of 70% formic acid in an Eppendorf tube and bubbled under nitrogen. A single crystal of CNBr is added (make sure it is colorless) and cleavage proceeds under nitrogen approximately 12 hours in the dark at room temperature. CAUTION: CNBr is highly toxic! The digest is diluted with water and dried down in a vacuum centrifuge (Speed-vac) to remove the CNBr and acid (use a KOH trap).

The Met residues are converted to homoserine or homoserine lactone. In subsequent handling, be aware that CNBr fragments often display poor solubility and may require strong solvents. Using formic acid as a solvent is not recommended because it often results in the formylation of primary amine groups. Aqueous trifluoroacetic acid may be substituted as the solvent.

Cleavages at Asn-Gly bonds with hydroxylamine (25) or at Asp-Pro bonds with dilute acetic acid (26) are also used occasionally. Numerous reactions have also been developed for cleavage at Trp, Cys, Asp, and others (27). Although these latter cleavages may be useful for specific applications, side reactions and poor yields make them impractical for general use.

3.2.2. ENZYMATIC METHODS

Many proteinases (proteases) are known and others are found every year. Listed in Table 2 are the most commonly used, commercially available proteinases. Comments and digestion conditions for several of these are provided. The use of volatile buffers is recommended so that their removal can easily be accomplished by lyophilization. Using immobilized enzymes facilitates removal of the enzyme from the digest and provides cleaner spectra (28), but less complete digestion usually results. Complete digestion often requires that all of the cleavage sites be readily accessible to the proteinase. For this reason, disulfide bonds should first be reduced and alkylated. Several procedures are available. One method involves reduction with dithiothreitol (DTT) and alkylation with 4-vinylpyridine (29). The most widely used method employs DTT as the reducing agent followed by alkylation with iodoacetic acid (30):

The protein is dissolved in 0.5 M Tris-HCl, 6 M guanidine-HCl, and 2 mM EDTA, pH 8.1, then bubbled under nitrogen and warmed to 37°C for 30 min. At the same

TABLE 2

Common Proteinases

Enzyme[a]	Specificity (C-terminal side of...)	Comments
Trypsin	Lys, Arg	
Chymotrypsin	Trp, Tyr, Phe, Leu, Met	
Pepsin	Phe, Met, Leu, Trp	To hydrophobic residues
Staph. aureus V8	Glu	Bicarbonate buffer
	Glu, Asp	Phosphate buffer
Lysine-C	Lys	
Post-proline cleaving enzyme	Pro	
Papain	Nonspecific	
Subtilisin	Nonspecific	
Pronase	Nonspecific	
Asp-N	N-terminal side of Asp	
Thermolysin	N-terminal side of Leu, Ile, Met, Phe, Val, Ala	

[a]Most enzymes do not cleave when the C-terminal bond is to Pro, for example, Lys-Pro.

time prepare a solution of DTT in the same Tris buffer, 1 mg/mL, and bubble under nitrogen at 37°C for 30 min. Add the DTT solution to the protein solution to give a 50-fold molar excess of DTT over protein. Incubate at 37°C for 30 min and cool. Make a solution of 5 mg/mL iodoacetic acid in the Tris buffer, add this to give a 5-fold excess over the DTT. Incubate at room temperature for 30 min, then acidify to pH 4 with glacial acetic acid. The reagents are then removed by gel filtration on a Biogel P-10 column in 0.01 M NH_4CO_3.

Trypsin cleaves at the C-terminus of Lys and Arg except for Lys-Pro and Arg-Pro bonds. Acidic residues on either side of Lys or Arg reduce the cleavage rate. This digestion is one of the most commonly used due to its specificity. As an added advantage for the mass spectrometrist, it primarily produces peptides that are below 3500 u in mass. Most trypsin preparations contain a chymotrypsin inhibitor (e.g., TPCK). Even so, chymotryptic fragments (see subsequent discussion) may be encountered in low abundance. The following reaction scheme (31) may be altered depending on the particular protein and its susceptibility to proteolysis:

The protein is dissolved in 100–200 μL of 0.1 M NH_4HCO_3, pH 8.5. Trypsin, dissolved in 0.1 M HCl at approximately the same concentration, is added to give an enzyme : substrate ratio of 1 : 100 and incubated at 37°C for 6 h. A second addition of an identical amount of trypsin solution is then made and incubation continued for 18 h more. The reaction is stopped by lyophilization, lowering the pH, or injection onto an HPLC system. The trypsin solution should always be freshly prepared to minimize autolysis.

Chymotrypsin cleaves at the C-terminus of hydrophilic residues, with the highest cleavage rates for Trp, Tyr, and Phe, and slightly slower rates for Leu and His. Because it is less specific than trypsin, the fragments are usually smaller and it is often used as a second digestion for aligning subsequences. The digestion conditions are identical to those given for trypsin.

Pepsin tends to cleave between two adjacent hydrophilic residues. Bonds to proline are not attacked. The specificity of pepsin for the most part is difficult to predict, however. One advantage of pepsin is its activity at low pH, making it useful for determining disulfide linkages (disulfide reduction and interchange are slow at low pH):

Dissolve the substrate in 99% formic acid. Add this solution slowly to twenty volumes of 1 mM HCl containing pepsin (1% by weight of the substrate). Incubate at 25°C for 2 h. The digestion can be stopped by addition of base or by lyophilizing (31).

3.3. SEPARATION OF PEPTIDES

Following cleavage, the peptide fragment mixture may be analyzed directly by mass spectrometry (see subsequent discussion). The desorption ionization techniques generally work best with single peptides or simple mixtures. For that reason, the peptide fragments are separated, most often by HPLC. The separation also removes the proteinase and chemical contaminants.

Because the desorption ionization is sensitive to salts, peptides should be separated by reverse phase HPLC using volatile buffers. A C-8 or C-18 large pore column (300–1000 Å) with a water/acetonitrile/TFA gradient is commonly used. Solvent A is 0.1% TFA in water, B is 0.07% TFA in acetonitrile, and the gradient is 0–60% B. A column of 4.6 mm diameter is commonly used but narrow bore (2 mm) columns allow more sensitive detection with smaller elution volumes and require little modification of most LC systems. Microbore columns (1 mm) allow for even better sensitivity and are rapidly becoming the choice for microseparations. Column lengths can be kept short because peptides tend to be retained at the front of the column until they are rapidly eluted at the proper mobile phase composition. Often separation into five or six fractions, rather than complete separation, is sufficient for analysis, thus saving time.

4. INSTRUMENTATION

The choice of instrumentation primarily depends on the ionization method to be used. For the GC–MS method and other EI-based analyses, most modern GC–MS instruments will prove satisfactory. Because FAB is the predominant ionization technique used for sequence determination, an instrument with a FAB source and an extended mass range is most desirable. Although sequence ions are limited in number for most peptides larger than 2000 Da with this technique, MH^+ ions of the intact peptide are more plentiful, and the ability to determine the molecular weight for peptides of 10,000 Da and higher is advantageous. (The ^{252}Cf plasma desorption instruments consistently give good results for peptides in the 1000–20,000 Da range.) Magnetic-sector instruments are available with mass ranges of up to 14,000 u at full accelerating voltage. Instruments of lower-mass range (at full accelerating voltage) can be used for larger masses by operating at decreased accelerating voltage, with the concomitant decrease in sensitivity. Proteins in excess of 20,000 u can be observed with magnetic-sector instruments when high-voltage ion guns are used for ionization [32]. A Wien filter with high-mass range is also in use and shows considerable promise [33]. The "zoom" capabilities of the Wien filter are especially useful, allowing rapid switching from wide-mass-range, low-resolution signal acquisition to narrow-range, high-resolution acquisition.

Peptide fragments produced by digestion with trypsin, one of the most popular proteolytic enzymes, are generally below 3500 Da in mass. Using the proper proteinase can reduce the need for instruments with a much wider mass range [34]. Indeed, smaller magnetic-sector instruments and quadrupole instruments with extended mass range are used successfully for this purpose. On the other hand, peptides in excess of this limit are often encountered. Many laboratories, for example, routinely use CNBr cleavage as the first step before sequencing. Therefore, digesting a peptide for the sole purpose of bringing its mass within the range of a smaller mass spectrometer is time consuming and may be of limited success, especially when very small quantities of peptide are available.

The utility of a mass range in excess of 20 kDa is often questioned. In the end, instrumentation is determined by the specific applications and by the available funding. Most researchers, while striving for bigger and better instruments, tend to utilize well the instrumentation that is available. Advances other than in instrumentation development, such as in sample handling, methodology development, and chemistry, will likely be of equal or greater importance in the future.

The instrument resolving power for molecular weight measurements is a critical issue. For peptides larger than 1500–2000 Da, the peak corresponding to the ^{12}C isotope mass (*monoisotopic mass*) is not the largest peak in the multiplet of peaks representing a given ion (35) (see Fig. 2). For larger peptides one must be careful in selecting the peak that represents MH^+. The most intense peak in Fig. 2 corresponds to a ^{13}C-isotope-containing ion. The *nominal mass*, based on the integral values of the most abundant isotopes, may be considerably less than the monoisotopic mass that is calculated from the exact atomic masses of the most abundant isotopes. The *average mass*, calculated from the atomic weights of each element, takes into account the distribution of the several isotopes.

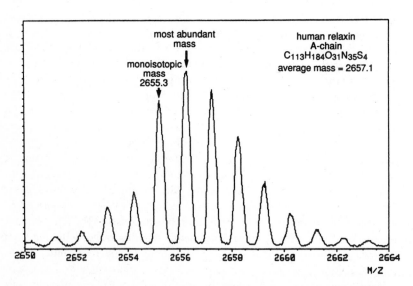

Fig. 2. The measured isotopic distribution for the MH^+ ion of the A-chain of human relaxin, resolution = 5000. The nominal mass (m/z 2654) is calculated from the integral atomic masses. The monoisotopic mass is the sum of the exact atomic mass for the lightest isotope of each element. The average mass is calculated from the component atomic weights. Owing to the large number of carbons and hydrogens, the monoisotopic mass is no longer represented by the largest peak. The peak intensities at m/z 2653 and 2654, not observed in the theoretical isotope distribution, are due to hydrogen loss from the more abundant ions.

Resolved isotopic clusters are helpful for distinguishing between peptides' of similar mass. For example, disulfide bond reduction leads to an increase of 2 u; partial reduction will yield two species with overlapping isotope clusters. Likewise, deamidation (a process that sometimes occurs in purification in which Asn or Gln are converted to Asp or Glu, respectively) produces a 1 u mass increase. When sufficient sample is available (>100 pmole), it is desirable to obtain fully resolved peaks for peptides <3500 Da so that homogeneity of the sample represented by the multiplet of isotope peaks can be verified.

The centroid mass of an unresolved isotopic cluster is equal to the calculated average mass of the ion. For large peptides, measurement of the average mass eliminates the need to determine which peak in an isotopic cluster is the monoisotopic mass. More importantly, much less sample is required when operating at low resolving power.

Tandem mass spectrometry has become an important aspect of peptide sequencing. Triple quadrupole instruments are used quite successfully (36), but are hampered by limited mass range. Newer triple quadrupole mass spectrometers as well as hybrid (BEQQ) instruments (37) do not have such a limitation. Two-sector instruments are also used for sequencing. Reverse geometry (BE) instruments can be operated in the E-scan mode, with fragmentation occurring between the sectors. In this mode the daughter ion spectra are of low resolution (<500), which makes sequencing of larger peptides difficult. Either BE or EB geometry instruments can be used for linked scans at constant B/E, with fragmentation occurring in the first field-free region. Such linked scans provide enhanced daughter ion resolution, but poor precursor ion selection likewise makes these instruments disadvantageous for larger peptides. Three- and four-sector instruments, as well as the hybrids, have the potential for higher resolution for precursor ion selection, and four-sector mass spectrometers can provide high-resolution daughter spectra (38). The recently developed tandem quadrupole Fourier transform mass spectrometer shows tremendous potential for providing sequence data at the low picomole level (39). More details on tandem mass spectrometry are given in Section 6.6.2.

5. MASS SPECTROMETRY OF VOLATILE DERIVATIVES

The earliest and, for many years, the only way to obtain the mass spectra of peptides was by making volatile derivatives of short peptides. Two principal approaches were developed: reduction to polyamino alcohols, and permethylation. The methodology for these approaches evolved considerably, but, owing to the requirements for small peptides, it was used primarily for sequencing small peptides and studying posttranslational modifications. The use of these derivatives has decreased since the introduction of FAB, but a few laboratories still make use of them. Advantages are the instrumental requirements for a low-cost, low-mass, low-resolution mass spectrometer, and the capacity to provide data complementary to that obtained by FAB. Applying low-resolution mass spectrometry to the quality control of recombinant proteins in the pharmaceutical industry is a useful application. In such cases, where sample quantity is not an issue, and the expected sequence is known, derivatization, followed by fully automated analysis to provide data for the entire sequence, is quite promising. More detailed discussions on derivatization methodology and applications can be found in an earlier review (40).

5.1. Electron Impact (EI)

5.1.1. POLYAMINO ALCOHOLS

As early as 1960 it was shown that *N*-acetyl peptide esters could be reduced to volatile polyamino alcohols suitable for analysis by gas chromatography (41). Using the refined technique with GC–MS provides a means of sequencing peptides (40, 42–44). The reaction scheme is given in Fig. 3a. The method

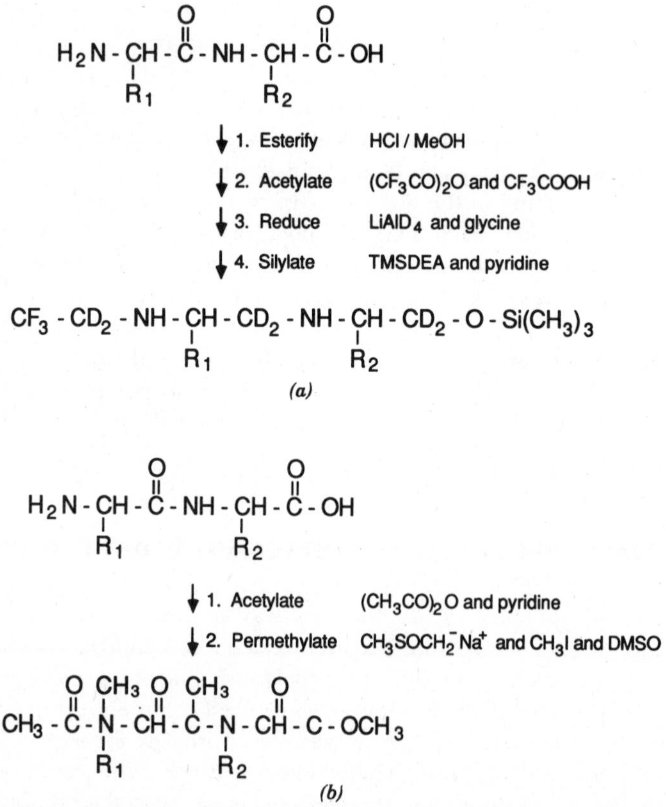

Fig. 3. Methodology for forming volatile derivatives of peptides. (*a*) Formation of *O*-trimethylsilyl polyamino alcohols. (*b*) Formation of *N*-acetyl-*N,O*-permethylated peptides.

requires di- to hexapeptides, which are obtained from larger peptides and proteins by enzymatic degradation or partial acid hydrolysis. These small peptides are derivatized as a mixture and then separated and analyzed by GC–MS. The derivatization procedure is lengthy and quite involved. However, starting with 50–100 nmole of peptide and using an optimized procedure make it possible to minimize problems with side chain modifications and low yields for certain amino acids (44). Using gas-phase reagent delivery (45) reportedly extends the sample requirements into the 100 pmole range.

A number of proteins have been analyzed by this technique, predominantly in the laboratory of Prof. K. Biemann at MIT, and usually in conjunction with other more traditional sequencing methods. The EI spectra of these derivatives exhibit fragmentations mainly in the peptide backbone between the side-chain-bearing carbon and the dideuterated methylene carbon.

One of the advantages of the GC–MS methodology is the ready adaptation to automation and computerized data interpretation. An algorithm, PEPALG, identifies polyamino alcohols from the GC–MS data (46). For quality control applications, customized libraries containing the spectra and retention times for a particular protein can be searched.

5.1.2. PERMETHYL DERIVATIVES

The second main class of volatile derivatives are the N-acetyl-N,O,S-permethylated peptides (47–52). These derivatives are generally applied to larger (5–10 residues) peptides, either as single components or a simple mixture, and are analyzed directly from a direct probe. The reaction scheme for their formation is shown in Fig. 3b. The procedure is less involved than the polyamino alcohol method, but careful attention to exact conditions must be made to minimize unwanted reactions with the residue side chains (53). The major fragment ions arise from cleavage on either the N- or C-terminal side of the backbone carbonyls to produce A_n or B_n ions, respectively, both of which retain the charge on the N-terminus of the molecule. The amount of material required is large (5–50 nmole) when compared with most modern methods.

The identification of gamma-carboxyglutamic acid, a modified amino acid found in some calcium binding proteins, was first made using the permethyl derivatives and mass spectrometry (54).

5.1.3. OTHER METHODS

Another approach to sequencing peptides via volatile derivatives is through dipeptides (55, 56). The peptide is cleaved enzymatically with either a dipeptidyl aminopeptidase or dipeptidyl carboxypeptidase. The trimethylsilyl derivatives are formed and the mixture analyzed by GC–MS. The dipeptides are aligned by a second identical experiment after removal or addition of one residue, known as "frame shifting." Identifying the two residues in each dipeptide is based on two ions in the EI spectrum, the $[M - CH_3]^+$ ion, and an ion corresponding to the amino-terminal moiety produced by cleavage at the CH–CO bond. The method has problems with side chain reactions during trimethylsilylation, and with cyclization. Despite these problems, it has been used successfully for characterization of a number of peptides, though widespread utilization has not occurred.

5.2. Chemical Ionization (CI)

Chemical ionization is often applied to analysis of N-acetyl-N,O,S-permethyl peptide derivatives. This method is more sensitive for CI because the $M + H^+$ ions formed in CI are more intense than the corresponding $M^{+\cdot}$ produced in EI. The derivatives tend to fragment at the amide bonds, forming either N-acylium ions or C-ammonium ions (57). The observed C-terminal ions complement the EI spectra in which few C-terminal ions are formed.

Negative-ion CI can be used in the analysis of other derivatized peptides (58). This procedure requires considerably less sample than EI or positive-ion CI. The spectra show different fragmentations, which complement EI spectra.

6. DESORPTION IONIZATION TECHNIQUES

Desorption ionization techniques have become increasingly popular in recent years for analyzing nonvolatile, thermally labile molecules such as peptides. Making volatile derivatives is undesirable because the process is time consuming, leads to unwanted by-products, and traditionally requires large amounts of sample. Furthermore, there is a mass limit above which not even derivatized peptides are volatile. The variety of available desorption ionization techniques generally eliminates the need for derivatization reactions and opens the door to direct analysis of even higher-mass compounds.

Each of the desorption ionization techniques has its particular advantages for certain applications. Although a thorough review of all the techniques is not possible here, the more useful ones will be discussed with emphasis on their applicability to specific problems.

6.1. Desorption Chemical Ionization (DCI)

Underivatized peptides can be desorbed and ionized by direct exposure of the sample to the ion plasma in a chemical ionization source (59). Few examples of applying DCI to the sequencing of peptides are available (60–63), but both molecular weight and extensive sequence information can be obtained from the spectra. The size of the peptide seems to limit its application. For molecular weights > 1000 Da, thermal degradation predominates, making it difficult to extend applications much beyond this barrier. For smaller peptides the simplicity of the technique, high sequence information in the spectra, and subnanomole sensitivity continue to make it a promising technique.

6.2. Field Desorption (FD)

Developed in the late 1960s, field desorption was for years the most popular method for obtaining molecular weights of underivatized peptides (64). Based on a combination of electron tunneling and thermal desorption at a heated high-voltage anode, field desorption is perhaps the softest of the desorption ionization techniques, producing little, if any, fragmentation. Predominantly protonated molecules, but also metal adduct ions, are formed. The sample is applied in solution to an "activated" emitter (a thin tungsten wire on which carbon whiskers or "dendrites" have been grown). The emitter is biased with several thousand volts and resistively heated by passing a current through it. The carbon dendrites not only provide a very large surface area, but their sharp points allow creation of incredibly large electric fields due to their proximity to the cathode. Unfortunately, the resulting ion signal can be transient. For this reason, FD remains a fairly specialized technique.

When applied to peptides, FD is only occasionally used for hydrophobic ones that exhibit limited solubility in polar solvents and thus perform poorly with FAB. Several hundred picomoles to a few nanomoles are required for analyzing peptides by FD.

Because FD produces limited fragmentation it became one of the first candidates for tandem mass spectrometry. Several examples have been published of FD–MS/MS (65–67).

Prior to the applications of MS/MS, several methods were devised utilizing consecutive steps of subtractive manual Edman degradation (68) (see Section 6.6.5) or endopeptidase digestion (69, 70). In these methods, one amino acid is removed from the intact peptide. The mass of the shortened peptide is measured. The difference in mass between this new peptide and the original peptide identifies the amino acid that was removed. This process is repeated multiple times to obtain the amino acid sequence. Unfortunately, repetitive yields for manual Edman degradation are low, and endopeptidases have widely varying hydrolysis rates for different amino acids. Thus, this process tends to be time-consuming, requires quite a bit of sample, and rarely provides the entire sequence.

6.3. Plasma Desorption Mass Spectrometry (PDMS)

Plasma desorption mass spectrometry is based on particle bombardment by fission fragments of californium-252 (71, 72). Upon spontaneous fission, ^{252}Cf produces a pair of nuclear fragments, for example, ^{142}Ba^{+18} and ^{106}Tc^{+22}, with MeV energies. These fragments move in opposite directions, one of which may be oriented to hit a sample that has been deposited on a thin film (73). The energy of the collision cascade desorbs and ionizes sample molecules from the film (74).

A typical spectrum is shown in Fig. 4. Peaks corresponding to ions of the intact molecule may be quite broad owing to metastable decompositions in the accelerating region and in the flight tube (75, 76). Protonated molecules are often observed for even very large molecules and for this reason it is called a soft

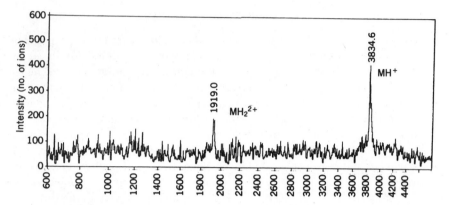

Fig. 4. PDMS spectrum of cecropin from *H. cecropia*, showing the MH^+ and MH_2^{+2} ions, $MH_{(calc)}^+ = 3835.7$. The signal was integrated for 30 min. A flat baseline is produced by background subtraction. Reprinted with permission from (87).

ionization technique. As with most of the desorption ionization techniques, there is, however, considerable fragmentation as evidenced by the large increase in signal at low masses. There are also substantial multiply charged ions [i.e., those for which the charge *(z)* is $+2$, $+3$, etc., and thus produce peaks at $\frac{1}{2}$, $\frac{1}{3}$, etc., the *m/z* value corresponding to the singly charged species] that serve as additional confirmation of molecular weight assignment. The width associated with peaks representing large, intact molecules, owing to large isotope distributions, metastable decompositions, and alkali metal contamination (adduct formation) may limit the precision of the mass determinations.

Samples are generally applied as a thin layer by electrospray onto a thin Mylar film (77), or they can be adsorbed to nitrocellulose-coated Mylar from solution (78). Rinsing the latter with solvent removes contaminants and gives enhanced signals (79). Adding glutathione to the sample also gives larger signals in some cases (80, 81).

Plasma desorption is frequently used for obtaining molecular weights of large peptides and small proteins. Chymotrypsin ($M_r = 35,000$) is the largest protein analyzed by PDMS (82). Owing to the low-flux pulsed nature of the fission-fragment production, its use is limited to time-of-flight analyzers (TOF) (71), and, more recently, Fourier transform instruments (83).

The simplicity of the PDMS–TOF system makes it an easy-to-operate, relatively inexpensive instrument. It is sensitive with detection limits usually in the low picomole range. Although signal must be integrated over time to obtain sufficient ion statistics, typical experiments for picomole amounts of peptide <10 kDa take less than an hour. The newest commercial versions of the instrument are automated so that up to eight samples can be loaded and analyzed unattended.

Numerous examples of PDMS spectra of different peptides and proteins are available (84–86). The lack of useful fragmentation by PDMS usually gives limited sequence information. However, combining analysis by PDMS with different approaches to peptide degradation, such as limited carboxypeptidase digestion, provides a useful strategy for C-terminal sequencing (87). Subjecting the protein layer on the nitrocellulose film directly to proteolytic digestion followed by PDMS of the resulting fragments provides an innovative approach (88). The use of PDMS for mapping protein fragments (89) further extends the utility of this technique. ("Mapping" involves enzymatically cleaving a protein, then matching the measured masses of these proteolytic fragments with the masses expected from a known or putative sequence. Unmatched masses point to modified peptides or errors in the sequence.)

As the quest continues toward larger and larger proteins, it remains to be seen whether the information provided by PDMS for peptides > 30 kDa is of any more practical utility than molecular weights determined by SDS–PAGE, a technique costing considerably less. If the mass precision is insufficient to distinguish one amino acid (< 50 Da), then there is little to be gained except to provide a second determination of mass for comparison (SDS–PAGE is highly dependent on the molecule's tertiary structure and composition, as well as its mass). For peptides < 20 kDa, however, PDMS has already shown its very significant value.

6.4. Laser Desorption (LD)

Peptides as well as a wide variety of other biomolecules can be analyzed by laser desorption mass spectrometry (LD–MS) (90). Samples are normally applied to metal substrates. Protonated or cationized molecules ($M + Na^+$ or $M + K^+$) are the predominant ions. Few fragments are observed at lower laser power (91), but substantial fragmentation can be generated at higher laser power (92). Some sequence ions can be found in peptide LD–MS spectra (93, 94). The technique has been demonstrated with only limited application. A dramatic improvement in high-mass laser desorption is observed when a UV-absorbing matrix (e.g., nicotinic acid) is added to the analyte (95). The molecular ion peak of bovine albumin at m/z 67,000 is easily observed for 10 pmole of sample with this approach. Some recent reports, in which laser desorption is used to desorb neutral molecules which are subsequently ionized by multiphoton ionization, also show great promise (96). The energy and intensity of the photoionization can be varied to change the "softness" of the ionization. Although laser desorption is not a commonly used technique for peptide analysis, these recent innovations will likely result in a dramatic increase in its use in the near future.

6.5. Secondary Ion Mass Spectrometry (SIMS)

Bombarding a surface with an ion beam produces secondary ions that are characteristic of that surface. If peptides or other organic molecules are applied to the surface, ions corresponding to the intact molecule [$(M + H)^+$, $(M − H)^-$] can be observed (97–99). This process, called secondary ion mass spectrometry (SIMS), is sensitive in the picomole range. One of the common problems with

SIMS is the surface damage caused by the primary ion beam, which limits the duration of the analytical signal. To overcome this problem, a number of groups use pulsed primary beams in combination with time-of-flight analyzers (100, 101). One instrument designed specifically for high sensitivity and high resolution gives MH^+ ions with femtomole levels of peptide (102).

Using a liquid matrix with SIMS enhances and prolongs the ion signal. This discovery was extremely important in the advancement of peptide analysis by mass spectrometry. This new technique is termed fast atom bombardment (FAB) because it was first demonstrated with a neutral-atom beam. Using a charged primary beam, liquid SIMS (LSIMS) (103), produces equivalent spectra. The term fast atom bombardment will be used through the remainder of this chapter to denote both FAB and LSIMS experiments.

6.6. Fast Atom Bombardment (FAB)

Fast atom bombardment provides for the first time a technique for ionizing nonvolatile samples that is both simple to use and gives reproducible results. This development plus the accompanying developments of higher-mass-range mass analyzers (104, 105) provided the impetus for explosive growth in the field of peptide analysis by mass spectrometry.

The original paper on FAB (106) showed as an example the spectrum of Met-Lys-Bradykinin with numerous sequence ions in abundance. Later papers (107–114) show the applicability of FAB to many different peptides and the generous amount of sequence information that could be derived from these spectra, although most were peptides of known sequence. Peptides of unknown sequence were quickly subjected to this procedure (111, 115).

FAB spectra of peptides show MH^+ as the predominant ion at the high-mass end (see Fig. 5). If approximately 1 nmole or more of peptide is used, the spectrum usually displays at least some sequence ions as will be defined in the next few paragraphs. The low-mass end of the spectrum is dominated by matrix ions. In the case of glycerol as the FAB matrix, oligomeric ions of the series $(92_n + 1)$ are often observed up to $n = 20$ and beyond.

Although the mechanism of desorption and ion formation in FAB is not completely understood, it is based on a combination of factors (116, 117). Among these mechanisms are desorption of preformed ions (118), including both protonated and metal ion (e.g., Na^+, K^+) adducts (119), and desorption of neutral molecules followed by gas-phase ionization (120, 121) in the high-pressure region ["selvedge" (122)] directly above the vacuum–solution interface. The mechanism that predominates depends in part on the matrix pH, the presence of metal ions or other contaminants, and the relative solution and gas-phase pK_a's of the matrix and analyte species. The desorption process also depends on sputtering from the matrix surface. Thus, the surface concentration of the peptide is an important factor as well (123). Hydrophobic peptides tend to provide better signals by FAB (124), although solubility in the matrix is required.

Peptide sequence information can be deduced by interpretation of the

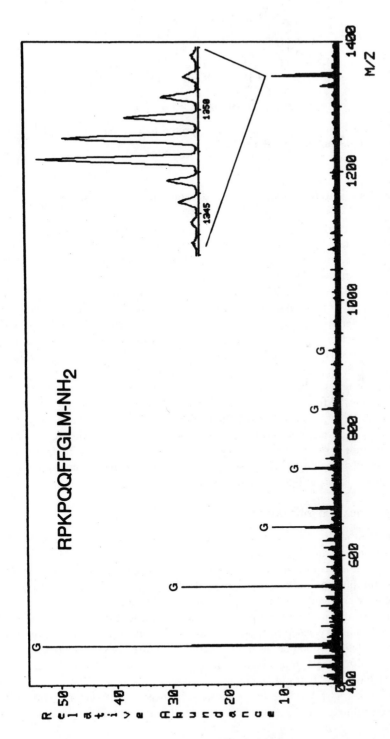

Fig. 5. FAB spectrum of Substance P, MH$^+$ = 1347.7. The glycerol matrix ions are labeled G. The MH$^+$ ion region is expanded to show the isotope peak envelope.

167

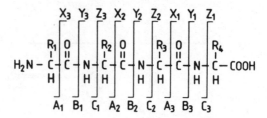

Fig. 6. Peptide fragment ion designations as proposed by Roepstorff and Fohlman. Reprinted with permission from Ref. 125.

fragmentation pattern. Fragment ion designations were first proposed by Roepstorff and Fohlman (see Fig. 6) (125). The fragment ion structures commonly observed in FAB mass spectra of peptides are shown in Fig. 7 (126). Their exact designations have undergone some change, for example, the y_n ions were originally termed Y'', the double-prime denoting addition of two hydrogens to the cleaved neutral peptide. A subsequent revision to y + 2 was suggested (127), then simply y (because ions with addition of two hydrogens were the only species commonly observed for this particular fragment). Lower case letters were adopted to differentiate them from the single-letter amino acid codes that are often used to identify single amino acid immonium ions or the loss of residue side chains from the MH^+ ion. It is important to differentiate between the N-terminal fragments (a, b, c) and the C-terminal fragments (x, y, z). Preferences for fragmentation will be discussed in a later section on spectral interpretation.

Negative ion FAB is used much less extensively for peptides. The $[M - H]^-$ ion is useful for confirmation of the molecular ion and the fragment ions give complementary data. However, for all but very acidic peptides, the signals tend to be less intense than the corresponding positive spectra. Negative ion fragments are also named according to Roepstorff and Fohlman. The predominant ions are the y, z, and c ions (no hydrogens are transferred) (128).

6.6.1. PRACTICAL CONSIDERATIONS

Fast atom bombardment is the most popular technique for analyzing peptides by mass spectrometry mainly because of the ease of obtaining usable spectra. However, certain aspects of the experimental procedure are worth noting, especially sample handling and matrix selection (129, 130). The quantity of sample required depends on the mass of the peptide, the mass resolution required, the cleanliness and purity of the peptide, and the characteristics of the peptide itself (hydrophobicity, isoelectric point). For unit-resolved peaks up to approximately mass 3500, 50–500 pmole may be required. Unresolved MH^+ peaks may be obtained with 10–50 pmole. Isotope peaks of samples larger than 3500 Da are seldom resolved; 20–2000 pmole are sufficient.

When applying FAB–MS to peptides, one needs to make a distinction between cleanliness and purity. The sample should contain nothing except

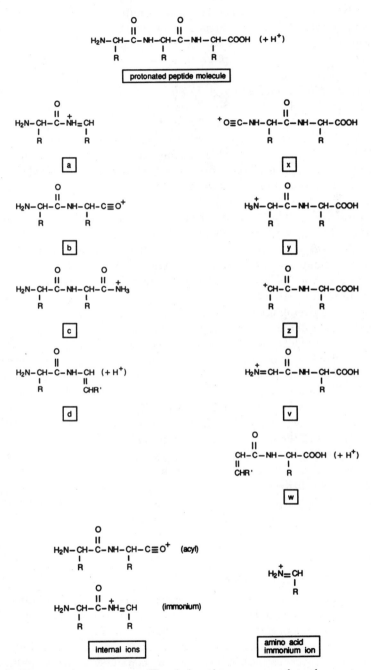

Fig. 7. Fragment ion structures. The designations correspond to the most commonly observed form of each fragment derived from Fig. 6. The d, v, and w ions are observed almost exclusively in high-energy collision-induced dissociation. Of the two types of internal ions, the acyl cation is observed more frequently.

peptide (cleanliness), but need not be a single component (purity). Mixtures of peptides do, however, display differences in spectrum intensity and the response of some peptides may be totally suppressed. The suppression is based on the surface concentration of each peptide (131), which correlates with the relative hydrophobicities of the peptides (124).

Samples should be purified by HPLC (or equivalent). To maintain cleanliness, peptides should be stored in plastic vials, *not* in glass. Peptides readily complex with metal ions that are easily leached from glass. Polyethylene "Eppendorf" tubes are most often used. Drying of peptides should be avoided because some losses due to irreversible adsorption to the tube walls is likely. When drying is necessary, such as on a Speed-Vac, heat should be avoided. Dried samples can be dissolved in several solvents such as dilute acetic, trifluoroacetic, hydrochloric, or formic acids, or DMSO. A particularly good solvent is $1:1$ water : acetonitrile with 0.1% TFA. The matrix should be added with the solvent (approximately $1:1$) and mixed thoroughly before applying to the FAB probe tip. Only $0.5-2~\mu L$ of sample may be applied to the probe, depending on the tip configuration. Studies of probe tip material seem to indicate that a gold-plated tip may provide the best sensitivity for small sample amounts (132).

Many different matrices are used with FAB (133, 134), but glycerol continues to be the best for overall use on unknown peptides. If the mass of a peptide under analysis is known, one should be sure to select a matrix that gives no interfering background ions. Thioglycerol use leads to enhanced signals for higher-mass peptides ($>2000\,\mathrm{Da}$), but its greater volatility has limited its widespread acceptance. If a cooled probe is used (135), the volatility of the matrix is not a problem and enhanced signals for tens of minutes are observed for thioglycerol (136). This is a distinct advantage for MS/MS experiments. More accurate isotope peak intensity ratios for the MH^+ ions of larger peptides can be obtained with thioglycerol as the matrix rather than glycerol (137). This effect is due to reduced attachment of radicals produced by radiation damage to the matrix. A $5:1$ eutectic mixture of dithiothreitol and dithioerythritol (138) has many of the characteristics of thioglycerol, but is less volatile. *m*-Nitrobenzyl alcohol is useful for more hydrophobic peptides (139) including high-mass peptides ($>8\,\mathrm{kDa}$) (32).

6.6.2. TANDEM MASS SPECTROMETRY

Direct determination of the amino acid sequences of peptides is possible with various desorption ionization techniques. However, the sequence-specific ions are often lacking or weak, and, especially in the case of FAB, background ions interfere at low mass. For this reason, tandem mass spectrometry is frequently used to produce sequence-specific ions from the peptide MH^+ ions (140).

Tandem mass spectrometry has the following advantages when the precursor ^{12}C-isotope ion is selected with unit resolution and the product ions are analyzed at unit resolution (141):

1. All fragment (daughter) ions are directly related to the peptide structure because they are derived from the precursor.

2. Matrix peaks are eliminated.

3. The spectrum is simplified because the ^{13}C-isotopic contribution is eliminated.

4. Fragmentation is enhanced by collision-induced dissociation.

5. Mixtures of peptides can be analyzed because MS1 selects the peptide of interest.

Fast atom bombardment is ideally suited to tandem mass spectrometry because signals are long-lived—10 min or more, typically. The continuous signal allows slow acquisition of the daughter scan or averaging of multiple scans to provide improved signal-to-noise ratios.

In a typical MS/MS experiment (142), a FAB spectrum of the peptide(s) is first obtained. The spectrum is examined to determine the mass(es) of the MH^+ ion(s). For example, a mixture of three peptides would produce MH^+ ions at three different mass values. The ions of interest are selected one mass at a time with MS1; the selected precursor (parent) ions undergo collision-induced dissociation (CID) (143) and the fragment ions are analyzed with MS2 (see Fig. 8). The MH^+ ^{12}C-isotope peak of the precursor ion cluster is chosen with unit resolution so that all daughter ions are monoisotopic. Daughter ions are analyzed at unit resolution to ensure reliable sequence information. For those instances when the daughter ion abundances are low, for example, small sample quantity or large precursor mass, less than unit resolution of the daughter ions may be necessary to enhance the signal. If the ^{12}C precursor ion is selected, there is little problem with reduced daughter ion resolution except when adjacent peaks occur at higher mass.

The ^{12}C selection becomes less practical for precursor ions of higher mass (>1800 u). In these cases, the ^{12}C isotopic peak is no longer the most intense peak in the isotope cluster, more resolving power is required to separate the ions, and the collision efficiency drops off. It may be necessary to reduce the resolving power of MS1 to accept the entire isotope multiplet. The daughter ions will then appear not at their monoisotopic mass or their average mass, but at a weighted average of their isotopic masses. If data interpretation is based on mass differences between peaks rather than on the precise mass of the ion, there is little problem.

Several different types of mass spectrometers are used successfully for peptide sequencing. Two-sector instruments are used with both B/E linked scans and electric sector scans for reverse geometry instruments (MIKES) (144). The former gives poor precursor ion resolution and the potential for artifact peaks. The latter yields poor daughter resolution. For peptides <500 u, either method provides acceptable results. Above approximately 500 u, the E-scan gives unacceptable resolving power for the daughter ion spectra owing to kinetic energy release (145). Kinetic energy loss during the collision process (146, 147) reduces the mass accuracy as well. The B/E linked scans continue to give usable spectra for higher precursor masses, but the poor parent ion resolution becomes a

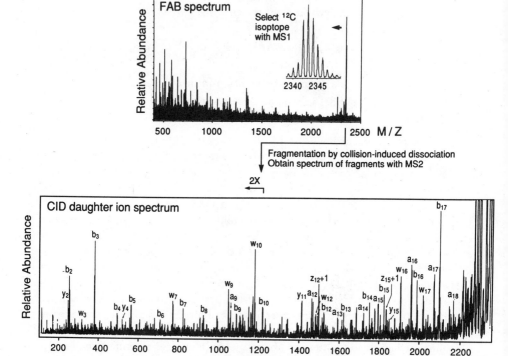

Fig. 8. Process for obtaining a CID daughter ion spectrum by MS/MS. The ^{12}C monoisotopic MH$^+$ ion is selected by MS1. The selected precursor (parent) ions are fragmented by CID and the product (daughter) ions are analyzed by MS2. The precursor is a tryptic peptide (LHQLAFDTYQEFEEAYIPK) from human growth hormone.

problem. Matrix-related daughter ions are frequently observed in the B/E-linked scans, especially for low sample quantities, owing to the poor precursor ion selection and the metastable ion contribution to the first field-free region decompositions.

For these reasons four-sector instruments are becoming more popular. [Three-sector instruments of EBE geometry have been used (148), but, when unit resolving power of the precursor is used for peptide sequencing, they provide little advantage over two-sector BE instruments.] Four-sector instruments allow unit resolution of both precursor and daughter ions. The double-focusing capabilities of MS2 correct for the kinetic energy loss from the CID process (149). The B/E-linked scan does not show the kinetic energy spread of the daughter ions so adequate resolution is possible. (Because the daughter ion energies are a fraction of the precursor mass, MS2 must be scanned at constant B/E.) The collision cell can be electrically floated to provide improved daughter ion resolution and enhanced transmission for low mass daughter ions (150). The recent introduction of electrooptical array detectors (151, 152) for MS2 promises to increase signal-to-noise ratios during analyses in the low picomole range (153, 154).

Use of four-sector instruments for many of the applications described above has been reported (155–158). The most ambitious of these applications has been the determination of the complete sequence of a thioredoxin, $M_r = 11,748$ (159).

Triple quadrupole instruments are also used for peptide sequencing (160). The low-energy collision process is different and so the spectra differ somewhat from the spectra produced by sector instruments. Fragmentations at the peptide bonds predominate and internal fragments are frequently observed. Until recently the mass range of quadrupoles was limited to 2000 u, so most work was restricted to this range. Newer instruments with mass ranges up to 4000 u are now available, but preliminary data from these and from hybrid instruments seem to indicate that the low-energy collision process becomes quite inefficient for precursor ions above 2000 u (161). The hybrid instruments (MS1 = sector instrument, MS2 = quadrupole) provide enhanced mass range and resolving power for MS1, but in practice do not provide any distinct advantage over triple quadrupole instruments for peptide sequencing.

The Fourier transform mass spectrometer with an external ion source (162, 163) has considerable potential for peptide sequencing (39, 164). Ions are formed by pulsed liquid SIMS, a quadrupole is operated in the rf-only cut-off mode to transmit ions above a certain mass, removing most of the matrix ions. A second quadrupole aids in transmission into the ion cyclotron resonance cell where the ions are trapped and all but the desired precursor ion is expelled. Then a pulse from an eximer laser (193 nm) induces photodissociation, followed by daughter ion analysis. The whole experiment requires only a few hundred milliseconds. Fragmentation from photodissociation depends on the laser intensity, but can be adjusted to yield fragmentation predominantly at the peptide bonds (165). Figure 9 demonstrates the results achievable with a 10 pmole sample of peptide. With continued improvements in FTMS in the offing, this technique will likely be heavily utilized in the future.

6.6.3. APPLICATIONS

A large number of peptides have been identified and sequenced in recent years. Extensive compilations of these are found in several excellent reviews (127, 166–169). Several of these applications are described in the following pages.

a. Posttranslation Modifications. One of the most important applications of mass spectrometry in peptide sequencing is the identification of posttranslational modifications (170). Because mass spectrometry provides direct evidence of the structure of the modification through mass and fragmentations, it is perhaps the best technique available to the protein chemist for characterizing that modification. Identifying amino-terminal blocking groups and sequencing the N-terminally blocked peptide are among the most important contributions of mass spectrometry to date (171–174). Figure 10 shows the CID spectrum (B/E-

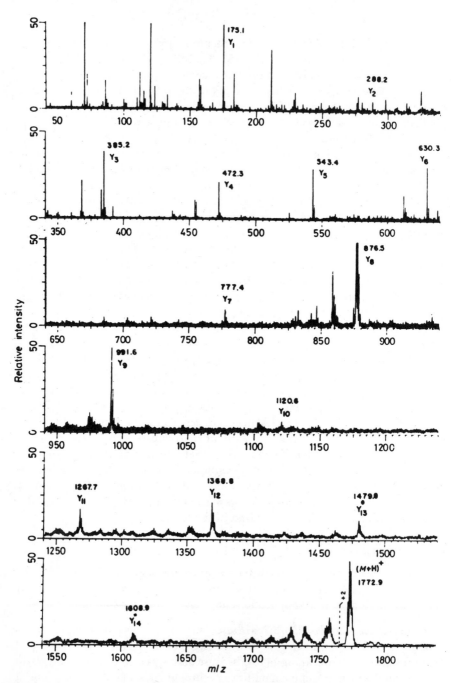

Fig. 9. Daughter ion spectrum of 10 pmole of a tryptic peptide from beef spleen purple acid phosphatase. The spectrum was obtained on a tandem quadrupole Fourier transform mass spectrometer using laser photodissociation. Ions show the complete sequence (FQETFEDVFSASPLR). The ion labeled Y_{14}^* is actually z_{14}. Reprinted with permission from (39).

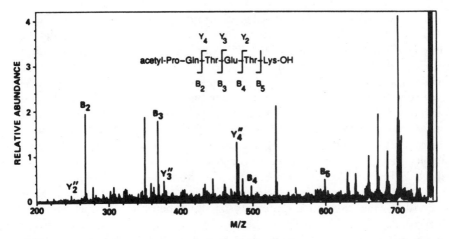

Fig. 10. CID daughter ion spectrum of MH^+ of the blocked N-terminal tryptic peptide of the large subunit of spinach ribulose bisphosphate carboxylase/oxygenase. The spectrum was obtained by a linked scan at constant B/E on a two-sector instrument. The unlabeled peaks (m/z 351 = $b_3 - H_2O$, 532 = w_5, 660 = w_6, 673 = Gln side chain loss, 701 = CO_2 loss) give further proof of the structure. Reprinted with permission from (175).

linked scan) of the MH^+ ion of the N-terminal peptide of spinach ribulose bisphosphate carboxylase/oxygenase (175). Attempts to sequence the peptide by automated Edman degradation failed, indicating that the peptide was likely blocked. The cDNA sequence was known. The CID spectrum showed an N-acetyl blocking group and revealed N-terminal processing.

Identifying phosphorylated side chains is also possible by mass spectrometry (176, 177). Facile hydrolysis of phosphate esters and poor stability of PTH-phosphoamino acids make analysis of phosphorylated peptides particularly problematic for Edman degradation. Reports of analyzing phosphorylation sites in spinach Photosystem II proteins (163), riboflavin-binding protein (178, 179), beta-casein (180), and phosphatase inhibitor-2 (181) demonstrate the variety of sequencing problems which were solved by mass spectrometry.

b. Glycoproteins. Determining the structure of glycoproteins is of great interest today because of their roles in immunology, intercellular recognition, and protein stability. Mass spectrometry is a technique that permits study of their protein sequence, assignment of glycosylation sites, and analysis of the corresponding carbohydrate. Usually the protein sequence is obtained and the glycosylation is studied at a later point. Carbohydrates are attached through the hydroxyl group of Ser or Thr, or at the amide nitrogen of Asn when it occurs in the sequence -Asn-X-Ser/Thr- (X = any amino acid except Pro). Any potential glycosylation site may or may not be glycosylated.

For analysis, the glycoprotein can be digested to yield glycopeptides, which are separated and analyzed (182). Fast atom bombardment tends, however, to

yield low sensitivity for underivatized glycopeptides owing to their hydrophilicity
(183). An ingenious method for mapping the attachment sites of Asn-linked
carbohydrates avoids this problem (184). The glycoprotein is digested with a
proteinase to give fragments that can be fitted to the known sequence. Part of the
digest is fractionated by HPLC. The remainder of the digest is treated with N-
glycanase [peptide-N^4-(N-acetyl-beta-glucosaminyl)asparagine amidase], then
fractionated by HPLC. N-Glycanase removes carbohydrate from Asn and
converts the Asn to Asp. FAB mass spectra for the pre- and postglycosidase-
treated HPLC fractions are compared. New signals in the glycosidase-treated
samples correspond to formerly glycosylated sites and are 1 u higher in mass than
expected (because Asn is converted to Asp) from the known sequence (see
Fig. 11). Glycopeptide peaks in the non-glycosidase-treated fraction often are not
observed, owing to their suppressed signals. When the glycopeptides are
observed, the mass shift in the peaks before and after deglycosylation provides the
composition of the carbohydrate. This method has been extended to provide
composition of each carbohydrate by FAB–MS following permethylation (185).
Linkage analysis for the carbohydrate is made by GC–MS after conversion of the
permethyl carbohydrate to the partially permethylated alditol acetates.

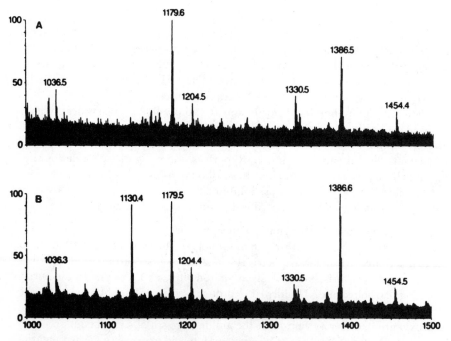

Fig. 11. Partial FAB spectrum of (A) the tryptic digest of reduced and carboxymethylated
tissue plasminogen activator, and (B) the same digest following incubation with N-
glycanase. The "extra" peak in (B) at m/z 1130.4 corresponds to a peptide to which an N-
linked carbohydrate had previously been attached. Taken with permission from (184).

*c. **Recombinant Peptides.*** Proteins produced by recombinant DNA techniques can also be readily analyzed by mass spectrometry (186, 187). Although many of the proteins are too large for direct analysis, cleavage into smaller fragments yields peptides that can be easily analyzed. The peptide mixture either can be analyzed directly or can be analyzed after fractionation by HPLC, depending on the complexity of the mixture. Such measurements are important for determining whether the expected protein has been expressed properly and whether any posttranslational modification or processing has occurred (188). Many proteins are expressed as fusion proteins, that is, the protein of interest is linked to another protein(s) in order to improve the expression. The extra protein is subsequently cleaved off to give the desired product. Using FAB mass spectrometry makes it possible to determine if the desired protein has, in fact, been produced.

*d. **Check of DNA Sequence.*** Molecular weight measurements are also used to check the sequence of a native protein against the cDNA-derived amino acid sequence (171, 186). This analysis is important as a check for errors in the DNA sequencing, but more important to check for posttranslational modification. The procedure involves cleaving the protein into smaller pieces by chemical or enzymatic means or both, then fractionating the mixture into four to six fractions. Each fraction is analyzed by FAB mass spectrometry. The molecular weights are compared with a table of expected weights. Differences are further analyzed to determine their origin. One or two steps of manual Edman degradation are used to confirm the N-terminal residue(s) of each peptide. Sometimes mass differences are due to substitutions of one amino acid for another due to a single base change. Table 3 is a list of mass differences corresponding to possible substitutions.

*e. **Synthetic Peptides.*** Synthetic peptides, commonly made by solid phase techniques utilizing t-BOC or FMOC chemistry (189), may be contaminated with peptides that arise from incomplete coupling of certain residues, resulting in missing residues (deletion peptides), or prematurely stopped peptides (amino-terminal acetylated). Protecting groups on many of the side chains may be partially cleaved or transferred to other side chains. Determining the molecular weight by mass spectrometry can easily confirm the proper sequence. Unexpected molecular weights can often be deduced from the mass difference and then checked by sequencing (190). Analysis of the by-product from the crude reaction mixture is useful for optimizing the synthesis conditions.

*f. **Disulfides.*** Disulfide linkages also can be determined by molecular weight measurements (191, 192). Determining the entire primary sequence is, however, a prerequisite for disulfide assignment. The protein should be cleaved, ideally, in such a way that each cysteine is separated along the linear chain, with disulfide bonds kept intact. The specific cleavages depend on the sequence of the particular protein. The cleaved peptides are then usually fractionated by HPLC and the molecular weights are determined experimentally by FAB–MS. Based on

TABLE 3

Mass Shifts for Amino Acid Substitutions

Mass Shift	Possible Substitution[a]
129	Gly > Trp
115	Ala > Trp
106	Gly > Tyr
99	Gly > Arg, Ser > Trp
92	Ala > Tyr
90	Gly > Phe
89	Pro > Trp
87	Val > Trp
85	Ala > Arg, Thr > Trp
83	Cys > Trp
80	Gly > His
76	Ser > Tyr, Ala > Phe
74	Gly > Met
73	Leu > Trp
72	Asn > Trp, Gly > Glu
71	Asp > Trp, Gly > Gln
69	Ser > Arg
66	Ala > His, Pro > Tyr
64	Val > Tyr
62	Thr > Tyr
60	Ala > Met, Cys > Tyr, Ser > Phe
59	Pro > Arg
58	Ala > Glu, Gly > Asp, Gln > Trp
57	Ala > Gln, Val > Arg, Gly > Asn, Glu > Trp
56	Gly > Leu
53	Cys > Arg
50	Ser > His, Leu > Tyr, Pro > Phe
49	Asn > Tyr, His > Trp
48	Asp > Tyr, Val > Phe
46	Gly > Cys, Thr > Phe
44	Ala > Asp, Cys > Phe, Gly > Thr, Ser > Met
43	Ala > Asn, Leu > Arg
42	Ala > Leu, Asn > Arg, Ser > Glu, Gly > Val
41	Asp > Arg, Ser > Gln
40	Gly > Pro, Pro > His
39	Phe > Trp
38	Val > His
36	Thr > His, Gln > Tyr
34	Cys > His, Leu > Phe, Glu > Tyr
33	Asn > Phe
32	Ala > Cys, Asp > Phe, Pro > Glu, Met > Tyr, Val > Met
31	Pro > Gln

Table 3 (*Continued*)

Mass Shift	Possible Substitution[a]
30	Ala > Thr, Arg > Trp, Gly > Ser, Thr > Met, Val > Glu
29	Val > Gln
28	Ala > Val, Gln > Arg, Ser > Asp, Cys > Met, Thr > Glu
27	Glu > Arg, Ser > Asn, Thr > Gln
26	Ala > Pro, Cys > Glu, Thr > His, Ser > Leu
25	Met > Arg, Cys > Gln
24	Leu > His
23	Asn > His, Tyr > Trp
22	Asp > His
19	His > Arg, Gln > Phe
18	Pro > Asp, Glu > Phe, Leu > Met
17	Pro > Asn, Asn > Met
16	Ala > Ser, Val > Asp, Asp > Met, Ser > Cys, Pro > Leu, Leu > Glu, Met > Phe, Phe > Tyr
15	Asn > Glu, Val > Asn, Leu > Gln
14	Gly > Ala, Asn > Gln, Thr > Asp, Val > Leu, Asp > Glu, Ser > Thr
13	Thr > Asn, Asp > Gln
12	Cys > Asp, Thr > Leu, Ser > Val
11	Cys > Asn
10	Cys > Leu, His > Phe, Ser > Pro
9	Phe > Arg, Gln > His
8	Glu > His
7	Arg > Tyr
6	Pro > Cys, Met > His
4	Val > Cys, Pro > Thr
3	Gln > Met
2	Leu > Asp, Thr > Cys, Glu > Met, Pro > Val, Val > Thr
1	Asn > Asp, Leu > Asn, Gln > Glu

[a]Leu/Ile and Gln/Lys are isomeric. The table only lists one of each pair.

knowledge of the cleavage conditions, molecular weights for all possible disulfide-linked peptides can be calculated and compared with the experimental results. Subsequent reduction and reanalysis of the peptides will show disappearance of peaks corresponding to the disulfide-linked peptides, with appearance of peaks for the two constituent peptides. Similar methodology may be applied to other types of protein cross-linkages (193).

Unfortunately, proteins with extensive disulfide linkages are often resistant to proteolytic digestions. This can sometimes be countered by carrying out the digestion under extreme conditions, for example, using long digestion time, adding 10–20% organic solvent, adding chaotropic agents (guanidine), or adding surfactants. However, some experimentation may be required. First, a delicate balance between breaking down the tertiary structure of the protein without inactivating the proteinase must be established. Second, basic conditions promote disulfide interchange, so acidic conditions are preferred. This leads to preferred use of CNBr or acetic acid cleavages, or digestion with Staph. V8 or pepsin. Analysis by SDS-PAGE may be used to determine the extent of cleavage.

Disulfide bonds can be slowly reduced by irradiation of the sample with the primary FAB beam (194). The gradual reduction can be used to identify disulfide-linked peptides (195). This phenomenon seems also to be applicable to other readily reduced groups, for example, on a quinone functionality of a protein prosthetic group (196). Care should be taken in acquiring and interpreting spectra of disulfide-linked peptides. The possibility for partial reduction also necessitates resolution of all isotopic peaks. Otherwise, for an unresolved peak multiplet, one would observe a weighted average of the two forms.

6.6.4. DERIVATIZATION

One of the chief advantages of fast atom bombardment, and of the other desorption ionzation techniques, is the ability to obtain useful spectra from nonvolatile compounds. This feature often eliminates the need for conversion to a volatile species as required for EI or CI experiments. Derivatization for FAB may prove useful, nonetheless, for altering the fragmentation or improving the sensitivity (197).

One of the primary types of derivatization reactions is that which leads to the formation of precharged ions, since they usually produce an increase in ion abundance (198). Such procedures are termed "reverse derivatization," since their goal is contrary to that of conventional derivatization. Attaching a quaternary ammonium group to the peptide N-terminus is possible (199, 200), but such a reaction is generally difficult to perform cleanly in high yield. Furthermore, lysine side chains are often also modified unless the lysine epsilon-amino groups are protected beforehand. Adding a precharged moiety also reduces or eliminates fragmentation if there are no other sites for charge attachment on the molecule.

Fragmentation can also be altered by removing or masking basic sites on the molecule (e.g., acetylating the N-terminus) or by adding a highly basic moiety to localize the charge. Adding a dansyl group to the N-terminus was successful (201). Fragment ions contain the added charged site, making sequence interpretation simpler. Formation of polyamino alcohols alters the fragmentation in FAB and provides complementary sequence information (202).

Often the N- or C-terminus of an aliquot of the peptide is modified. FAB spectra of the modified and unmodified peptides are then compared. Shifts in mass reveal which fragment ions are derived from which end of the molecule. Most often the N-terminus in acetylated with acetic anhydride (N-terminal fragments shift $+42$ u). The C-terminus can be esterified with methanolic HCl (C-terminal fragments shift $+14$ u) (36). Acetylation with $1:1$ $(CH_3CO)_2O:(C^2H_3CO)_2O$ gives N-terminal fragments that are represented by easily recognized "goalposts" 3 u apart (109).

Adding lipophilic moieties such as hydrocarbon chains to peptides (131) alters the surface activity. The more surface active (hydrophobic) species in a mixture of peptides tend to be observed preferentially (124). Therefore, adding hydrophobic groups tends to enhance the surface activity of smaller peptides, since the hydrophobicity of larger peptides is not changed significantly by this procedure.

The MS/MS spectra of peptides can also be altered considerably by derivatization (202, 203). A highly basic or quaternary ammonium group retains the charge during fragmentation. Collision spectra are generally simpler as a result, making sequence interpretation more facile. Simplifying the fragmentation can be especially important for high-energy collision spectra of unknowns where several ion series are present. Fewer fragment series make for easier interpretation plus the ion current is spread over fewer ions, yielding a rise in ion abundances.

6.6.5. MANUAL EDMAN DEGRADATION

When mass spectrometry is used to identify a peptide on the basis of molecular weight, confirmation of this identification is recommended. The peptide structure could be confirmed by amino acid analysis, sequencing of the first one to three residues by automated Edman degradation, or additional mass measurement after shortening the peptide chain. For the latter method, manual Edman degradation is used for removing a single amino acid from the amino terminus of a peptide. The reaction works equally well with a single peptide or mixtures of peptides, making it well suited to the FAB mapping technique described above. For sequence confirmation, one or two steps of manual Edman degradation are usually sufficient.

> The peptide(s) is dried in an Eppendorf tube, then dissolved in $50\,\mu L$ of 25% trimethylamine in water and purged with nitrogen. Add $50\,\mu L$ of 10% phenylisothiocyanate (PITC) in pyridine. Incubate for 10 min at 50°C. Wash twice with 2 : 1 heptane : ethyl acetate. Vacuum dry. Add $50\,\mu L$ of anhydrous trifluoroacetic acid (TFA) and incubate for 20 min at 50°C. Add $50\,\mu L$ of water and vacuum dry (KOH trap!).

The preceding procedure is a simplified adaptation of Tarr (204) and Hemling (205), which works for larger quantities (>500 pmole) of peptide. For smaller amounts and when repetitive cleavages are to be performed, more rigorous attention to many steps is necessary (e.g., exclusion of oxygen, purity of solvents, etc.). Several highly detailed procedures have been developed and should be consulted (11, 204).

7. ON-LINE HPLC TECHNIQUES

Several LC interfaces are useful for peptide analysis. The first, thermospray, produces protonated molecules with little fragmentation. Peptides up to several thousand daltons that were eluted in an ammonium acetate buffer (206) have been identified. To obtain sequence information, thermospray may be combined with on-line digestion (trypsin and carboxypeptidase Y) and HPLC separation (207, 208). The technique appears promising but the amount of sample required for analysis (> 1 nmole) puts it outside the range of many applications in protein chemistry.

A second technique, involving continuous flow introduction with FAB, was developed simultaneously by two groups, using either a stainless-steel frit (209) or an open capillary tube (210). The operation and performance of each appear to be similar. The mobile phase containing 1–5% glycerol is introduced at a rate of 5–10 μL/min. This low flow requires use of microbore or capillary HPLC, or a flow splitter for conventional analytical systems. Protonated molecules for peptides up to 6000 u have been measured (211, 212). Flow FAB has two advantages with respect to conventional FAB: suppression of matrix background ions (213) and reduction of competitive ionization that is due to hydrophobicity differences in peptide mixtures (214). Since FAB spectra often give limited sequence data, the flow FAB technique may be combined with carboxypeptidase digestion to produce sequence information (215, 216).

The same type of flow-FAB interface has also been adapted for use with capillary zone electrophoresis (CZE) for the detection of peptides (217). This interface, as well as a CZE–electrospray ionization interface (218), are just beginning to show utility for capillary electrophoresis, which is rapidly gaining popularity as a powerful separation technique for peptides and proteins.

8. SPECTRAL INTERPRETATION

8.1. Preferences for Fragmentation

The mechanism of formation of the fragments is the subject of some debate (109, 110, 219–222). It is generally accepted that fragmentations occur at and are induced by the site of protonation on the precursor ion (223). Molecules with fixed charges, such as peptides modified with quaternary ammonium groups, also yield abundant fragmentations in CID daughter ion spectra (203), attributed to remote-site fragmentations (224). Fortunately for interpretation, cleavages at the amide bonds predominate in most spectra.

It is, for the most part, difficult to predict a priori what the fragmentation of a particular peptide will be. An in-depth study correlating the fragmentations with the sequences of a large number of unrelated peptides remains to be done, although there are indications that fragmentation patterns may be partially predicted (225, 226). It is likely that the three-dimensional structure in solution (and in the gas phase) may play a significant role in the fragmentations, as evidenced by reports of fragmentations of peptide M + Na$^+$ ions (227).

Several generalizations can be made concerning structural features that promote fragmentation. Proline, which has a highly basic secondary amine, tends to produce intense y (and y$_{-2}$) ions at its amino terminus (36). Fragmentations at glycine often result in peaks of low intensity. Basic residues, when located near either end of a peptide, tend to cause retention of the charge at that end and thus direct fragmentation (225). For example, tryptic peptides have either Lys or Arg at the C-terminus and produce spectra in which the y and z ion series (and w ion series in CID spectra) are prominent. Loss of water from ions with Ser or Thr positioned at either end of the fragment is also commonly observed. In addition, the lack of a full understanding of fragmentations precludes giving much value to fragment peak intensities.

Low mass fragment ions include the immonium ions (see Fig. 7), which are representative of the amino acids within the peptide. Presence of particular immonium ions are predictive of the presence of those residues within the peptide. Absence of particular immonium ions, however, does not preclude the existence of those residues within the peptide. Likewise, loss of side-chain residues from the MH^+ ion is indicative of the presence of specific residues, but not a necessary occurrence. Loss of side-chain pieces is also observed (e.g., H_2O, NH_3, CO_2, $HCOOH$, CH_3CONH_2). Finally, internal fragments, that is, those where residues from both ends of the peptide are lost, may also be observed.

The question of differentiation of Gln/Lys and Leu/Ile is often raised, because each pair has identical mass. Lysine can be easily derivatized with PITC to form the corresponding epsilon-amino PTC-lysine. A mass shift indicates the presence of Lys and shows how many lysines are present. For certain peptides, for example, tryptic fragments, one can initially assume that the C-terminal residue is Lys if the residue mass is 128. (The assignment should be verified to eliminate the possibility of Gln at the protein carboxy terminus.) Discrimination between leucine and isoleucine is much more difficult. The best method (aside from amino acid analysis) is the appearance of the appropriate w ions in the high energy CID spectra (126, 228). The w ions correspond to cleavage at the beta-carbon on the amino acid side chain (see Fig. 7). Ile gives two possibilities that are different in mass from the single fragment for Leu.

8.2. Interpretation Strategies

Interpreting spectra usually requires far more time and effort than acquiring the actual data. Deducing the amino acid sequence of a peptide from a mass spectrum is very much like solving a puzzle. The sequence ions, like puzzle pieces, must be connected together properly to show the sequence. The process is made easier if additional information is known, for example, amino acid composition, source of peptide (tryptic peptides have either Lys or Arg at the C-terminus, for example), or homology to other peptides. Sequencing can also be simplified if the N- and C-terminal fragments can be differentiated, for example, by N-terminal acetylation or C-terminal esterification as already mentioned.

The masses of the amino acid residues are listed in Table 4 along with the masses of their corresponding immonium ions and masses of side-chains that may be lost from the MH^+ ion. Table 5 lists all possible dipeptide masses, which may prove useful when a single residue mass does not fit as the interpretation

TABLE 4

Amino Acid Residue Masses[a,b]

Amino Acid	Residue Mass	Immonium Ion Mass	Side-Chain Mass
Gly	57	30	—
Ala	71	44	15
Ser	87	60	31
Pro	97	70	—
Val	99	72	43
Thr	101	74	45
Cys	103	76	47
Leu	113	86	57
Ile	113	86	57
Asn	114	87	58
Asp	115	88	59
Lys	128	101	72
Gln	128	101	72
Glu	129	102	73
Met	131	104	75
His	137	110	81
Phe	147	120	91
Arg	156	129	100
Tyr	163	136	107
Trp	186	159	130
CM-Cys	161	134	105
Hser	101	74	45
Hser-Lac	83	—	—
pGlu	112	—	—

[a]By definition, —NH—CHR—CO— is the generalized structure for an amino acid residue.
[b]CM-Cys = carboxymethylcysteine, Hser = homoserine, Hser-Lac = homoserine lactone, pGlu = pyroglutamic acid.

progresses. Note that there are dipeptides which have identical masses to single amino acids. One must be careful to eliminate these dipeptide possibilities when sequencing, especially when a glycine-containing dipeptide is a possibility.

Two general approaches to interpretation can be taken. For either approach, one should first examine the low-mass end of the spectrum to identify candidate immonium ions. These ions serve to provide a partial amino acid composition. (Note that the peak height provides little information about how many of a particular amino acid are present in a peptide.) Likewise, one should examine the region near the MH^+ ion for side-chain losses.

In the first approach (229), one calculates the mass difference between the MH^+ ion and any fragment ion that could correspond to loss of one residue, for

TABLE 5

Dipeptide Residue Masses

	Gly	Ala	Ser	Pro	Val	Thr	Cys	Leu/Ile	Asn	Asp	Lys/Gln	Glu	Met	His	Phe	Arg	Tyr	Trp	CM-Cys
Gly	114																		
Ala	128	142																	
Ser	144	158	174																
Pro	154	168	184	194															
Val	156	170	186	196	198														
Thr	158	172	188	198	200	202													
Cys	160	174	190	200	202	204	206												
Leu/Ile	170	184	200	210	212	214	216	226											
Asn	171	185	201	211	213	215	217	227	228										
Asp	172	186	202	212	214	216	218	228	229	230									
Lys/Gln	185	199	215	225	227	229	231	241	242	243	256								
Glu	186	200	216	226	228	230	232	242	243	244	257	258							
Met	188	202	218	228	230	232	234	244	245	246	259	260	262						
His	194	208	224	234	236	238	240	250	251	252	265	266	268	274					
Phe	204	218	234	244	246	248	250	260	261	262	275	276	278	284	294				
Arg	213	227	243	253	255	257	259	269	270	271	284	285	287	293	303	312			
Tyr	220	234	250	260	262	264	266	276	277	278	291	292	294	300	310	319	326		
Trp	243	257	273	283	285	287	289	299	300	301	314	315	317	323	333	342	349	372	
CM-Cys	218	232	248	258	260	262	264	274	275	276	289	290	292	298	308	317	324	347	322

example, between MH^+ and $MH^+ - 71$. Those with mass differences that exactly match a residue mass (e.g., $71 = Ala$, from Table 4) are candidates for the y_{n-1} ion. There will likely be several of these. For each of the y_{n-1} candidates, one searches for the next residue mass loss that could correspond to y_{n-2}. For example, if there were peaks corresponding to MH^+, $MH^+ - 71$, $MH^+ - 71 - 101$, and so forth, the mass differences would correspond to Ala, Thr, and so forth. These data then suggest an amino acid sequence starting at the N-terminus of Ala-Thr-$\cdots$. Constructing a table or tree diagram makes it easy to keep track of the candidate sequences. The best candidate(s) are those for which the data produce the longest sequence. A second check of the validity of y-ion assignment is identification of accompanying z, $z+1$, or $z+2$ ions, which would appear 17, 16, or 15 u lower in mass, respectively, then the corresponding y ion (although z ions do not always accompany y ions). In the ideal case, there will be a single set of y ions that provide the entire sequence. More likely, there will be several partial sequences, and in the worst case, numerous short sequences that give no information.

After finding several possible y-ion series, one can next look for the N-terminal fragments. The b series starts 18 u below the MH^+ ion mass, which would be b_n (n is the number of residues in the peptide). Search for a peak that corresponds to $MH^+ - (18 + residue)$; this peak corresponds to the b_{n-1} ion. As with the y ions, look for residue mass losses from the b_{n-1} candidate(s) and continue until one or a few members of a long b-ion series are found. One can follow the identical process for the a-ion series, where a_n is 46 u below the MH^+ ion mass. The c-ion series, also found by the same process, begins with c_n which, if it existed, would be 1 u below the MH^+ mass. The c series is generally not observed if neither the a nor the b series is found. As a slightly different tact, when a putative b ion is found, the existence of an a or c ion can be checked by looking for an ion 28 u below or 17 u above, respectively. With a certain amount of experience and oftentimes considerable luck, one will have one or two sequences that match the data. Make sure all the major peaks are assigned. If not, one needs to find possible identities for these: internal fragments, rearrangement ions, matrix-related peaks, contaminants, water losses, and so forth. Major peaks that cannot be assigned a reasonable structure may be a clue that the putative sequence is incorrect, even if most of the other peaks match.

A second approach to interpreting a spectrum begins at the middle or lower-mass end. One picks a fairly intense peak and looks for higher-mass peaks that are separated by the mass of one of the amino acid residues. For all matches found, one tries to continue the series up to the MH^+ ion. The identity of the series may not be known until the MH^+ ion is reached, when one must recall where the different ions series, a_n, b_n, c_n, begin (see previous approach). One may also be able to determine the series identity by finding related ions 15, 18, or 28 u different. This approach works less well with FAB spectra that have interfering matrix peaks at lower mass. It is superior to the previous approach for peptides that produce numerous fragment ions in the middle of the peptide, but few at either end.

An example is provided to demonstrate peptide sequence interpretation. Figure 12 is the CID daughter spectrum of a tryptic peptide, $MH^+ = 693.4$. Amino acid analysis yields the following composition: Gly-1, Thr-1, Ile-1, Lys-1, Glx-1, and Phe-1. Glx could be either Gln or Glu, since acid hydrolysis changes Gln to Glu. The sum of the residue masses of each of these amino acids $+ 18(H_2O) + 1(H^+)$ equals 693, showing that Glx = Gln, and confirming that no other residues nor any posttranslational modifications are present. Often amino acid analysis is not possible for every sample, especially when limited quantity is available. Composition is not necessary for deriving the sequence from a spectrum, although it does make interpretation simpler and gives additional support to the derived sequence.

One generally begins by looking for low-mass immonium ions, although in this example the amino acid composition is already known. The immonium ions are: m/z 74—Thr; 86—Leu/Ile; 101—Lys/Gln; 120—Phe; 129—Arg; and 159—Trp. The latter two masses obviously represent some other structure. In addition, we know that m/z 86 corresponds to Ile, and m/z 101 to both Lys and Gln. One also checks for side-chain losses from MH^+. These are m/z 648 = $MH^+ - 45 = $ Thr, 636 = $MH^+ - 57 = $ Ile/Leu, and 621 = $MH^+ - 72 = $ Lys/Gln. The peak at m/z 675 is due to the loss of water.

Sequencing begins by looking for losses from MH^+ that correspond to an amino acid residue mass. These are the candidates for y_5: 636 = $MH^+ - 57 = $ Gly, 592 = $MH^+ - 101 = $ Thr. Since either residue is possible, one looks for losses from these two candidates that would give the y_4

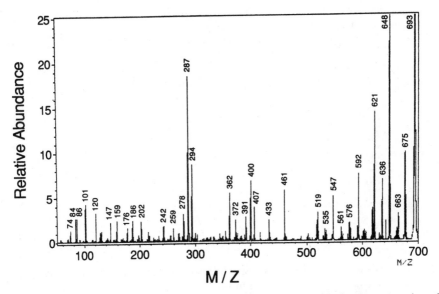

Fig. 12. CID daughter spectrum of an "unknown" tryptic peptide for demonstration of sequence interpretation. $MH^+ = 693.4$.

candidates: $535 = 636 - 101 =$ Thr, $535 = 592 - 57 =$ Gly, and $461 = 592 - 131 =$ Met. (Figure 13 shows a tree diagram which helps keep track of these assignments.) Since Met was not found in the amino acid analysis, that sequencing route is not followed any further. So far two sequences are possible, Gly-Thr—, or Thr-Gly—. Let us continue. From m/z 535 there are two candidates for y_3: $407 = 535 - 128 =$ Lys/Gln, $372 = 535 - 163 =$ Tyr. Since

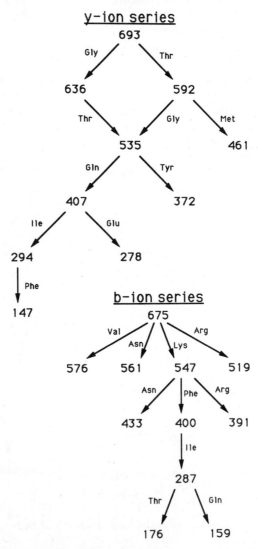

Fig. 13. Mass difference "tree" for peaks from Fig. 12 that correspond to amino acid masses. Where no arrow continues, no further matches could be found, or the sequence does not match the amino acid composition.

Tyr is not possible and Lys should be at the C-terminus (tryptic peptide), the next residue is Gln. From m/z 407, there are two candidates for y_2: $294 = 407 - 113 = $ Leu/Ile, $278 = 407 - 129 = $ Glu. Only Ile is possible from the composition. From m/z 294, there is only one possibility: $147 = 294 - 147 = $ Phe. The y_1 ion for Lys appears at m/z 147 [$= 128$(residue) $+ 17$(OH) $+ 2$(H's); see Fig. 7].

There are two possible sequences: Gly-Thr-Gln-Ile-Phe-Lys or Thr-Gly-Gln-Ile-Phe-Lys. Examining the z-ion series helps this analysis: m/z $278 = z_2 + 1$, $391 = z_3 + 1$, $519 = z_4 + 1$, $576 = z_5 + 1$ (for Thr-Gly-Gln-Ile-Phe-Lys) (or m/z $621 = z_5$ for Gly-Thr-Gln-Ile-Phe-Lys). Because the $z + 1$ series is more prevalent, Thr-Gly-Gln-Ile-Phe-Lys is more likely, but the other cannot be ruled out yet.

An examination of the b-ion series gives further evidence and provides confirmation of the putative sequence. The b_6 ion is 18 u below MH^+, m/z 675. Figure 13 shows the possible sequences given by the b-ion series. The C-terminal residue is expected to be Lys or Arg because the peptide is a tryptic peptide. The amino acid composition eliminates Arg and the other possibilities. No b_1 ion is found, so the amino terminal residue is still in question.

Other peaks in the spectrum that can be assigned based on the putative sequence are $a_3 = 259$, $a_4 = 372$, $a_5 = 519$, $d_3 = 202$, $w_3 = 362$, $w_4 = 461$, $x_3 = 433$, and $x_4 = 561$. One can decide between the two candidate sequences by checking to see which, if either, leaves the least number of unassigned peaks. The sequence Gly-Thr-Gln-Ile-Phe-Lys leaves m/z 576 and 592, unassigned while Thr-Gly-Gln-Ile-Phe-Lys assigns these two peaks to $z_5 + 1$ and y_5, respectively. Thus, Thr-Gly-Gln-Ile-Phe-Lys is most likely and is, in fact, the true sequence. One could obtain further confirmation by performing a single step of manual Edman degradation and subsequently measuring the mass of the shortened peptide.

A second example is provided to demonstrate peptide sequence interpretation from a FAB spectrum. The reader might first try this example independently before reading on. Figure 14 is the FAB spectrum of an "unknown" peptide, $MH^+ = 900.6$. The glycerol matrix peaks are labeled with an "*." One begins by checking the immonium ions for likely amino acids. These are m/z 87—Asn (or matrix); 104—Met; 120—Phe; and 136—Tyr. Examination of side-chain losses from the MH^+ ion only yields 793—Tyr. The ions corresponding to $-CH_3$ (m/z 885) and $-HCOOH$ (m/z 854) are found for many peptides. One can start interpretation from m/z 900 and check for ions that differ by exactly one amino acid residue mass. The peaks at m/z 786 ($-114 = $ Asn) or m/z 737 ($-163 = $ Tyr) are the only candidates for y_{n-1} ions (i.e., loss of the N-terminal amino acid residue from MH^+). From each of these candidates, look for the next possible residue loss (see Fig. 15). For m/z 786: $729 = 786 - 57 = $ Gly, $623 = 786 - 163 = $ Tyr. For m/z 737: $680 = 737 - 57 = $ Gly, $623 = 737 - 114 = $ Asn, $608 = 737 - 129 = $ Glu. At this point, one can continue looking for the next possible residue loss from each of the candidates for y_{n-2}, or try to continue as far as

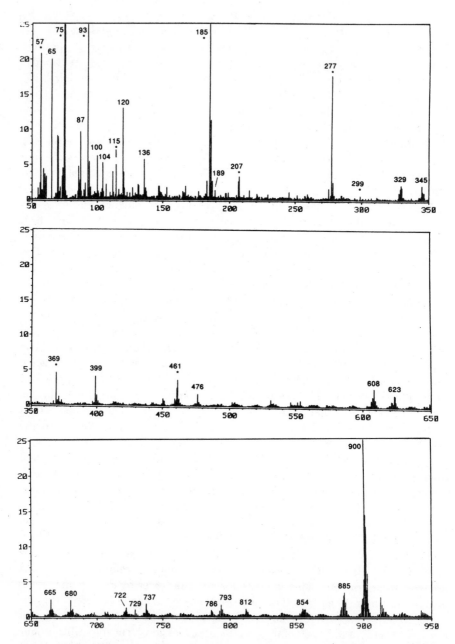

Fig. 14. FAB spectrum of an "unknown" peptide for demonstration of sequence interpretation (see text). The glycerol matrix ions are identified by "*."

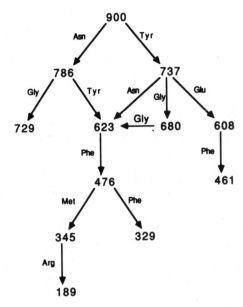

Fig. 15. Mass difference "tree" for peaks from Fig. 14 that correspond to amino acid masses. Where no arrow continues, no further matches could be found.

possible with just one of the sequences. At some point one should look for the z, $z + 1$, or $z + 2$ ions that are sometimes associated with the y ions. These would be 17, 16, or 15 u lower in mass, respectively. Of the masses checked so far, masses 722, 665, 608, and 461, are all 15 u lower than the respective y ions. Observing this accompanying set of z ions gives credence to the sequence Tyr-Gly-Gly over Tyr-Asn or Asn-Tyr. If one continues down from 476, the sequence becomes Tyr-Gly-Gly-Phe-Met-Arg. Below m/z 189 there are numerous peaks so it may be easier to check possible dipeptides. The dipeptide masses in Table 5 are simple sums of the component residue masses. As such, one must subtract 19 u from the corresponding y ion mass (due to the structure of the y ion) to obtain the appropriate dipeptide mass. Dipeptides that correspond to $189 - 19 = 170$ are Leu-Gly, Ile-Gly, or Val-Arg. One also can look for N-terminal ions that might help choose between these possibilities. No a or b ions correspond, but $c_7 = 786 = 899 - 113$ and $c_6 = 729 = 786 - 57$ indicate that the carboxy-terminus is either Gly-Leu or Gly-Ile. No distinction can be made between Leu and Ile in the FAB spectrum. (The Leu/Ile question could be answered by amino acid analysis.) Thus, the likely sequence is Tyr-Gly-Gly-Phe-Met-Arg-Gly-Leu/Ile.

One can be confident in this sequence because most major nonmatrix ions are assigned (m/z 399 is likely a contaminant). One could check the sequence by going through one or two cycles of manual Edman degradation. Any other putative sequences that were derived during interpretation should be checked to eliminate these other possibilities.

An equivalent strategy can be used for an MS/MS daughter spectrum. Interpreting these spectra is usually easier because interferences from matrix ions, isotope peaks, and contaminants are eliminated.

8.3.   Computer Aids to Interpretation

Manual interpretation of spectra is time-consuming and may not produce all possible sequences that fit the spectral data. Computer interpretation programs are designed to minimize both of these problems. Although most of the programs described work with either FAB or MS/MS spectra, the matrix ions in the FAB spectra limit the use of some.

The simplest method is to calculate the fragment ion masses for all possible amino acid sequences that match the MH^+ mass, then determine which set(s) best fit the experimental data (230–233). The chief drawback to these programs is the inordinate amount of computer time and memory required, effectively limiting this approach to peptides < 1000 u. Limiting the number of possibilities by input of the amino acid composition extends the usefulness of these programs, but necessitates an additional experimental procedure.

Another approach is based upon manual interpretation strategies, namely starting from the MH^+ ion (234, 235) or a low-mass fragment (236, 237) and finding ions whose neutral loss or gain matches an amino acid residue mass. These approaches extend the possible mass range considerably, since only the observed sequence ion masses are used. This approach has been adapted for use with cyclic peptides (238), and for high-energy CID spectra by including additional ion types (e.g., d, v, and w) (239).

A third approach is an interactive graphics display of mass differences that correspond to amino acid residue masses (141). The mass differences between all peaks in the spectrum are calculated. Those differences that match amino acid residue masses and that extend at least two residues are saved in a table. Labeled connections between those peaks are shown on a graphics display, subject to an adjustable intensity threshold.

This approach follows most closely the manual interpretation of the data. As such it may not yield all possible sequences that are consistent with the data. But if used in combination with one of the other programs described above, it should provide the best overall approach to data interpretation.

8.4.   A General Approach to Sequence Determination

The plan of attack for any particular sequencing problem depends on a large number of factors:

1. What is desired—the complete primary structure of an unknown? a partial sequence for constructing oligonucleotide probes? confirmation of cDNA sequence?

2. What is known about the protein/peptide—size? amino acid composition? putative sequence? is it glycosylated?

3. How much material is available?

4. What is its purity?

The list could go on and on. The process becomes more straightforward and the outcome more certain if one can find out as much as possible about the sample before starting.

A general outline for sequencing by mass spectrometry is shown in Fig. 16. If possible, one should determine the molecular weight of the peptide or protein. This is possible with FAB or PDMS for up to 20 kDa. The mass, if it is to within 1 u accuracy, is used in the end to tell whether the entire sequence was determined accurately and whether posttranslational modifications are present.

The protein is cleaved into several large pieces, usually by CNBr digestion. After separation, the mass of each of these pieces is determined, and each is subjected to further digestion (e.g., trypsin) to give fragments from which sequence ions can be obtained. These fragments are separated and a FAB spectrum of each fragment is obtained. The sequence may then be obtained directly from the FAB spectra. However, it is normally necessary to get further sequence data by MS/MS experiments, manual Edman degradation, or car-

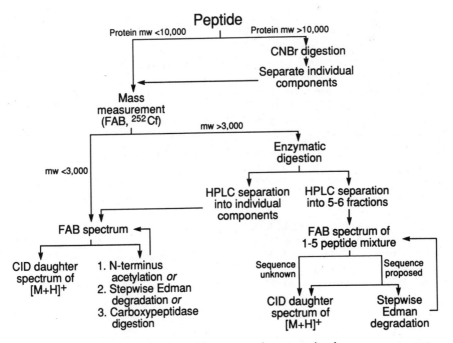

Fig. 16. A general approach to peptide sequence interpretation by mass spectrometry. The exact strategy depends on what is already known about the peptide, what information is desired, and how much peptide is available.

boxypeptidase digestion. From these data a number of unconnected subsequences will be obtained. Subsequent digestion of the intact protein and/or the CNBr fragments, with sequencing of these pieces provides overlap data to fit the entire sequence together.

While this approach relies totally on mass spectrometry and has been used successfully (159), the process would likely be more efficient if conventional Edman microsequencing were used in conjunction with mass spectrometry. Because the two techniques are complementary, one benefits from the strengths of each.

As mass spectrometry evolves, its use as an essential technique in protein chemistry will no doubt increase. Judging from the progress that has been made in mass spectrometry in the last 6–8 years, the growth in this area will continue at a rapid pace.

References

1. F. Wold, *Ann. Rev. Biochem.* **50**, 783–814 (1981).
2. F. Wold and K. Moldave, Eds., *Methods Enzymol.* **106** and **107** (1984).
3. B. C. Johnson, Ed., *Posttranslational Covalent Modifications of Proteins,* Academic Press, New York, 1983.
4. C. W. Ward, in A. Darbre, Ed., *Practical Protein Chemistry—A Handbook,* Wiley, New York, 1986, pp. 491–525.
5. H.-W. Lahm, D. H. Hawke, J. E. Shively, and C. W. Todd, in K. A. Walsh, Ed., *Methods in Protein Sequence Analysis,* Humana Press, Clifton, NJ, 1987, pp. 357–364.
6. R. P. Ambler, *Methods Enzymol.* **25**, 143 (1972); **25**, 262 (1972).
7. R. Hayashi, in Ajit S. Bhown, Ed., *Protein/Peptide Sequence Analysis: Current Methodologies,* CRC Press, Boca Raton, FL, 1988, pp. 145–159.
8. B. N. Jones, in J. E. Shively, Ed., *Methods of Protein Microcharacterization: A Practical Handbook,* Humana Press, Clifton, NJ, 1986, pp. 337–361.
9. R. M. Caprioli and T. Fan, *Anal. Biochem.* **154**, 596–603 (1986).
10. P. Edman, *Acta Chem. Scand.* **4**, 238–293 (1950).
11. G. E. Tarr, in J. E. Shively, Ed., *Methods of Protein Microcharacterization: A Practical Handbook,* Humana Press, Clifton, NJ, 1986, pp. 155–194.
12. P. Edman and G. Begg, *Eur. J. Biochem.* **1**, 80 (1967).
13. T. M. Hewick, M. W. Hunkapiller, L. E. Hood, and W. H. Dreyer, *J. Biol. Chem.* **256**, 7990–7997 (1981).
14. A. S. Bhown and J. C. Bennet, in A. S. Bhown, Ed., *Protein/Peptide Sequence Analysis: Current Methodologies,* CRC Press, Boca Raton, FL, 1988, pp. 49–71.
15. J. J. L'Italien, in J. E. Shively, Ed., *Methods of Protein Microcharacterization: A Practical Handbook,* Humana Press, Clifton, NJ, 1986, pp. 279–314.
16. A. J. H. Smith, *Meth. Enzymol.* **65**, 560–580 (1980).
17. A. M. Maxam and W. Gilbert, *Meth. Enzymol.* **65**, 499–560 (1980).
18. L. M. Smith, J. Sanders, T. Kaiser, P. Hughes, C. Dodd, and L. E. Hood, *Nature* **321**, 674–679 (1986).
19. J. M. Prober, G. L. Trainor, R. J. Dam, F. W. Hobbs, C. W. Robertson, R. J. Zagursky, A. J. Cocuzza, M. A. Jensen, and K. Baumeister, *Science* **238**, 336–341 (1987).
20. R. K. Scopes, *Protein Purification: Principles and Practice,* 2nd ed., Springer-Verlag, New York, 1987.

21. G. Allen, *Sequencing of Proteins and Peptides*, Elsevier, Amsterdam, 1981.

22. J. E. Shively, Ed., *Methods of Protein Microcharacterization: A Practical Handbook*, Humana Press, Clifton, NJ, 1986.

23. A. Darbre, Ed., *Practical Protein Chemistry—A Handbook*, Wiley, New York, 1986.

24. E. Gross, *Meth. Enzymol.* **11**, 238–255 (1967).

25. P. Bornstein and G. Balian, *Meth. Enzymol.* **47**, 145–149 (1977).

26. M. Landon, *Meth. Enzymol.* **47**, 145–149 (1977).

27. A. Fontana and E. Gross, in A. Darbre, Ed., *Practical Protein Chemistry—A Handbook*, Wiley, New York, 1986, pp. 67–120.

28. R. M. Wagner and B. A. Fraser, *Biomed. Environ. Mass Spectrom.* **14**, 235–239 (1987).

29. P. C. Andrews and J. E. Dixon, *J. Biol. Chem.* **256**, 8367–8270 (1981).

30. W. Konigsberg, *Meth. Enzymol.* **25**, 185–188 (1972).

31. G. Allen, *Sequencing of Protein and Peptides*, Elsevier, Amsterdam, 1981, pp. 43–70.

32. M. Barber and B. N. Green, *Rapid Commun. Mass Spectrom.* **1**, 80–83 (1987).

33. W. Aberth, *Int. J. Mass Spectrom. Ion Processes* **68**, 209–212 (1986).

34. H. R. Morris, in C. J. McNeal, Ed., *Mass Spectrometry in the Analysis of Large Molecules*, Wiley, New York, 1986, pp. 121–129.

35. J. Yergey, D. Heller, G. Hansen, R. J. Cotter, and C. Fenselau, *Anal. Chem.* **55**, 353–356 (1983).

36. D. F. Hunt, J. R. Yates III, J. Shabanowitz, S. Winston, and C. R. Hauser, *Proc. Natl. Acad. Sci. USA* **83**, 6233–6237 (1986).

37. A. E. Schoen, J. W. Amy, J. D. Ciupek, R. G. Cooks, P. Dobberstein, and G. Jung, *Int. J. Mass Spectrom. Ion Processes* **65**, 125–140 (1985).

38. K. Biemann, S. A. Martin, H. A. Scoble, R. S. Johnson, I. A. Papayannopoulos, J. E. Biller, and C. E. Costello, in C. J. McNeal, Ed., *Mass Spectrometry in the Analysis of Large Molecules*, Wiley, New York, 1986, pp. 131–149.

39. D. F. Hunt, J. Shabanowitz, and J. R. Yates III, *J. Chem. Soc. Chem. Commun.* 548–550 (1987).

40. K. Biemann, in G. R. Waller and O. C. Dermer, Eds., *Biomedical Applications of Mass Spectrometry*, First Supplementary Volume, Wiley, New York, 1980, pp. 469–525.

41. K. Biemann and W. Vetter, *Biochem. Biophys. Res. Commun.* **3**, 578–584 (1960).

42. J. A. Kelley, H. Nau, H.-J. Forster, and K. Biemann, *Biomed. Mass Spectrom.* **2**, 313–325 (1975).

43. H. Nau, H.-J. Forster, J. A. Kelley, and K. Biemann, *Biomed. Mass Spectrom.* **2**, 326–339 (1975).

44. S. A. Carr, W. C. Herlihy, and K. Biemann, *Biomed. Mass Spectrom.* **8**, 51–61 (1981).

45. J. E. Vath and K. Biemann, presented at the 35th ASMS Conf., Denver, 1987, pp. 570–571.

46. W. Herlihy and K. Biemann, *Biomed. Mass Spectrom.* **8**, 70–77 (1981).

47. H.-K. Wipf, P. Irving, M. McCamish, R. VenKataraghavan, and F. W. McLafferty, *J. Am. Chem. Soc.* **95**, 3369–3375 (1973).

48. H. R. Morris, *FEBS Lett.* **22**, 257–260 (1972).

49. K. Rose, M. G. Simona, and R. E. Offord, *Biochem. J.* **215**, 261–272 (1983).

50. M. L. Polan, W. J. McMurray, S. R. Lipsky, and S. J. Lande, *J. Am. Chem. Soc.* **94**, 2847–2850 (1972).

51. A. Dell and H. R. Morris, *Biomed. Mass. Spectrom.* **8**, 128–136 (1981).

52. P. J. Arpino and F. W. McLafferty, in F. C. Nachod, J. J. Zuckerman, and E. W. Randall, Eds., *Determination of Organic Structures by Physical Methods*, Academic Press, New York, 1976, Vol. 6, pp. 1–89.

53. H. R. Morris, *Nature* **286**, 447–452 (1980).

54. S. Magnusson, L. Sottrup-Jensen, T. E. Petersen, H. R. Morris, and A. Dell, *FEBS Lett.* **44**, 189–193 (1974).

55. H. C. Krutzch and J. J. Pisano, *Biochemistry* **17**, 2791–2797 (1978).

56. H. C. Krutzch, in J. E. Shively, Ed., *Methods of Protein Microcharacterization: A Practical Handbook*, Humana Press, Clifton, NJ, 1986.

57. A. A. Kiryushkin, H. M. Fales, T. Axenrod, E. J. Gilbert, and G. W. A. Milne, *Org. Mass Spectrom.* **5**, 19–31 (1971).

58. D. F. Hunt, G. C. Stafford, F. W. Crow, and J. W. Russel, *Anal. Chem.* **48**, 2098–2105 (1976).

59. M. A. Baldwin and F. W. McLafferty, *Org. Mass Spectrom.* **7**, 1353–1356 (1973).

60. V. N. Reinhold and S. A. Carr, *Anal. Chem.* **54**, 499–503 (1982).

61. S. A. Carr and V. N. Reinhold, in M. Elzinga, Ed., *Methods of Protein Sequence Analysis*, Humana Press, Clifton, NJ, 1982, pp. 263–270.

62. S. A. Carr, K. Biemann, S. Shoji, D. C. Parmelee, and K. Titani, *Proc. Natl. Acad. Sci. USA* **79**, 6128–6131 (1982).

63. N. Takeda, K. Harada, M. Suzuki, and A. Tatematsu, *Org. Mass Spectrom.* **20**, 236–242 (1985).

64. H. U. Winkler and H. D. Beckey, *Biochem. Biophys. Res. Commun.* **46**, 391–397 (1972).

65. T. Matsuo, H. Matsuda, I. Katakuse, Y. Shimonishi, Y. Maruyama, T. Higuchi, and E. Kubota, *Anal. Chem.* **53**, 416–421 (1981).

66. T. Matsuo, H. Matsuda, S. Aimoto, Y. Shimonishi, T. Higuchi, and Y. Maruyama, *Int. J. Mass Spectrom. Ion Processes* **46**, 423–426 (1983).

67. D. M. Desiderio and J. E. Sabbatini, *Biomed. Mass Spectrom.* **8**, 565–568 (1981).

68. Y. Shimonishi, Y.-M. Hong, T. Kitagishi, T. Matsuo, H. Matsuda, and I. Katakuse, *Eur. J. Biochem.* **112**, 251–264 (1980).

69. Y.-M. Hong, T. Takao, S. Aimoto, and Y. Shimonishi, *Biomed. Mass Spectrom.* **10**, 450–457 (1983).

70. A. Tsugita, R. VanDenBroek, and M. Przybylski, *FEBS Lett.* **137**, 19–24 (1982).

71. R. D. Macfarlane and D. F. Torgerson, *Science* **191**, 920–925 (1976).

72. R. D. Macfarlane and D. F. Torgerson, *Int. J. Mass Spectrom. Ion Processes* **21**, 81–92 (1976).

73. B. Sundqvist and R. D. Macfarlane, *Mass Spectrom. Rev.* **4**, 421–460 (1985).

74. D. A. Kidwell, M. M. Ross, and R. J. Colton, *Int. J. Mass Spectrom. Ion Processes* **78**, 315–328 (1987).

75. B. T. Chait and F. H. Field, *Int. J. Mass Spectrom. Ion Processes* **41**, 17–29 (1981).

76. B. T. Chait, *Int. J. Mass Spectrom. Ion Processes* **53**, 227–242 (1983).

77. C. J. McNeal, R. C. Macfarlane, and E. L. Thurston, *Anal. Chem.* **57**, 2036 (1979).

78. G. P. Jonsson, A. B. Hedin, P. L. Hakansson, B. U. R. Sundqvist, B. G. S. Save, P. F. Nielsen, P. Roepstorff, K. E. Johansson, I. Kamensky, and M. L. S. Lindberg, *Anal. Chem.* **58**, 1084 (1986).

79. P. Roepstorff, P. F. Nielsen, B. U. R. Sundqvist, P. Hakansson, and G. Jonsson, *Int. J. Mass Spectrom. Ion Processes* **78**, 229–236 (1987).

80. M. Alai, P. Demirev, C. Fenselau, and R. J. Cotter, *Anal. Chem.* **58**, 1303–1307 (1986).

81. I. Jardine, G. F. Scanlan, A. Tsarbopoulos, and D. J. Liberato, *Anal. Chem.* **60**, 1086–1088 (1988).

82. A. G. Craig, A. Engstrom, H. Bennich, and I. Kamensky, 35th ASMS Conference, Denver, 1987, pp. 528–529.

83. J. A. Loo, E. R. Williams, J. J. P. Furlong, B. H. Wang, and F. W. McLafferty, *Int. J. Mass Spectrom. Ion Processes* **78**, 305–313 (1987).

84. B. Sundqvist, P. Roepstorff, J. Fohlman, A. Hedin, P. Hakansson, I. Kamensky, M. Lindberg, M. Salepour, and G. Save, *Science* **226**, 696–698 (1984).

85. B. Sundqvist, I. Kamensky, P. Hakansson, J. Kjellberg, M. Sadehpour, S. Widdiyasekera, J. Fohlman, P. A. Peterson, and P. Roepstorff, *Biomed. Mass Spectrom.* **11**, 242–257 (1984).

86. B. Sundqvist and R. D. Macfarlane, *Mass Spectrom. Rev.* **4**, 421–460 (1985).

87. A. G. Craig, A. Engstrom, H. Bennich, and I. Kamensky, *Biomed. Environ. Mass Spectrom.* **14**, 669–673 (1987).

88. B. T. Chait and F. H. Field, *Biochem. Biophys. Res. Commun.* **134**, 420–426 (1986).

89. A. Tsarbopoulos, G. W. Becker, J. L. Occolowitz, and I. Jardine, *Anal. Biochem.* **171**, 113–129 (1988).

90. M. A. Posthumus, P. G. Kistemaker, H. L. C. Meuzelaar, and M. C. Ten Noever de Brauw, *Anal. Chem.* **50**, 985–991 (1978).

91. D. A. McCrery, E. B. Ledford Jr., and M. L. Gross, *Anal. Chem.* **54**, 1435–1437 (1982).

92. Ch. Shiller, K.-D. Kupka, and F. Hillenkamp, *Fresenius Z. Anal. Chem.* **308**, 304–308 (1981).

93. J.-C. Tabet and R. J. Cotter, *Anal. Chem.* **56**, 1662–1667 (1984).

94. C. L. Wilkins, D. A. Weil, C. L. C. Yang, and C. F. Ijames, *Anal. Chem.* **57**, 520–524 (1985).

95. M. Karas and F. Hillenkamp, *Anal. Chem.* **60**, 2301–2303 (1988).

96. J. Grotemeyer and E. W. Schlag, *Org. Mass Spectrom.* **23**, 388–396 (1988).

97. A. Benninghoven and W. K. Sichtermann, *Org. Mass Spectrom.* **12**, 595–597 (1977).

98. A. Benninghoven and W. K. Sichtermann, *Anal. Chem.* **50**, 1180–1184 (1978).

99. H. Kambara, S. Hishida, and H. Naganawa, *Org. Mass Spectrom.* **17**, 67–73 (1982).

100. B. T. Chait and K. G. Standing, *Int. J. Mass Spectrom. Ion Processes* **40**, 185–193 (1981).

101. J. B. Westmore, W. Ens, and K. G. Standing, *Biomed. Mass Spectrom.* **9**, 119–124 (1982).

102. A. Benninghoven, E. Niehuis, T. Friese, D. Griefendorf, and P. Steffens, *Org. Mass. Spectrom.* **19**, 346 (1984).

103. W. Aberth, K. M. Straub, and A. L. Burlingame, *Anal. Chem.* **54**, 2029 (1982).

104. A. Dell and G. W. Taylor, *Mass Spectrom. Rev.* **3**, 357–394 (1984).

105. J. S. Cottrell and R. J. Greathead, *Mass Spectrom. Rev.* **5**, 215–247 (1986).

106. M. Barber, R. S. Bordoli, R. D. Sedgewick, and A. N. Tyler, *J. Chem. Soc. Chem. Commun.*, 325–327 (1981).

107. M. Barber, R. S. Bordoli, R. D. Sedgewick, and A. N. Tyler, *Nature* **293**, 270–275 (1981).

108. M. Barber, R. S. Bordoli, R. D. Sedgewick, A. N. Tyler, and E. T. Whalley, *Biomed. Mass Spectrom.* **8**, 337–342 (1981).

109. H. R. Morris, M. Panico, M. Barber, R. S. Bordoli, R. D. Sedgewick, and A. N. Tyler, *Biochem. Biophys. Res. Commun.* **101**, 623–631 (1981).

110. D. H. Williams, C. Bradley, G. Bojesen, S. Santikarn, and L. C. E. Taylor, *J. Am. Chem. Soc.* **103**, 5700–5704 (1981).

111. K. L. Rinehart, L. A. Gaudioso, M. L. Moore, R. C. Pandley, J. C. Cook, Jr., M. Barber, R. D. Sedgewick, R. S. Bordoli, A. N. Tyler, and B. N. Green, *J. Am. Chem. Soc.* **103**, 6517–6520 (1981).

112. M. Barber, R. S. Bordoli, G. V. Garner, D. B. Gordon, R. D. Sedgewick, L. W. Tetler, and A. N. Tyler, *Biochem. J.* **197**, 401–404 (1981).

113. M. Barber, R. S. Bordoli, R. D. Sedgewick, A. N. Tyler, and B. W. Bycroft, *Biochem. Biophys. Res. Commun.* **101**, 632–638 (1981).

114. A. Dell, H. R. Morris, M. D. Levin, and S. M. Hecht, *Biochem. Biophys. Res. Commun.* **102**, 730–738 (1981).

115. H. R. Morris, M. Panico, A. Karplus, P. E. Lloyd, and B. Riniker, *Nature* **300**, 643–645 (1982).

116. C. Fenselau and R. J. Cotter, *Chem. Rev.* **87**, 501–512 (1987).

117. S. J. Pachuta and R. G. Cooks, *Chem. Rev.* **87**, 647–669 (1987).

118. B. D. Musselman, J. T. Watson, and C. K. Chang, *Org. Mass Spectrom.* **21**, 215–219 (1986).

119. T. Keough, *Anal. Chem.* **57**, 2027–2034 (1985).

120. J. A. Sunner, R. Kulatunga, and P. Kebarle, *Anal. Chem.* **58**, 1312–1316 (1986).

121. J. A. Sunner, R. Kulatunga, and P. Kebarle, *Anal. Chem.* **58**, 2009–2014 (1986).

122. R. G. Cooks and K. L. Busch, *Int. J. Mass Spectrom. Ion Processes* **53**, 111–124 (1983).

123. W. V. Ligon, Jr and S. B. Dorn, *Int. J. Mass Spectrom. Ion Processes* **78**, 99–113 (1986).

124. S. Naylor, A. F. Findeis, B. W. Gibson, and D. H. Williams, *J. Am. Chem. Soc.* **108**, 6359–6363 (1986).

125. P. Roepstorff and J. Fohlmann, *Biomed. Mass Spectrom* **11**, 601 (1984).

126. R. S. Johnson, S. A. Martin, K. Biemann, J. T. Stults, and J. T. Watson, *Anal. Chem.* **59**, 2621–2625 (1987).

127. K. Biemann and S. A. Martin, *Mass Spectrom. Rev.* **6**, 1–76 (1987).

128. K. Ishikawa and Y. Niwa, *Biomed. Environ. Mass Spectrom.* **13**, 373–380 (1986).

129. T. D. Lee, in J. E. Shively, Ed., *Methods of Protein Microcharacterization: A Practical Handbook*, Humana Press, Clifton, NJ, 1986, pp. 403–441.

130. W. Kausler, K. Schneider, and G. Spiteller, *Biomed. Environ. Mass Spectrom.* **17**, 15–19 (1988).

131. W. Ligon, Jr., *Anal. Chem.* **58**, 485–487 (1986).

132. A. M. Buko, L. R. Phillips, and B. A. Fraser, *Biomed. Mass Spectrom.* **10**, 324–333 (1983).

133. J. L. Gower, *Biomed. Mass Spectrom.* **12**, 191–196 (1985).

134. E. Depauw, *Mass Spectrom. Rev.* **5**, 191–212 (1986).

135. A. M. Falick, F. C. Walls, and R. A. Laine, *Anal. Biochem.* **159**, 132–137 (1986).

136. S. A. Martin, J. A. Hill, and K. Biemann, 36th ASMS Conf., San Francisco, 1988.

137. B. D. Musselman and J. T. Watson, *Biomed. Environ. Mass Spectrom.* **14**, 247–248 (1987).

138. J. L. Witten, M. H. Shaffer, M. O'Shea, J. C. Cook, M. E. Hemling, and K. L. Rinehart, Jr., *Biochem. Biophys. Res. Commun.* **124**, 350–358 (1984).

139. J. Meili and J. Seibl, *Org. Mass Spectrom.* **19**, 581 (1984).

140. S. A. Martin and K. Biemann, *Int. J. Mass Spectrom. Ion Processes* **78**, 213–228 (1987).

141. H. A. Scoble, J. E. Biller, and K. Biemann, *Fresenius Z. Anal. Chem.* **327**, 239–245 (1987).

142. H. A. Scoble and K. Biemann, *Science* **237**, 992–998 (1987).

143. M. M. Sheil and P. J. Derrick, in S. J. Gaskell, Ed., *Mass Spectrometry in Biomedical Research*, Wiley, New York, 1986, pp. 251–268.

144. W. Heerma, J. P. Kamerling, A. J. Slotboom, G. J. M. Scharrenberg, B. N. Green, and I. A. S. Lewis, *Biomed. Mass Spectrom.* **10**, 13–16 (1983).

145. R. G. Cooks, J. H. Beynon, R. M. Caprioli, and G. R. Lester, *Metastable Ions*, Elsevier, Amsterdam, 1973.

146. G. M. Neumann and P. J. Derrick, *Org. Mass Spectrom.* **19**, 165–170 (1984).

147. D. L. Bricker and D. H. Russel, *J. Am. Chem. Soc.* **108**, 6174–6179 (1986).

148. K. B. Tomer, M. L. Gross, H. Zappey, R. H. Fokkens, and N. M. M. Nibbering, *Biomed. Environ. Mass Spectrom.* **15**, 649–657 (1988).

149. K. Sato, T. Asada, M. Ishihara, F. Kunihiro, Y. Kammei, E. Kubota, C. Costello, S. A. Martin, H. A. Scoble, and K. Biemann, *Anal. Chem.* **59**, 1652–1659 (1987).

150. R. K. Boyd, *Int. J. Mass Spectrom. Ion Processes* **75**, 243–264 (1987).

151. H. G. Boettger, C. E. Giffin, and D. D. Norris, in Y. Talmi, Ed., *Multichannel Image Detectors*, ACS Symposium Series 102, American Chemical Society, Washington, DC, 1979, pp. 291–318.

152. J. S. Cottrell and S. Evans, *Anal. Chem.* **59**, 1990–1995 (1987).

153. J. A. Hill, S. A. Martin, and K. Biemann, 36th ASMS Conf., San Francisco, 1988.

154. G. Elliot, R. Gallagher, S. Evans, A. Ashcroft, and G. Gooch, 36th ASMS Conf., San Francisco, 1988.

155. J. W. Crabb, L. G. Armes, S. A. Carr, C. M. Johnson, G. D. Roberts, R. S. Bordoli, and W. L. McKeehan, *Biochemistry* **25**, 4988–4993 (1986).

156. D. J. Harvan, J. R. Hass, W. E. Wilson, C. Hamm, R. K. Boyd, H. Yajima, and D. G. Klapper, *Biomed. Environ. Mass Spectrom.* **14**, 281–287 (1987).

157. W. R. Mathews, R. S. Johnson, K. L. Cornwell, T. C. Johnson, B. B. Buchanan, and K. Biemann, *J. Biol. Chem.* **262**, 7537–7575 (1987).

158. R. J. Anderegg, S. A. Carr, I. Y. Huang, R. A. Hiipakka, C. Chang, and S. Liao, *Biochemistry* **27**, 4214–4221 (1988).

159. R. S. Johnson and K. Biemann, *Biochemistry* **26**, 1209–1214 (1987).

160. D. F. Hunt, J. R. Yates III, J. Shabanowitz, S. Winston, and C. R. Hauer, *Proc. Natl. Acad. Sci. USA* **83**, 6233–6237 (1986).

161. S. J. Gaskell, M. H. Reilly, S. A. Carr, M. Bean, and R. Vickers, 36th ASMS Conf., San Francisco, 1988.

162. D. F. Hunt, J. Shabanowitz, J. R. Yates III, R. T. McIver, Jr., R. L. Hunter, J. E. P. Syka, and J. Amy, *Anal. Chem.* **57**, 2728–2733 (1985).

163. D. F. Hunt, J. Shabanowitz, J. R. Yates, N.-Z. Zhu, and D. H. Russel, *Proc. Natl. Acad. Sci. USA* **84**, 620–623 (1987).

164. H. Michel, D. F. Hunt, J. Shabanowitz, and J. Bennett, *J. Biol. Chem.* **263**, 1123–1130 (1988).

165. W. D. Bowers, S.-S. Delbert, R. L. Hunter, and R. T. McIver, Jr., *J. Am. Chem. Soc.* **106**, 7288–7289 (1984).

166. A. L. Burlingame, J. O. Whitney, and D. H. Russel, *Anal. Chem.* **56**, 417R–467R (1984).

167. A. L. Burlingame, T. A. Baille, and P. J. Derrick, *Anal. Chem.* **58**, 165R–211R (1986).

168. A. L. Burlingame, D. Maltby, D. H. Russel, and P. T. Holland, *Anal. Chem.* **60**, 294R–342R (1988).

169. M. E. Hemling, *Pharm. Res.* **4**, 5–15 (1987).

170. S. A. Carr and K. Biemann, *Methods Enzymol.* **106**, 29–58 (1984).

171. B. W. Gibson and K. Biemann, *Proc. Natl. Acad. Sci. USA* **81**, 1956–1960 (1984).

172. B. W. Gibson, D. J. Daley, and D. H. Williams, *Anal. Biochem.* **169**, 217–226 (1988).

173. B. W. Gibson, Z. Yu, W. Aberth, A. L. Burlingame, and N. M. Bass, *J. Biol. Chem.* **263**, 4182–4185 (1988).

174. P. C. Andrews, R. Nichols, and J. E. Dixon, *J. Biol. Chem.* **262**, 12692–12699 (1987).

175. M. Mulligan, R. L. Houtz, and N. E. Tolbert, *Proc. Natl. Acad. Sci. USA* **85**, 1513–1517 (1988).

176. B. W. Gibson, A. M. Falick, A. L. Burlingame, G. L. Kenyon, L. Poulter, D. H. Williams, and P. Cohen, in K. A. Walsh, Ed., *Methods in Protein Sequence Analysis*, Humana Press, Clifton, NJ, 1986, pp. 463–478.

177. B. W. Gibson, A. M. Falick, A. L. Burlingame, L. Nadasdi, A. C. Nguyen, and G. L. Kenyon, *J. Am. Chem. Soc.* **109**, 5343–5348 (1987).

178. C. Fenselau, D. H. Heller, M. S. Miller, and H. B. White III, *Anal. Biochem.* **150**, 309–314 (1985).

179. V. L. Vaughn, R. Wong, C. Fenselau, and H. B. White III, *Biochem. Biophys. Res. Commun.* **147**, 115–119 (1987).

180. P. Petrilli, P. Pucci, H. R. Morris, and F. Addeo, *Biochem. Biophys. Res. Commun.* **140**, 28–37 (1986).

181. C. F. B. Holmes, N. K. Tonks, H. Major, and P. Cohen, *Biochim. Biophys. Acta* **929**, 208–219 (1987).

182. R. Townsend, M. Alai, M. R. Hardy, and C. C. Fenselau, *Anal. Biochem.* **171**, 180–191 (1988).

183. S. Naylor, N. J. Skelton, and D. H. Williams, *J. Chem. Soc. Chem. Commun.* 1619–1621 (1986).

184. S. A. Carr and G. D. Roberts, *Anal. Biochem.* **157**, 396–406 (1986).

185. S. A. Carr, G. D. Roberts, A. Jurewicz, B. Frederick, and M. Vettese, 36th ASMS Conf., San Francisco, 1988.

186. H. R. Morris, M. Panico, and G. W. Taylor, *Biochem. Biophys. Res. Commun.* **117**, 299–305 (1983).

187. M. E. Hemling, S. A. Carr, C. Capiau, and J. Petre, *Biochemistry* **27**, 699–705 (1988).

188. F. Raschdorf, R. Dahinden, B. Domon, D. Mueller, and W. J. Richter, in C. J. McNeal, Ed., *Mass Spectrometry in the Analysis of Large Molecules*, Wiley, New York, 1986, pp. 49–65.

189. J. M. Stewart and J. D. Young, *Solid Phase Peptide Synthesis*, 2nd ed., Pierce Chemical Company, Rockford, IL, 1984.

190. E. Canova-Davis, R. C. Chloupek, I. P. Baldonado, J. E. Battersby, M. W. Spellman, L. J. Basa, B. O'Connor, R. Pearlman, C. Quan, J. A. Chakel, J. T. Stults, and W. S. Hancock, *Am. Biotechnol. Lab.* **6**, 8–17 (1988).

191. H. R. Morris and P. Pucci, *Biochem. Biophys. Res. Commun.* **126**, 1122–1128 (1985).

192. R. Yazdanparast, P. C. Andrews, D. L. Smith, and J. E. Dixon, *J. Biol. Chem.* **262**, 2507–2517 (1987).

193. P. Toren, D. Smith, R. Chance, and J. Hoffman, *Anal. Biochem.* **169**, 287–299 (1988).

194. A. M. Buko and B. A. Fraser, *Biomed. Mass Spectrom.* **12**, 577–585 (1985).

195. R. Yazdanparast, P. Andrews, D. L. Smith, and J. E. Dixon, *Anal. Biochem.* **153**, 348–353 (1986).

196. W. S. McIntire and J. T. Stults, *Biochem. Biophys. Res. Commun.* **141**, 562–568 (1986).

197. R. J. Anderegg, *Mass Spectrom. Rev.* **7**, 395–424 (1988).

198. K. L. Busch, S. E. Unger, A. Vincze, R. G. Cooks, and T. Keough, *J. Am. Chem. Soc.* **104**, 1507–1511 (1982).

199. D. A. Kidwell, M. M. Ross, and R. J. Colton, *J. Am. Chem. Soc.* **106**, 2219–2220 (1984).

200. D. Renner and G. Spiteller, *Biomed. Environ. Mass Spectrom.* **13**, 405–410 (1986).

201. D. Renner and G. Spiteller, *Angew. Chem. Int. Ed. Engl.* **24**, 408–409 (1985).

202. D. L. Lippstreu-Fisher and M. L. Gross, *Anal. Chem.* **57**, 1174–1180 (1985).

203. R. S. Johnson and K. Biemann, 35th ASMS Conf., Denver, 1987, pp. 556–557.

204. G. E. Tarr, *Methods Enzymol.* **47**, 335–357 (1977).

205. M. E. Hemling, S. A. Carr, C. Capiau, and J. Petre, *Biochemistry* **27**, 699–705 (1988).

206. D. Pilosof, H. Y. Kim, D. F. Dyckes, and M. L. Vestal, *Anal. Chem.* **56**, 1236–1240 (1984).

207. H. Y. Kim, D. Pilosof, D. F. Dyckes, and M. L. Vestal, *J. Am. Chem. Soc.* **100**, 7304–7309 (1984).

208. K. Stachowiak, C. Wilder, M. L. Vestal, and D. F. Dyckes, *J. Am. Chem. Soc.* **110**, 1758–1765 (1988).

209. Y. Ito, T. Takeuchi, D. Ishii, and M. Goto, *J. Chromatogr.* **346**, 161–166 (1985).

210. R. M. Caprioli, T. Fan, and J. S. Cottrell, *Anal. Chem.* **58**, 2949–2954 (1986).

211. T. Minuzo, T. Kobayashi, Y. Ito, and D. Ishii, *Mass Spectrom.* **35**, 9–13 (1987).

212. R. M. Caprioli, B. DaGue, T. Fan, and W. T. Moore, *Biochem. Biophys. Res. Commun.* **146**, 291–299 (1987).

213. R. M. Caprioli and T. Fan, *Biochem. Biophys. Res. Commun.* **141**, 1058 (1986).

214. R. M. Caprioli, W. T. Moore, and R. Fan, *Rapid Commun. Mass Spectrom.* **1**, 15–18 (1987).

215. A. E. Ashcroft, J. R. Chapman, and J. S. Cottrell, *J. Chromatogr.* **394**, 15–20 (1987).

216. R. M. Caprioli, *Biochemistry* **27**, 513–521 (1988).

217. R. D. Minard, E. Long, P. Curry, Jr., and A. Ewing, 36th ASMS Conf., San Francisco, 1988.

218. R. D. Smith, J. A. Olivares, N. T. Nguyen, and H. R. Udseth, *Anal. Chem.* **60**, 436–441 (1988).

219. D. H. Williams, C. V. Bradley, S. Santikarn, and G. Bojesen, *Biochem. J.* **201**, 105–117 (1982).

220. D. Renner and G. Spiteller, *Biomed. Environ. Mass Spectrom.* **15**, 75–77 (1988).

221. D. R. Mueller, M. Eckersley, and W.-J. Richter, *Org. Mass Spectrom.* **23**, 217–222 (1988).

222. C. Dass and D. M. Desiderio, *Anal. Biochem.* **163**, 52–66 (1987).

223. D. Renner and G. Spiteller, *Biomed. Environ. Mass Spectrom.* **13**, 405–410 (1986).

224. N. J. Jensen, K. B. Tomer, and M. L. Gross, *J. Am. Chem. Soc.* **107**, 1863–1868 (1985).

225. C. E. Costello, S. A. Martin, and K. Biemann, 33rd ASMS Conf., San Diego, 1985, pp. 190–191.

226. P. Roepstorff, P. Hojrup, and J. Moller, *Biomed. Mass Spectrom.* **12**, 181–189 (1985).

227. L. M. Mallis and D. H. Russel, *Anal. Chem.* **58**, 1076–1080 (1986).

228. J. T. Stults and J. T. Watson, *Biomed. Environ. Mass Spectrom.* **14**, 583–586 (1987).

229. S. Seki, H. Kambara, and H. Naoki, *Org. Mass Spectrom.* **20**, 18–24 (1985).

230. T. Matsuo, H. Matsuda, and I. Katakuse, *Biomed. Mass Spectrom.* **8**, 137–143 (1981).

231. T. Matsuo, T. Sakurai, H. Matsuda, H. Wollnick, and I. Katakuse, *Biomed. Mass Spectrom.* **10**, 57–60 (1983).

232. T. Sakurai, T. Matsuo, H. Matsuda, and I. Katakuse, *Biomed. Mass Spectrom.* **11**, 396–399 (1984).

233. C. W. Hamm, W. E. Wilson, and D. J. Harvan, *Comput. Appl. Biosci.* **2**, 115–118 (1986).

234. T. D. Lee and V. Spayth, 33rd ASMS Conf., San Diego, 1985, pp. 266–267.

235. T. D. Lee, V. Spayth, and K. Legesse, 34th ASMS Conf., Cincinnati, 1986, pp. 842–843.

236. K. Ishikawa and Y. Niwa, *Biomed. Environ. Mass Spectrom.* **13**, 373–380 (1986).

237. M. M. Siegel and N. Bauman, *Biomed. Environ. Mass Spectrom.* **15**, 333–343 (1988).

238. K. Ishikawa, Y. Niwa, K. Hatakeda, and T. Gotoh, *Org. Mass Spectrom.* **23**, 290–291 (1988).

239. R. S. Johnson and K. Biemann, 36th ASMS Conf., San Francisco, 1988.

Mass Spectrometry of Nucleic Acid Components

KARL H. SCHRAM, *College of Pharmacy, University of Arizona, Tucson, Arizona*

---

1. INTRODUCTION

Since publication of the first spectrum of a nucleoside more than 25 years ago (1), mass spectrometry has successfully been applied to a wide variety of problems in nucleic acid chemistry. The areas in which mass spectrometry has found greatest application are (in approximate order of literature citations): (1) the structure elucidation of nucleic acid components isolated from biological sources, especially the identification of modified nucleosides in tRNA hydrolysates, nucleoside antibiotics, and nucleosides or nucleic acid bases or both in human urine; (2) for the quantitation of nucleic acid analogs (antimetabolites) of medicinal importance in the treatment of cancer and other diseases; and, (3) most recently, the determination of the structure of complexes formed between the nucleic acids and drugs or suspected carcinogens.

Information obtained in each of these three areas has had a significant impact on the knowledge of nucleic acid chemistry, ranging from a better understanding of the biochemical processes involved in nucleic acid biosynthesis to improving the clinical utility and design of antitumor agents, and other classes of medicinal agents that are analogs of naturally occurring nucleic acid components.

A number of factors are responsible for the continuing, and increasingly important, role of mass spectrometry in the analysis of nucleic acid components. First, of all currently available analytical techniques, only mass spectrometry combines the sensitivity and specificity needed for the analysis of microgram (μg) and submicrogram quantities of sample with the highly informative, structurally specific information contained in the mass spectrum. The value of mass spectrometry in the structure elucidation of an unknown nucleoside is evident in the many literature citations where the total amount of material available for analysis is in the low microgram range. Likewise, the sensitivity and specificity of mass spectrometry is of primary importance in the quantitation of nanogram (ng) and subnanogram levels of potent nucleoside antitumor agents in the blood of cancer patients.

A second factor in the expansion of the application of mass spectrometry in the study of nucleic acids is a result of recent developments in mass-spectrometry instrumentation. Until the introduction of fast atom bombardment (FAB) in 1981 (2), analysis of nucleic acid components was restricted to a mass range of approximately 1200 daltons because of limited sample volatility, even following the preparation of derivatives. Relative to the nucleosides and bases, the analysis of mononucleotides was more difficult and analysis of dinucleotide monophosphates was about the limit of volatility of the trimethylsilyl (TMS) derivatives; analysis of more polar samples, for example, nucleoside di- and triphosphates and polynucleotides, was not possible. Although some of these more intractable samples could be ionized by field desorption techniques, this approach was difficult and costly and required considerable expertise to perform a successful analysis. The introduction of FAB was, then, a step of fundamental importance for the mass spectral analysis of nucleic acid components, since, for the first time, the analysis of underivatized nucleosides, nucleotides, and small polynucleotides was possible in a fairly simple, reproducible manner.

Coincident with, or possibly because of the introduction of FAB, new magnet technology was introduced that, when coupled with FAB, expanded the application of mass spectrometry to the analysis of samples with molecular weights exceeding 2000 Daltons on a "standard" type magnetic instrument. Other techniques, that is, desorption chemical ionization (DCI) and ^{252}Cf plasma desorption (PD) have also made contributions to the analysis of nucleic acid components intractable to the standard EI and CI methods, but the potential of these methods has not as yet been exploited to the same degree as that of FAB.

A third important factor was the introduction of the thermospray (TSP) method (3) of coupling a liquid chromatograph (LC) to a mass spectrometer to provide an LC–MS system compatible with the chromatographic conditions required for the separation of nucleic acid bases, nucleosides, and nucleotides. Of equal importance as an interface was that TSP also provided a new method of producing ions from nonvolatile, underivatized nucleic acid components. Previous LC–MS systems, that is, the moving-belt and direct-liquid-injection (DLI) interfaces were capable of ion production using only standard EI and CI conditions; thus, sample volatility was somewhat of a limitation with these earlier LC–MS interfaces.

Other developments that have expanded capabilities for the mass spectral analysis of nucleic acid components include the development of new or more functional mass analyzers such as the hybrid mass spectrometers, three- and four-sector magnetic instruments, and the triple quadrupole. Coupled with advances in computer design and software availability, such techniques as mass spectrometry/mass spectrometry (MS/MS) with collisionally induced dissociation (CID) are proving to be, or have the potential of becoming, tools of fundamental importance in solving problems of biochemical and biomedical interest concerning the nucleic acids.

The intent of this review is to provide both the novice and advanced researcher with an overview of the current status of the role of mass spectrometry in the analysis of nucleic acid components of all classes. The first topic to be discussed is sample preparation prior to GC–MS analysis, because even with the powerful tools available in a modern mass-spectrometry laboratory, sample preparation remains the key to a successful analysis. The next section will present structure–fragmentation relationships for interpretation of EI spectra of nucleosides and other nucleic acid components. A number of examples will illustrate the continuing importance EI in structure elucidation and quantitative problems. The importance of CI, particularly in obtaining data of clinical significance, will follow. Newer methods of analyzing nucleic acid components, especially very polar and high-molecular-weight samples, for example, nucleotides and polynucleotides, will be described in the section on desorption methods. The application of LC–MS to the analysis of nucleic acid bases and nucleosides will then be discussed. Throughout, attention will be given to practical considerations of these analytical techniques, and the value of MS/MS, CID, and other methods will be shown. The chapter will close with some observations and thoughts as to the future of mass spectrometry in the analysis of nucleic acid components.

A number of fundamental review articles/chapters/papers on the topic of the application of mass spectrometry to the analysis of nucleic acid components have appeared over the years. These references should be considered as mandatory reading for those who are new to the field; these articles also will be of considerable utility to established researchers who wish to review the fundamentals or have at hand ready reference material. The fundamental reference to the mass spectrometry of nucleic acid components is McCloskey's chapter in *Nucleic Acid Chemistry* (4). This chapter describes the basic structure–fragmentation rules for the interpretation of the mass spectra of nucleic acid bases, nucleosides, and nucleotides and the important derivatives of these compound classes, and provides a literature review to approximately 1972. The literature through mid-1979 is thoroughly covered in the chapters by Hignite in *Biochemical Applications of Mass Spectrometry* and the supplementary volume to this book (5, 6). The surveys by Burlingame et al. (7) are also valuable aids for searching the current literature. These articles appear every 2 years and are very thorough in their citations. Finally, a comprehensive, general review of the field, emphasizing the clinical aspects of the mass spectrometry has recently been published (8).

More selective reviews or articles on the mass spectrometry of nucleic acid components have covered the major topics of experimental approaches and sample preparation (9, 10), derivatization (11–15), analysis of tRNA hydrolysates (16, 17), DNA adducts (18), and the use of FAB (19–21), FD (22), PD (23), and LC–MS (24) in the analysis of nucleic acid components.

2. SAMPLE PREPARATION

A number of factors must be considered in designing a method for the preparation of a sample containing a nucleic acid component prior to analysis using mass spectrometry. Broadly speaking, three questions must be asked in planning a sample preparation scheme: (1) What are the capabilities of the mass spectrometer(s) that will be used in the experiment? (2) What is the complexity of the sample to be analyzed? (3) What is the sensitivity level needed to obtain the desired information? Although answers to these questions may be individually determined, the overall design of the sample preparation scheme will depend on the mutual interdependence of the answers. Since few researchers have access to all needed equipment, instrumental capability is, probably, the limiting factor in designing a method of sample preparation.

2.1. Type of Mass Spectrometer Needed for Analysis of Nucleic Acid Components

Nucleic acids and their components may be divided into the following classes: nucleic acid bases, nucleosides, nucleotides, oligonucleotides, and intact RNA and DNA. The range of physical properties, for example, solubility, volatility, polarity, and molecular weight, represented by these compound classes is extremely wide. Because of this diversity in physical properties, a single mass spectrometer does not have the capability of performing the analytical functions needed to solve all problems of interest in nucleic acid chemistry.

Most problems in nucleic acid chemistry can be approached using commercially available magnetic or quadrupole mass analyzers and would, in general, permit the analysis of the first three compound classes listed previously. For example, either of these two instrument types would solve a majority of the problems encountered in a synthetic, biochemical, or clinical laboratory. For the clinical laboratory involved in quantitation of antimetabolites, the quadrupole may offer advantages in terms of initial purchase price, upkeep, and operator training. On the other hand, even though more expensive and requiring greater expertise in operation, the magnetic-sector instruments offer the powerful advantage of being able to determine exact mass values, measurement of which are needed to assign elemental compositions to the ions in the mass spectra of compounds of unknown structure, including drug metabolites, that may be encountered in a biological matrix.

For general work in the area of nucleic acid bases and nucleosides, the required mass-spectrometry capabilities include a solids probe, a gas chromatograph coupled to the mass spectrometer, ionization by EI and CI, and a mass range of at least 1000 Daltons. If the identification of any unknowns is anticipated, the additional cost of the magnetic-sector instrument may be justified.

Alternative approaches or exceptions to the standard instrument previously described would include situations where the same samples are being analyzed on a routine basis, for example, in a pharmacokinetic study of a low-molecular-weight compound amenable to GC–MS analysis. In this case, a "bench-top"-type instrument, either a quadrupole or ion-trap mass spectrometer, would suffice. The advantage of a mass spectrometer, relative to FID, EC, or NPD, as a

GC detector in these, or any, applications, is in increased specificity and sensitivity.

The more polar and higher-molecular-weight nucleic acid compound classes will require analysis using more sophisticated techniques. If the analysis of free nucleotides or intact oligonucleotides is required, the first approach would be analysis using FAB ionization. This method will provide molecular weight and some structural information in a relatively simple manner. Mass range requirements are, obviously, determined by the molecular weight of the sample and, at least historically, a magnetic instrument would be preferred—although quadrupole mass filters are now available with a mass range to 3000 Daltons. Because of significant contamination of the source from the continued presence of a matrix, FAB experiments should be performed on a dedicated mass spectrometer; instrument downtime for maintenance will increase significantly if all ionization modes are performed on a single instrument, especially if the instrument is used for high-resolution mass measurements. A similar argument applies to LC–MS, that is, an instrument needs to be dedicated to this mode of operation. The analysis of nucleic acid components by LC–MS, except the most simple bases and nucleosides, is *not* a routine matter with any of the currently available interfaces. However, considerable research is being done in this area.

As stated earlier, most applications of mass spectrometry to the analysis of nucleic acids and their components are possible using standard magnetic-sector or quadrupole mass spectrometers. More sophisticated techniques like MS/MS and LC–MS are still in the experimental stages and are not yet considered routine. Likewise, newer techniques, such as continuous-flow FAB, have not yet been applied to a wide variety of problems and are not readily available in most laboratories. These more advanced techniques are discussed in later sections.

For purposes of illustration, a "standard" mass spectrometer needed for analysis of compound classes ranging from nucleic acid bases through small oligonucleotides will have the following characteristics: a double-focusing magnetic-sector instrument with a mass range of 2000 Daltons with ionization by EI, CI, and FAB, with the latter technique being available on a second mass spectrometer, if possible. Inlet systems will include a solids probe, FAB probe, and capillary gas chromatograph. Software and hardware will be available for performing both low- and high-resolution mass measurements. Metastable ion spectra may be acquired using daughter, parent, or neutral loss scans. Such an instrument will permit the analysis of most nucleic-acid-related samples of interest to the synthetic chemist wishing to characterize a newly prepared nucleoside, the biochemist attempting to identify a modified nucleoside isolated from tRNA, or the clinician studying the pharmacokinetics of a new nucleic-acid-related antimetabolite used in the treatment of cancer, AIDS, or other diseases.

2.2. Sample Class and Complexity

The complexity of a nucleic-acid-related sample may range from a single component, for example, a starting material in a synthetic reaction, to a complex mixture of 20 or more nucleosides in a urine sample or tRNA hydrolysate. Mixtures containing a small number of components may be analyzed directly using careful control of the heating rate of the direct probe to effect fractional distillation of the components. However, in all except the most simple of cases, some form of chromatography will be required to separate the components. (Direct analysis of mixtures can also be achieved using MS/MS techniques, but such experiments require access to a hybrid mass spectrometer, a triple quadrupole, or a multisector mass spectrometer. These instruments and their application to the analysis of nucleic acid components will be described subsequently.) Assuming sufficient sample is available, components of a mixture may be isolated using paper (25), thin layer (TLC) (26), or high-pressure liquid chromatography (HPLC) (27) to fractionate the more complex samples prior to mass spectrometry. The purified components can then be analyzed by EI, CI, or FAB using the probe inlet or, after derivatization, GC (EI and CI only).

In many situations, the class of nucleic acid component, that is, base, nucleoside, nucleotide, or oligonucleotide, is fixed and no decisions need be made concerning the form in which to analyze the sample. For example, the characterization of natural products should proceed in such a manner that the structure of the sample is not altered. Thus, the novel nucleoside antibiotic A201A (1), produced by *Streptomyces capreolus* and showing high *in vivo* activity against Gram-positive bacteria, was isolated by a combination of extraction and chromatographic techniques, and the structure determined using mass spectrometry [EI (low and high resolution) and field desorption], NMR, and chemical techniques (28). Similar situations exist, that is, the class of the target compound is fixed, when the analytical objective is the identification or quantitation of naturally occurring pyrimidine (29) and purine (30) bases in

1, A201A

biological materials, for monitoring the excretion of methylated purines (31), or for determination of drug levels in urine or blood samples during clinical studies, for example, theophylline (**2**) (32), allopurinol (**3**) (33), 6-mercaptopurine (**4**) (34, 35), and arabinocytidine (**5**) (36, 37). However, when the objective of the analysis is to determine the structure of a component in RNA, quantitate a base in DNA, or to identify the structure of a DNA adduct, a decision must be made as to the class of nucleic acid component that will provide the greatest structural information, the best sensitivity and most simple procedure of sample preparation.

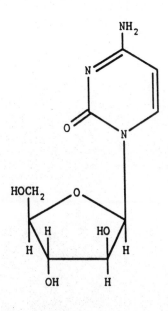

2, Theophylline

3, Allopurinol

4, 6-Mercaptopurine

5, Cytosine arabinoside

2.2.1. HYDROLYSIS OF tRNA

When the identification or quantitation of components of nucleic acids is the objective, a decision to perform the analysis at the base, nucleoside, or mononucleotide stage must be made. The analysis of RNA, especially tRNA, for modified components is best performed at the nucleoside stage for three principal reasons (9). First, the experimental details of the enzymatic degradation of the RNA have been well studied (38, 39) and a variety of enzyme systems are available that provide quantitative release of nucleosides from tRNA under mild conditions. Thus, treatment of RNA with venom phosphodiestrase or nuclease P_1 will produce mononucleotides from which the phosphate groups are then cleaved by exposure to alkaline phosphatase. As an example (taken directly from Ref. 38), tRNA (40 μg) in 40 μL of water is incubated with 1 u of RNase T_2 for 12 h at 37°C in a screw-capped vial. Triethylammonium bicarbonate (0.2 M, 4 μL), alkaline phosphatase (1 u) and snake venom phosphodiesterase (1 u, 1 μL) are added and the mixture incubated at pH8 for 6 h at 37°C. The hydrolysate reaction mixture is then dried under vacuum over P_2O_5 and converted to the TMS derivative for separation and analysis by GC–MS (see subsequent discussion).

A similar approach, that is, the enzymatic conversion of a nucleotide to a nucleoside, has been used for the quantitative analysis of the nucleotides isolated from the blood of cancer patients receiving 6-mercaptopurine (4) (6-MP) treatment (40). *In vivo*, 6-MP is enzymatically converted to a mixture of 6-mercaptopurine riboside monophosphate (6-MPRP) (6) and 6-methylmercaptopurine riboside monophosphate (6-MMPRP) (7).

Because the chromatographic separation of nucleosides is more easily performed than the analysis of the nucleotides, alkaline phosphatase is used to cleave the nucleotides (previously separated from other compounds) to the nucleosides 8 and 9, which are then analyzed by GC–MS after derivatization.

6-MP $\xrightarrow{\text{in vivo}}$ 6-MPRP + 6-MMPRP $\xrightarrow[\text{phosphatase}]{\text{alkaline}}$

4   6   7

8, 6-Mercaptopurine riboside; R = H

9, 6-Methylmercaptopurine riboside; R = CH₃

The second argument for analysis of tRNA hydrolysates at the nucleoside level is that, in contrast to DNA, RNA contains a 2'-hydroxyl group, which may be methylated. Hydrolysis to the base stage would not reveal 2'-O-methylation and important information concerning the posttranscriptional modifications present in the tRNA would not be detected. Finally, the mass spectrum of a nucleoside contains the same structural information as the spectrum of the nucleotide, but without the complication of structurally uninformative phosphate ions diluting the ion current of structurally relevant ions.

Additional details of tRNA isolation, source of reagents and significance of tRNA modifications may be found in the original literature cited in the above section.

2.2.2. HYDROLYSIS OF DNA

In contrast to RNA, DNA does not undergo sugar modification. Therefore, hydrolysis of DNA to the base stage does not result in the loss of information and the base level is preferred for the analysis of modified bases in DNA. Both enzymatic and chemical degradation may be used to free the nucleic acid bases from the DNA chain. The following enzymatic approach has been used for the preparation of DNA for analysis of the modified bases resulting from the free radical radiation-induced damage to DNA (41): 1 mg of radiation-exposed DNA is dissolved in 0.5 mL of 10 mM Tris-HCl buffer (pH 8.5) containing 2 mM magnesium chloride. This solution is incubated with DNase I (100 u), spleen exonuclease (0.01 u), snake venom exonuclease (0.5 u), and alkaline phosphatase (10 u) for 24 h at 37°C. The sample is then lyophilized and the TMS derivative prepared prior to analysis by GC–MS.

A chemical method for hydrolysis of DNA to the base stage has been described for the quantitation of 5-methylcytosine (**10**) by isotope dilution methods (42): DNA is prepared for hydrolysis by placing aliquots (typically 0.02 A$_{260}$ unit) in a 500 μL polyethylene centrifuge tube, followed by addition of the appropriate amount of internal standard. After careful mixing, the DNA solution is transferred by syringe to a 5 cm × 4 mm o.d. tube fashioned from thoroughly

10, 5-Methylcytosine

cleaned Pyrex tubing. Solutions are dried *in vacuo* and hydrolysis carried out in 10–15 μL of distilled formic acid (adjusted to 98% with distilled H_2O) for 1 h at 175°C. After digestion, formic acid volume is reduced on an 80°C sand bath and residual acid removed *in vacuo*. The residue is then derivatized for quantitation by GC–MS.

2.2.3. URINE SAMPLES

The identification and quantitation of nucleic acid bases and nucleosides in normal and pathogenic human urine is of considerable interest because elevated, or depressed, levels of these compounds have potential utility as "biological markers" of disease states that are characterized by abnormal nucleic acid metabolism. By monitoring the excretion levels of selected modified nucleosides in urine, the diagnosis of such diseases as cancer (43, 44), immunodeficiency disorders (45), and AIDS (46, 47) may be possible. Levels of these nucleosides may also provide a means of monitoring a course of therapy, since, if the disease is responding to treatment, a change in the urinary levels of these compounds should be observed.

Methods for the isolation of the nucleoside fraction of human urine are based, primarily, on the work of high-performance liquid chromatographers, modifications to which are applicable to mass spectrometry. The major problem with most of the published sample preparation methods (48, 49) is the use of phosphate buffers, which, being nonvolatile, will remain admixed with the sample and interfere with the subsequent derivatization step. The use of volatile buffers (50, 51) should, however, eliminate these problems. In addition, the use of volatile buffers is a requirement for the separation of mixtures by LC–MS (see subsequent discussion).

A rapid method for the preparation of urine and serum samples for analysis of modified nucleosides involves the use of a Radial-Pak cartridge (52): An aliquot of the sample (0.5 mL) is transferred to a 1.5 mL microfuge tube, 300 μL of 2.5 M ammonium acetate buffer (pH 9.5) are added and the sample mixed intermittently for 5 min with a Vortex mixer. The sample is centrifuged at 12,000 g for 5 min and the supernatant is transferred onto a phenyl boronate affinity column (4.5 cm × 0.7 cm) after equilibration with 0.25 M ammonium acetate buffer (pH 8.8). The nucleosides are eluted with 10 mL of 0.1 M formic acid. The eluate is transferred to glass tubes and lyophilized. The lyophilized material is reconstituted in 2.0 mL of an aqueous solution containing an internal standard and analyzed, in this case, using HPLC. Derivatization prior to reconstitution should provide a sample amenable to analysis by GC–MS. A similar approach is used for the isolation of the nucleoside fraction of serum.

One problem with the use of boronate columns is that nucleosides modified in the sugar by methylation of the 2′-hydroxyl group are not retained on the column and the presence of these compounds may be overlooked. An alternative procedure using charcoal adsorption (53, 54) avoids this difficulty. This large-scale method (54) proceeds in the following manner: A 24 h pooled urine sample is adjusted to pH3 and passed through a column (2.54 cm × 50 cm) of charcoal-celite (50 g each). The column is washed with water (3 L) until the washings are chloride free and the column-bound material eluted with 2 N NH$_4$OH in 50% aqueous ethanol (3 L). The eluate is concentrated to a small volume (50 mL) and applied to a column (2.54 cm × 35 cm) of 125 g of AG-1X formate resin. The column is washed with 2.5 L of water and the wash concentrated to about 50 mL and then passed through a column of DEAE cellulose equilibrated with 0.14 M boric acid. The DEAE column is first washed with 3 L of 0.14 boric acid and then eluted with 4 L of 0.70 boric acid to obtain the nucleoside fraction. The urinary nucleoside fraction is then carried through additional chromatographic steps for the isolation of the target compound.

Both of the above methods are valuable in the separation of nucleosides of both known and unknown structures from human urine. However, caution should be exercised with any isolation scheme to prevent decomposition of the sample. For example, 3-methyluridine (**11**), recently confirmed by GC–MS to be a component of human urine (55), will decompose upon exposure to boronate columns (pH 9) (56) and the presence of this nucleoside in human urine could, thus, be overlooked.

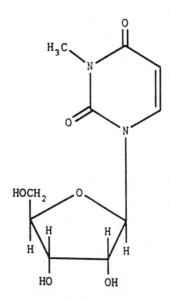

11, 3-Methyluridine

2.2.4. EXTRACTION OF NUCLEIC ACID COMPONENTS FROM CELLS

Analysis of cellular nucleic acid components is more difficult than that of most other biological sources, because of the complexity of the medium, and more extensive sample preparation schemes must be used. As an example, a ^{13}C-tracer method developed to study *de novo* pyrimidine biosynthesis *in vitro* and *in vivo* involved preparation of samples for analysis by GC–MS in the following manner (57): L1210 cultured cells growing in RPMI 1630 plus L-glutamine and 5% fetal calf serum were diluted to a concentration of 0.6×10^6 cells/mL and grown in fresh medium for 24 h prior to the experiment to achieve concentrations between 1.2 and 1.7×10^6 cells/mL. The samples were immediately placed on ice and sedimented at 100 g for 10 min at 4°C. The media were discarded, the cell pellets were resuspended in 1 mL phosphate-buffered saline, and the internal standard added. The cell proteins were denatured with 10% trichloroacetic acid (TCA) (1 mL) and the precipitate sedimented at 300 g for 20 min. Excess TCA was removed by washing twice with 2 mL of 1,2-trichlorotrifluoroethane : n-trioctylamine (2:1, freshly prepared). Uracil nucleotides in the acid-soluble fraction were then enzymatically degraded to uridine by incubating the samples with phosphodiesterase 1 Type IV and alkaline phosphatase type 1-S for 30 min. The samples were then lyophilized and the permethyl derivative prepared for GC–MS experiments.

2.2.5.   OTHER BIOLOGICAL SAMPLES

The literature is extensive in methods for the preliminary isolation of nucleic acid components, primarily nucleic acid bases, from other biological media. Examples include the analysis of orotic acid (**12**) and uracil (**13**) in amniotic fluid (58), the extraction of 5-fluorouracil (5-FU) (**14**) (59) from plasma, and the isolation of cytokinins from plant materials (60–63). For a more thorough coverage of the literature in this area see Ref. 8.

12, Orotic acid   13, Uracil   14, 5-Fluorouracil

2.3.   Derivatization

The analysis of complex mixtures of bases and nucleosides, especially samples derived from a biological matrix, is best achieved using a capillary gas chromatograph. However, because of the polar nature of the nucleic acid bases and nucleosides, derivatization is necessary. Although a number of examples of the gas chromatography of free bases have appeared in the literature, the extra step of derivatization is preferred for a number of reasons. First, the potential of degradation of the sample during chromatography is significantly reduced because the derivative, being more volatile, elutes at a lower temperature and spends less time on the column. Second, peak shape is improved by elimination of tailing of the sample caused by interaction with the stationary phase. Finally, the increased molecular weight of the derivative helps to eliminate interfering background ions at lower mass values by shifting the molecular ion to higher mass, thus providing a cleaner mass spectrum.

2.3.1. TRIMETHYLSILYL DERIVATIVES

A variety of functional groups are used to overcome the nonvolatile character of the nucleic acid components, with the most generally useful being the trimethylsilyl (TMS) derivative (9–11). Major advantages of this derivative include good chromatographic peak shape permitting resolution of closely related samples (64), availability of excellent molecular weight and structural information from the mass spectrum (4, 12) (discussed in the next section), and ease of sample preparation. Use of the TMS derivative is applicable to all classes of nucleic acid components; these derivatives have been characterized by both GC and MS for nucleic acid bases (65), nucleosides (11), and nucleotides (66, 67). In addition, reagents for the preparation of the TMS-($^2H_9$) are commercially available and analysis of the mass spectrum of this C^2H_3-analog provides additional information helpful in the interpretation of the spectra of unknowns (68). Finally, since this is the most commonly used derivative for mass spectral analysis of nucleic acid components, an extensive library of mass spectral data has accumulated over the years (69).

The procedure for preparation of the TMS derivatives of nucleic acid bases, nucleosides, and, in general, nucleotides is as follows (12): After *thorough* drying, a 50 μg sample of the nucleoside is heated in a sealed microreaction vial with N,O-bis(trimethylsilyl)triflouroacetamide (BSTFA), trimethylchlorosilane (TMCS), and pyridine (100 : 1 : 10) at 100°C for 1 h. A 1 μL sample is then injected onto the gas chromatographic inlet and the mass spectrum acquired. Lesser quantities of samples may be used, depending on the sensitivity of the mass spectrometer.

Chromatographic conditions are extremely variable with a variety of column sizes and types being described in the literature. Chromatographic conditions are thus not critical but column selection should be based on the highest possible operating temperature with the least amount of column bleed. Typical operating conditions used in the author's laboratory for the separation of complex nucleoside mixtures are a DB-5 capillary column (30 m × 0.25 mm, 0.25-μm film thickness). An initial temperature of 180°C with a program rate of 4 deg/min to 300°C and a 5-min hold time provides good results for the separation of urinary nucleoside mixtures.

Different chromatographic conditions have been used for the GC separation of various nucleic acid components (as their TMS derivatives) such as radiation-damaged (70) and other (71) DNA bases, cytokinins (72), and nucleosides in tRNA hydrolysates (73). The exact experimental conditions needed to effect a particular separation may be empirical, but a literature search (5, 7, 8, 11, 12) should lead to appropriate conditions, or to conditions that may be easily modified to suit the problem.

In general, the TMS moiety replaces all exchangeable hydrogens in both the sugar and base, with some exceptions. Thus, uridine will produce the uridine(TMS)$_4$ analog **15** (74), as the predominant derivative. Compounds with exocyclic amino groups will add only one TMS function due to the steric hindrance resulting from the presence of a second TMS group, for example, guanosine(TMS)$_5$ (**16**).

15, Uridine(TMS)$_4$ 16, Guanosine(TMS)$_5$

The derivatization reaction proceeds smoothly in most cases, but abnormal products have been reported. For example, the addition of an oxygen atom to the C-8 position of 7-alkylated purine nucleosides will occur unless atmospheric oxygen is excluded (75), alkylated exocyclic amino groups do not add a TMS group and thymidine and 5-fluorouridine do not react in the base portion of the molecule. An additional problem is encountered with cytidine and its analogs which produces broad peaks in the chromatogram, and alternative approaches must be used for the gas chromatography of these compounds, for example, formation of an etheno analog (76) or use of a TMS-acetate mixed derivative (77). The TMS derivatives are, however, susceptible to hydrolysis and complete replacement of all exchangeable hydrogens may not be observed.

2.3.2. PERALKYL DERIVATIVES

Of the peralkyl derivatives of nucleic acid bases, nucleosides, and nucleotides, the permethyl analog has been most widely studied (14, 78). The permethyl derivatives offer a number of advantages relative to the TMS derivatives. First, the methyl ether bond is considerably more stable to hydrolysis relative to the TMS and other silyl-based derivatives. Second, except for the most complex of the hypermodified nucleosides, full replacement of exchangeable hydrogens is observed during the derivatization reaction; substitution on exocyclic amino groups is useful for distinguishing free from substituted amino groups. Finally, the mass of each added functional group is only 14 mass units verṣus 72 mass units for the TMS derivative. Although the mass increase of the TMS derivative is not a major consideration with magnetic and higher-mass-range quadrupole instruments, the mass range of the "bench-top" instruments may be a consideration in selecting the appropriate derivative.

At least five different procedures for the preparation of permethyl derivatives of nucleic acid bases, nucleosides, and nucleotides have been described and reviewed (14). The two most commonly used methods of preparing these derivatives are the methylsulfinyl carbanion method (78) and an "on-column" procedure using trimethylanilinium hydroxide (TMAH) (14, 79–83).

In the methylsulfinyl carbanion procedure, sodium hydride (NaH) in an oil suspension is rinsed with anhydrous ether to remove the oil. The NaH is then added to dry dimethyl sulfoxide (DMSO) and the mixture stirred rapidly, with heating to 65°C in an argon atmosphere, until the evolution of hydrogen ceases. The anion solution is used without further purification and is stored under nitrogen in an airtight container at 4°C for future use. For the preparation of the permethyl derivative of a nucleoside, 50 μg of the sample is dissolved in dry DMSO (100 μL), a 10-fold excess of the anion solution is added, and the reaction kept at room temperature for 30 min. An equimolar amount of methyl iodide is added and the reaction allowed to proceed for 2 h at room temperature. Excess anion is destroyed by addition of water (1 mL). The permethylated nucleoside is extracted with chloroform, dried over sodium sulfate and an aliquot (0.5–1 μL) injected onto the gas chromatograph. If sample quantity is limited, the chloroform layer may be evaporated to provide a more concentrated sample.

The TMAH procedure (14, 79–83) is experimentally simple and much faster than the anion method. The nucleoside sample (50 μg) is dissolved in a 0.2 M solution of TMAH in methanol (100 μL) and a 1 μL sample of the solution is injected into the hot (300°C) injection port of the gas chromatograph. The trimethylanilinium hydroxide in methanol reagent is commercially available (MethElute™, Pierce Chemical Co., Rockford, IL), and a method for the preparation of deuterium-labeled TMAH has been described (83). Use of the deuterium-labeled methylating reagent parallels that of the labeled TMS derivatives.

A problem with the permethyl derivatives is the formation of isomers for guanosine and cytidine (78). With guanosine, two products are formed in approximately equal proportion while cytidine produces a minor peak in the chromatogram followed by a major component. The structures of these four products have been established as **17–20**, based on examination of reference compounds (78).

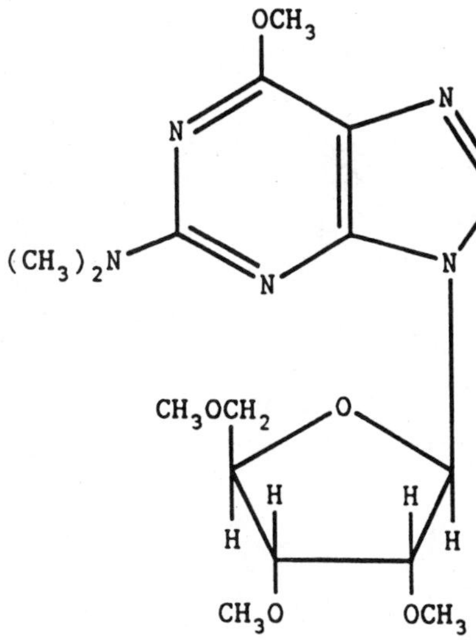

17

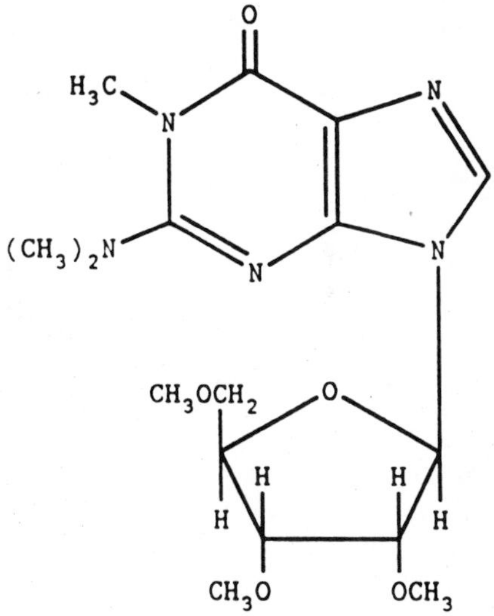

18

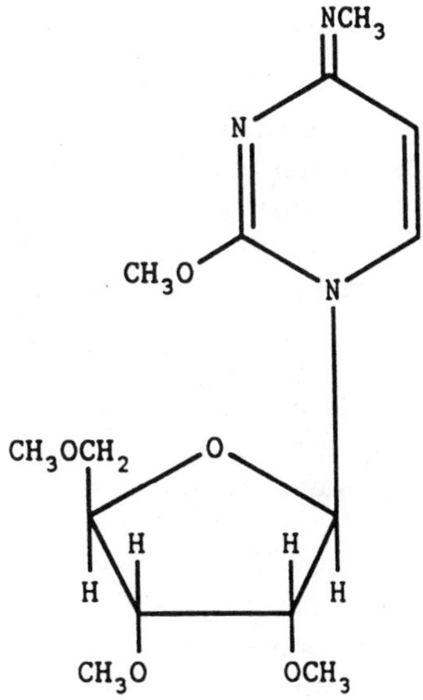

19

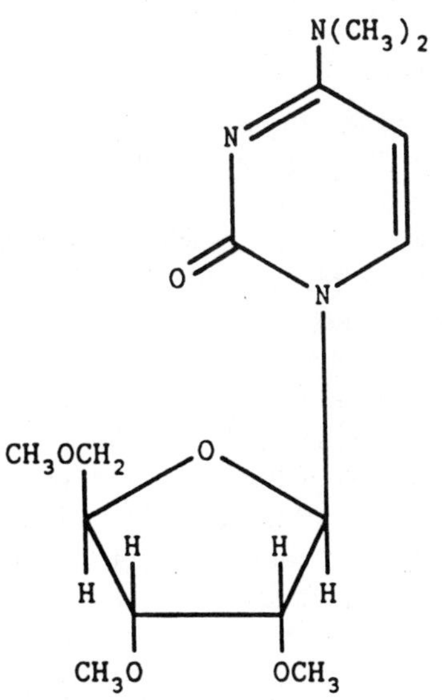

20

A unique reaction is observed between 5,6-dihydropyrimidine nucleosides and methylsulfinyl anion–methyl iodide that produces the 3,5,5-trimethyl analogs, for example, **21** (84). Thus, in spite of offering the advantages in terms of stability and complete derivatization of exocyclic amino groups, a number of side reactions occur during permethylation that could complicate the identification or quantitation of nucleosides in a mixture.

21

Although use of the permethylation reaction to form a volatile derivative of nucleic acid components has not been as widely used as the TMS derivatives, literature reports describe the analysis of permethyl derivatives in studies of the pyrimidine *de novo* pathway (57), for the determination of nucleic acid bases in human plasma and urine samples (63), and for the quantitation of nucleic acid bases and nucleosides in cancer patient plasma (85).

Closely related to the permethyl derivatives are the perethyl analogs that find utility in the chromatographic separation of cytosine, adenine, and guanine bases, either as the perethyl derivatives or as a mixed derivative of ethyl and acetate functions (86). Preparation of these derivatives was explored because the compounds mentioned previously can, as the TMS derivative, show tailing and humps in the baseline of the chromatogram. The TMS derivatives of cytosine and 5-methylcytosine are also poorly resolved during gas chromatography. The ethyl and ethyl-acetate derivatives show good chromatographic characteristics and the cytosine/5-methylcytosine resolution is significantly enhanced with this derivative. These perethyl, or mixed, derivatives may find utility in the separation of DNA hydrolysates since they are easily prepared with ethyl iodide being substituted for methyl iodide in the reaction, and show good chromatographic properties.

2.3.3. STERICALLY CROWDED TRIALKYLSILYL DERIVATIVES

Several alternatives to the TMS derivative have been examined in an effort to produce a derivative that possesses the excellent gas chromatographic properties of the TMS derivatives but which are not as susceptible to hydrolysis. A number of such derivatives have been examined in detail and include the *tert*-butyldimethylsilyl (TBDMS), cyclotetramethyleneisopropylsilyl (TMIPS), cyclotetramethylene-*tert*-butylsilyl (TMTBS) (13), and vinyldimethylsilyl (VDMS) (87) groups. Of these, the only one to emerge with value in GC–MS studies is the TBDMS analog.

The advantages of the TBDMS derivative, relative to those of the TMS derivative, include a significantly greater stability to hydrolysis (this derivative was in fact first used as a blocking group in nucleoside and nucleotide synthesis and may be recrystallized) and the presence of a strong M-57 ion that dominates the mass spectrum, in most cases. Because of the size of the TBDMS group, not all exchangeable hydrogens are displaced and a mixture of derivatives is formed in the case of nucleosides (13). The use of a TMS–TBDMS mixed derivative has overcome, to some extent, this difficulty while retaining the powerful fragmentation-directing capability of the *tert*-butyldimethylsilyl group. The TBDMS or TMS–TBDMS mixed derivative finds utility in the low-level quantitation of 5-methylcytosine in DNA hydrolysates (42), where the M-57 ion carries approximately 40% of the total ion current, and in a GC–MS study to identify and quantify the metabolic incorporation of stable isotope-labeled adenine into cytokinins (88). The TBDMS derivative has also been applied to the mass spectral analysis of cytokinin bases (89). However, it should be noted that, owing to the potential for rearrangement reactions during gas chromatography, the use of the mixed derivative is recommended (90).

Preparation of the TBDMS derivative of 5-methylcytosine and thymidine proceeds as follows (42): 10 μL of a 1 : 1 mixture of pyridine and *N*-methyl-*n*-(*tert*-butyl)dimethylsilyl)trifluoroacetamide containing 1% *tert*-butyldimethylchlorosilane is added to a dry DNA digest in the original hydrolysis tube. The solution is heated in a sealed tube for 20 min at 120°C, after which time the derivatization is essentially complete. (Distillation of the reagents was necessary prior to use to remove trace contaminants which interfered with the analysis of DNA containing low levels of 5-methylcytosine.) The recent commercial availability (Regis Chemical Co., Morton Grove, IL) of the reagents needed for preparation of the TBDMS derivative should stimulate the use of this blocking group, especially for cases where enhanced detection limits are needed.

2.3.4. FLUORINATED DERIVATIVES

The final class of derivatives of interest are those containing fluorine that are used primarily in cases where low-level detection or quantitation studies are being conducted. In general, these derivatives are used in conjunction with electron-capture negative-ionization (EC–NI) mass spectrometry to provide the lowest possible detection limits.

Trifluoroacetate (TFA) derivatives of ribosides and deoxyribosides are superior to the simple acetate derivatives in terms of both their chromatographic and mass spectrometric properties (15). Hydroxyl groups on both the base and sugar are easily reacted and amino groups with exchangeable hydrogens will add one or two TFA functions. In contrast to the TMS derivatives, however, enolizable carbonyl groups and carboxyl groups do not react. Even in positive ion EI mass spectrometry, the detection limits are very low for some sample classes, as evidenced by the detection of 1 pg of various cytokinins examined using this derivative (91).

TFA derivatives are prepared in the following manner (15): A sample (50–100 μg or proportionally less) of the nucleoside or deoxynucleoside mixture from a DNA hydrolysate is heated with 100 μL of CH_2Cl_2 and 7 μL of trifluoroacetic anhydride in a sealed ampoule for 30 min at 100°. Derivatizing guanosine and related compounds requires heating at 150°C, which causes some cleavage of the glycosidic bonds.

Lowest detection limits are realized, however, by analysis of these fluoro derivatives in the EC–NI mode. For example, detection limits down to 50 fg are reported for the pentafluorobenzyl derivative of 5-fluoro- and 5-chlorouracil (92), and the pentafluorobenzoyl derivatives of 5-methylcytosine and cytosine are detected at the 1 fg level (93). A mixed heptafluorobutryl–pentafluorobenzyl derivative is used in quantitation of the excretion levels of 7-methylguanine following administration of alkylating agents to rats (94), where the derivative has structure **22**.

22

In spite of the fact that a considerable amount of work has been done on the preparation of volatile derivatives of the nucleic acid bases, nucleosides, and, to a lesser degree, the nucleotides, no ideal derivative has yet been developed. For the simple bases and nucleosides, GC–MS is a relatively routine procedure. However, problems still exist in the GC analysis of the hypermodified nucleosides and nucleotides, and other means for the identification and quantitation of the more polar and higher-molecular-weight compounds of this class are being developed, that is, desorption methods of ionization of the free compounds and LC–MS. However, for the identification of a new nucleoside from a natural source, whether that source is a microbial fermentation broth, a tRNA hydrolysate, or the metabolite of an antitumor agent, the first mass spectrometry experiment will most likely be a standard EI analysis, either from the probe or by GC–MS.

3. ELECTRON IMPACT IONIZATION

Electron-impact mass spectrometry remains *the* fundamental ionization mode for the structural elucidation of an unknown nucleic acid component. Even with the assortment of sophisticated approaches to the analysis of nucleosides and nucleotides, the amouht of structural information in the low- and high-resolution EI mass spectrum far exceeds that of any of the other ionization modes. Techniques such as CI, FAB, and thermospray LC–MS should be considered complementary to EI, except in those cases where volatility, following derivatization, is limited and no other approaches using EI are successful.

3.1. Nucleic Acid Bases

The EI mass spectra of the primary nucleic acid bases adenine (**23**), uracil (**13**), guanine (**24**), and cytosine (**25**) and their analogs have been examined in detail, both as the free compounds (4, 95, 96) and as their TMS derivatives (65, 97). In general, the mass spectra of the TMS derivatives of the nucleic acid bases are dominated by peaks representing the M^+ and $(M - 15)^+$ ions and, although some structural information is available, few basic fragmentations are common to all members of a given class of heterocycles. Thus, the interpretation of the mass spectrum of a new modified base is a somewhat unique endeavor, with the observed fragmentation pattern being highly dependent on the site and extent of modification to the basic ring system. Structural assignments in the mass spectrum of a new base are dependent to a significant degree on high-resolution

23, Adenine   24, Guanine

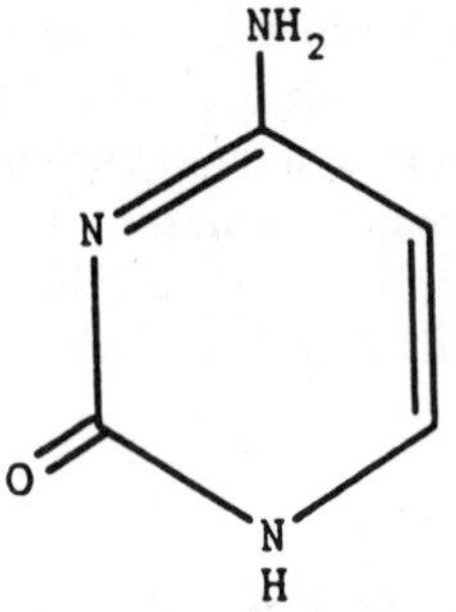

25, Cytosine

mass measurements, on the use of stable isotope-labeled derivatives, and on the knowledge and intuition of the investigator. In spite of this, a number of important qualitative and quantitative applications of EI mass spectrometry, primarily GC–MS studies, have been described.

One of the major applications of GC–MS using EI in the nucleic acid base area to emerge recently has been the identification of changes in DNA structure resulting from interaction with radiation or by reaction of DNA with other organic molecules. Studies in this area are of considerable importance because modifications in DNA structure to any extent, from whatever source, are implicated in mutagenesis, carcinogenesis, and cell death.

Applying GC–MS with EI to the characterization of DNA base damage resulting from an exposure of aqueous solutions of bases, deoxynucleosides or higher-order analogs, including DNA, to ionizing radiation is described in a recent review paper (98). Starting with simple systems, for example, the irradiation of an aqueous solution of thymine (**26**) by a ^{60}Co-γ-source, models have been developed that are applicable to the identification and quantitation of damaged bases in DNA. The complexity of the mixtures formed in such reactions is surprising, even with very simple systems. For example, the capillary gas

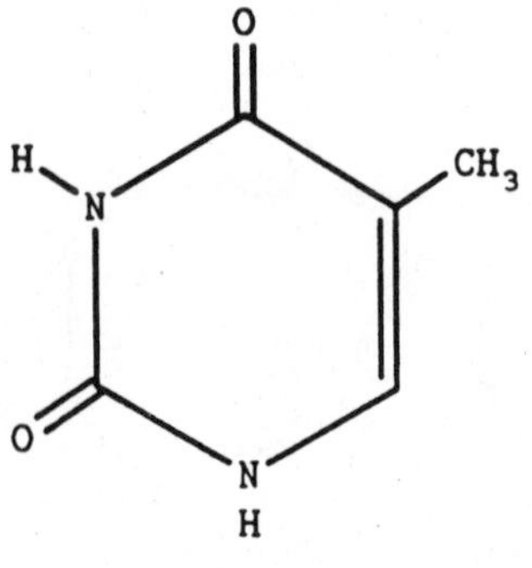

26, Thymine

chromatogram of the products of the thymine experiment (99) shows more than 30 peaks, 18 of which were assigned structures based on the low-resolution mass spectra of the TMS derivatives. Most of the modified bases, including a number of dimeric species, could be accounted for on the basis of either attack by OH· on the C-5 or C-6 positions, or by abstraction of a hydrogen atom from the methyl group, to form the radical intermediates 27–29. Of particular interest are the products formed by pairing any two of the radicals leading to dimers with structures like 30, formed by combination of two of the 27 species. Examining the

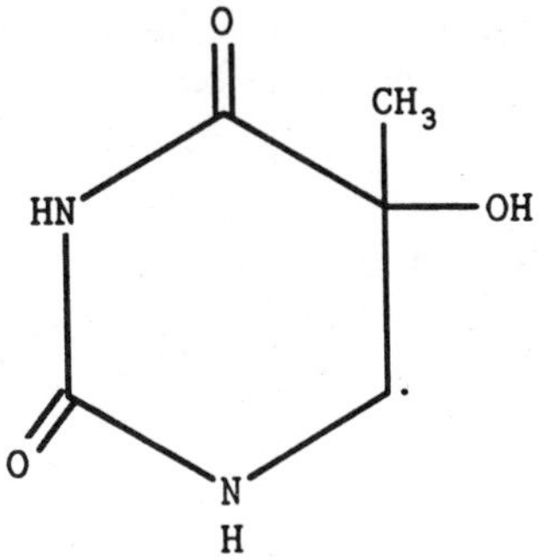

27

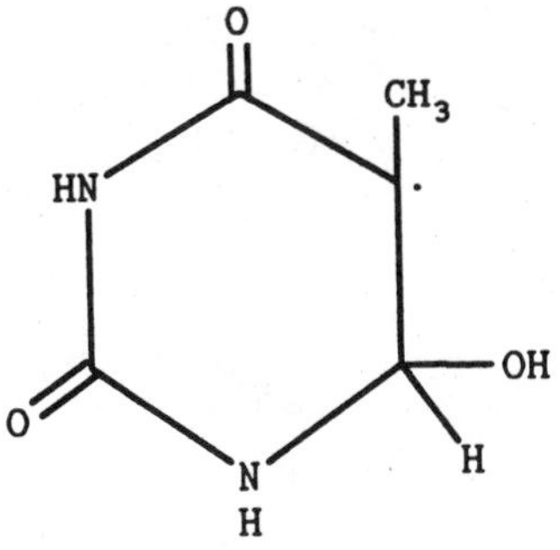

28

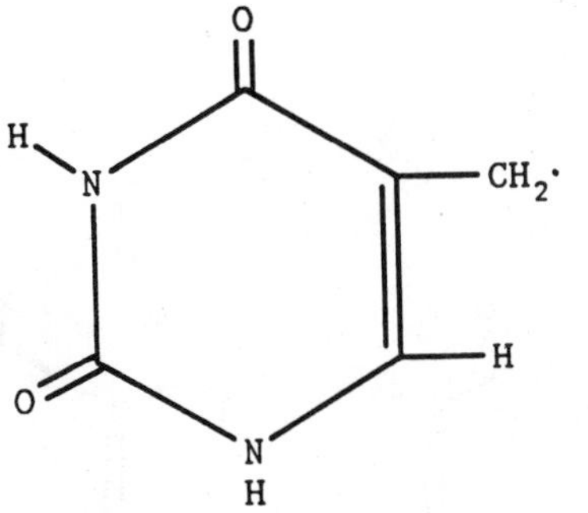

29

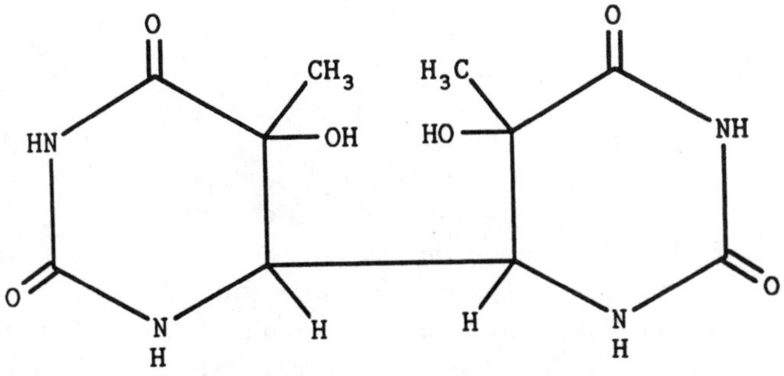

30

mass spectra for each of the GC peaks reveals five components having essentially identical spectra, with characteristic peaks at m/z 718 (M^+) and 703 ($M - 15$), corresponding to isomers of **30** (as its TMS_6 derivative). Further complicating the analysis, however, is that **30**, and its isomers, may eliminate H_2O to form **31** (and isomers). Elimination of a second H_2O can, in turn, lead to **32**. Unfortunately, the stage at which the water molecules are lost is not known and, thus, some confusion arises as to which of the products are formed by the ionizing radiation and which are artifacts of isolation, derivatization, or chromatography. For the analysis of more complex systems, for example, the irradiation of oligodeoxynucleotides or intact DNA, the oligomer is hydrolyzed using formic acid or an appropriate enzyme system to provide the modified bases amenable to analysis by GC–MS.

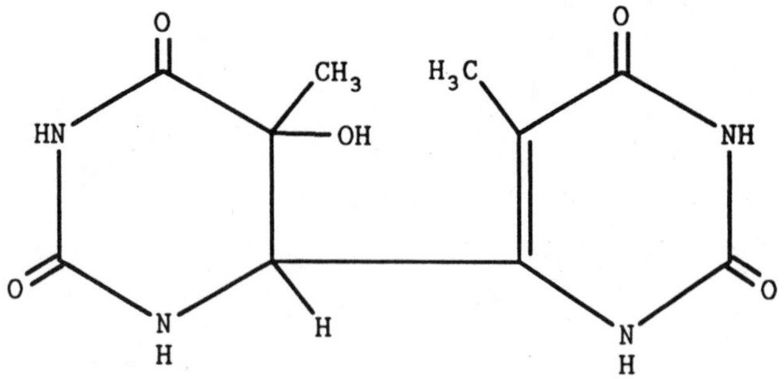

31

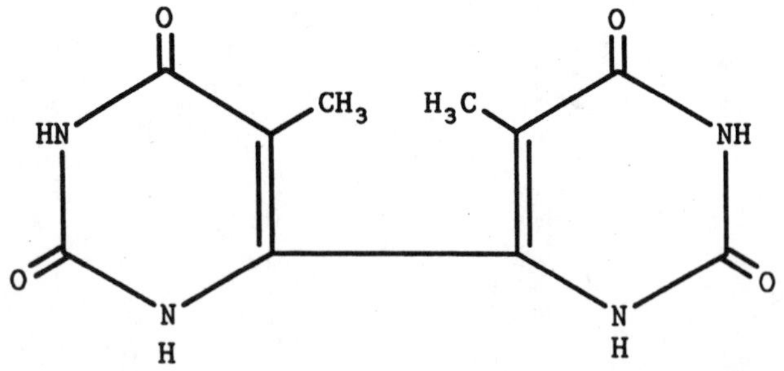

32

Mass spectrometry has been used to identify products formed in the reaction of DNA with the antitumor compound BCNU (N,N'-bis(2-chloroethyl-N-nitrosourea) (**33**) (100). Among the compounds identified following selective release and HPLC separation of 7-substituted purines were 7-(β-chloroethyl)guanine (**34**) and a product resulting from cross-linking, 1,2-(diguan-7-yl)ethane (**35**). Mass spectrometry of the HPLC fraction containing **34** displayed a peak for the molecular ion at m/z 213 with a second isotope peak of

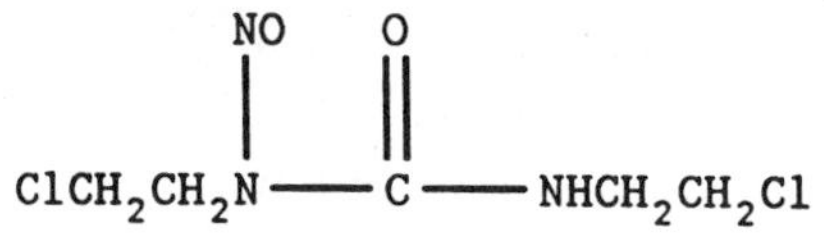

$$\text{ClCH}_2\text{CH}_2\overset{\overset{\displaystyle NO}{|}}{N}\text{---}\overset{\overset{\displaystyle O}{\|}}{C}\text{---}\text{NHCH}_2\text{CH}_2\text{Cl}$$

33, BCNU

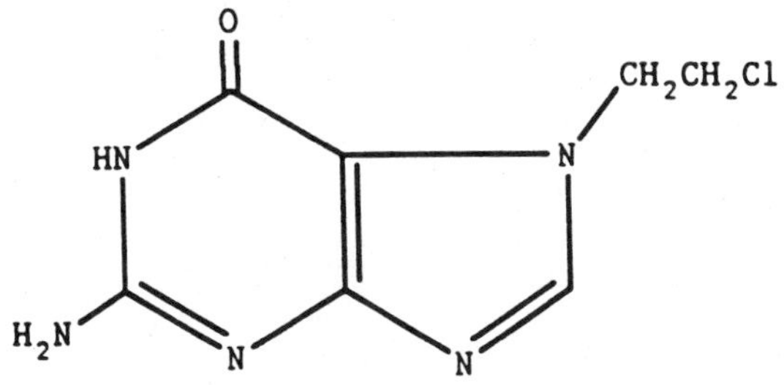

34, 7-(β-chloroethyl)guanine

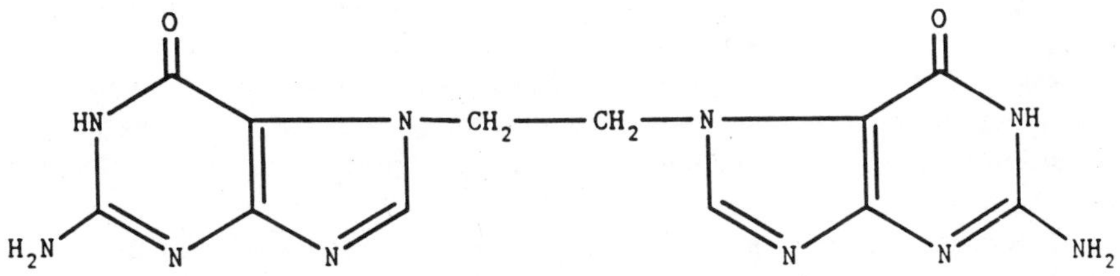

35

correct intensity indicating the presence of ^{37}Cl. Other peaks used in assigning structure were at m/z 177 (M − 36) for the loss of HCl and an M − 49 peak representing the loss of a CH$_2$Cl radical. Fragment ion peaks are also observed at m/z 151, for protonated guanine, and ribose, m/z 133. (An explanation of the origin or significance of the latter peak is not given.) No mass spectrometry is presented for the cross-linked base, which was identified by HPLC and UV based on comparison with a synthetically prepared reference sample. The identification of **35** adds support for the hypothesis that formation of cross-linked DNA species is an important aspect of the antitumor activity of nitrosoureas and the nitrogen mustards.

Another example of cross-link formation of nucleic acid bases and nucleosides is the formation of methylene-bridged adenine and adenosine compounds, for example, **36**, upon reaction with formaldehyde (101). The principal ions in the

36

mass spectrum of the permethylated cross-linked adenine compound (**36**) show fragmentations associated with cleavages along the methylene bridge. A comparison of the spectra of the C^2H_3-derivative with that of the unlabeled analog permitted elucidation of mechanisms of formation for the major ions observed in the spectrum. The spectra of the cross-linked nucleoside analogs display a distinctive pattern of two major clusters of peaks, with the major ions arising from cleavage of the methylene bridge in a manner analogous to that shown for **36**. The other cluster of peaks is associated with the presence of one or both of the ribose entities and to ions related to the general fragmentation of permethylated nucleosides.

Mass spectrometry is also used in more clinically oriented studies involving the identification of drug metabolites and as a tool in pharmacokinetic studies.

Of considerable current interest are drugs that may be of value in treating acquired or genetically determined deficiencies in cell-mediated immune function. The metabolites of one such drug currently in clinical trials, erythro-9-(2-hydroxy-3-nonyl)hypoxanthine (NPT 15392) (**37**) (102), have been isolated from the urine of rats, rabbits, dogs, and monkeys, and their structures determined using GC–MS. Identifying and separating the drug and its metabolites, designated M-1 to M-5, was aided by administration of **27** labeled in the C-8 position with ^{14}C. Following isolation of pure drug and metabolites by TLC and HPLC, the TMS derivatives were prepared and analyzed by GC–MS. Metabolite structures were assigned based on observation of fragment ion peaks in the mass spectrum of **37**, stable isotope incorporation into selected sites of some metabolites, and confirmation by exact mass measurement. Fragmentation leading to major ions represented in the spectrum of **37** and the structures of five of the metabolites are shown subsequently. In all cases, the hypoxanthine base remains unchanged with oxidative metabolism being limited to alteration of the nonyl side chain. Differences in metabolic products are noted between species.

$$37, \text{ NPT } 15392, \quad R = CH_3CH_2CH_2-$$

$$M-1, \quad R = CH_3CH(OH)CH_2-$$

$$M-2, \quad R = HOC(O)CH_2-$$

$$M-3, \quad R = HOC(O)-$$

$$M-4, \quad R = CH_3C(O)CH_2-$$

$$M-5, \quad R = HOC(O)CH_2-$$

The alcohol, ketone, and acid metabolites are present in all species and glucuronide conjugates of the starting drug and the alcohol metabolite are present in most species. The rat produces shorter side chain acid derivative than the other species and no glucuronides are detected in the rat urine. The monkey excretes both glucuronides while the dog produces only the glucuronide of **37**. The identification of these metabolic products in various animal species should aid in the design of similar experiments in humans.

An excellent example of the application of stable isotope methodology to a clinical problem is given in a pharmacokinetic study of the interaction of theophylline (**2**) and cimetidine (103). The methodology for this study requires oral administration of unlabeled **2** with concurrent intravenous infusion of (1,3-$^{15}N_2$, 2-^{13}C)theophylline (**38**) and the subsequent quantitation of both of these compounds with $(C^2H_3)_2$-theophylline (**39**) as the internal standard. Preparing a sample requires extraction of plasma using a four-component organic phase followed by HPLC purification of the fractions of interest. Mass spectrometry is performed by sublimation of the samples from a glass rod inserted directly into the source of the mass spectrometer. Selected ion monitoring is then performed by monitoring M^+ ions characteristic for each of the compounds at m/z 180, 183, and 186. Quantitation is achieved using calibration curves of peak height ratios

38   39

generated from plasma blanks. Although the level of isotope label is high, correction for the isotopic contribution of **2** at m/z 183 from the ^{15}N-containing analog **38** is necessary. The practical limit of detection for the assay is about 10 ng/mL of **2**. Analysis of the initial clinical data indicates that cimetidine reduces the clearance of **2** by 39% and increases the half-life by one-third, with no significant effect on the volume of distribution, absorption rate, or absolute bioavailability.

As the preceding study shows, the combined use of mass spectrometry with stable isotope-labeled materials for performing pharmacokinetic studies has a number of advantages over other methods. First, a complete pharmacokinetic profile may be determined under steady-state conditions without interfering with the patient's normal therapeutic regimen. Second, the pharmacokinetics of drug interactions may be determined without exposing the patient to radioactive materials or potentially dangerous levels of a drug. Finally, this approach permits the oral administration of the readily available, unlabeled drug while the more scarce isotopically labeled materials may be infused in small quantities.

3.2. Nucleosides

Adding a sugar group to the aglycone of a nucleic acid base significantly increases not only the complexity of the mass spectrum but also the experimental procedures for sample preparation. Although modifications of the sugar portion of nucleotides in DNA are not known, a wide diversity in structure becomes possible for nucleosides isolated from other biological sources. Because of the likely limitation in sample quantity of materials isolated from natural sources, mass spectrometry is widely used in determination of the structures of nucleosides obtained from, for example, tRNA, human urine, and bacterial cell cultures. In order to begin a structural assignment, some knowledge of the general features of the mass spectrum of a nucleoside is needed.

3.2.1. STRUCTURE–FRAGMENTATION RELATIONSHIPS

In general, the structural/fragmentation relationships of nucleosides are well established (4). Although variations and exceptions exist to a number of these general rules, some information concerning the structure of the unknown nucleoside is available following a quick perusal of the mass spectrum.

a. Mass Spectra of Free Nucleosides. Structures of the important ions in the mass spectrum of a free nucleoside will be described in reference to the EI spectrum of uridine (**40**) shown in Fig. 1.

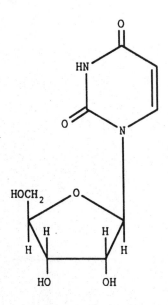

40, Uridine

Molecular ion. [M^+]: A molecular ion peak (104) is observed at m/z 244 and represents the intact molecule. If the abundance of this ion permits exact mass measurements, considerable information will be gained concerning the elemental composition of the molecule. The abundance of the molecular ion is highly variable and dependent on nucleoside structure (4–6, 105), but little information is available on the basis of abundance alone.

Base and Sugar Ions [B^+, BH^+, BH_2^+, S^+]. Among the most important ions in the spectrum, this series provides direct information concerning the identity of the aglycone and sugar portions of the molecule. The most abundant of the ion series related to the aglycone, the BH_2^+ ion is represented by the most intense peak (m/z 113) in the spectrum of uridine. The peak at m/z 112 represents the BH^+ ion. In general, the BH_2^+ ion is of greater abundance in the spectra of ribosides relative to those of deoxyribosides and in the spectra of pyrimidines compared to

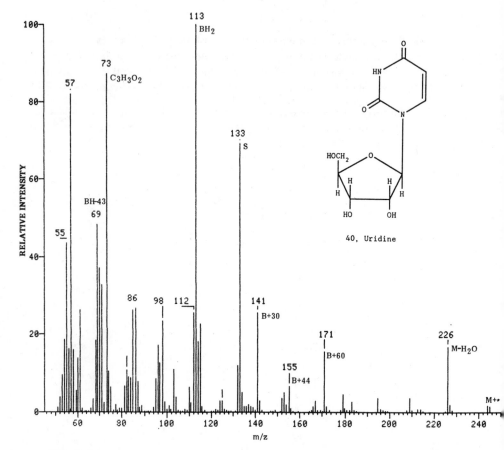

Fig. 1. Low-resolution, 70-eV electron ionization mass spectrum of uridine obtained by direct probe introduction of the sample. Major ion designations are described in the text.

those of purines (4). The S^+ ion representing the ribose moiety is evident in the spectrum of uridine at m/z 133, but may be weak or absent in the spectra of purine nucleosides.

Ions Related to the Base with Portions of the Sugar Ring attached [B + 30, B + 44, B + 60]. A number of ions are related to the aglycone with portions of the sugar ring attached. These ions provide structural information concerning the site of modification in the sugar ring; they also provide confirmation of the identity of base-related ions because one or more of these ions are present in all nucleoside spectra obtained using EI.

B + 30: This ion, represented by a peak at m/z 141 in the spectrum of uridine, corresponds to the base with the anomeric carbon of the sugar, the substituent at the 1′ position, the sugar ring oxygen, and has the following structure:

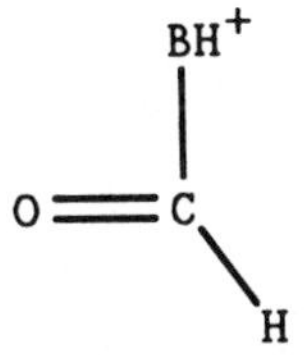

BH$^+$

O $=$ C

H

B + 30

Any substitutions in the elements comprising this ion are evident in appropriate shifts in the B + 30 ion. For example, substituting a sulfur for the oxygen of the ribose ring shifts the B + 30 ion from m/z 164 in the spectrum of adensonine to m/z 180 in the spectrum of 4'-thioadenosine (**41**) (105).

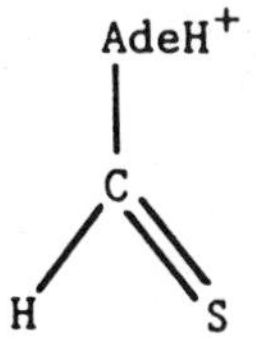

AdeH$^+$

C

H   S

41

The abundance of the B + 30 ion is used as an indicator of the presence of a carbon–carbon bond between the aglycone and sugar moiety in C-nucleosides, with the mass spectra of the C-nucleosides pseudouridine (**42**) (106) and formycin (**43**) (107) displaying the B + 30 ion as the base peak in their spectra.

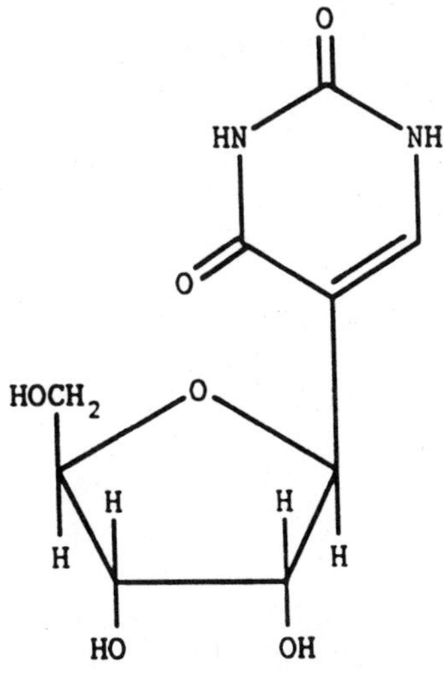

42, Pseudouridine

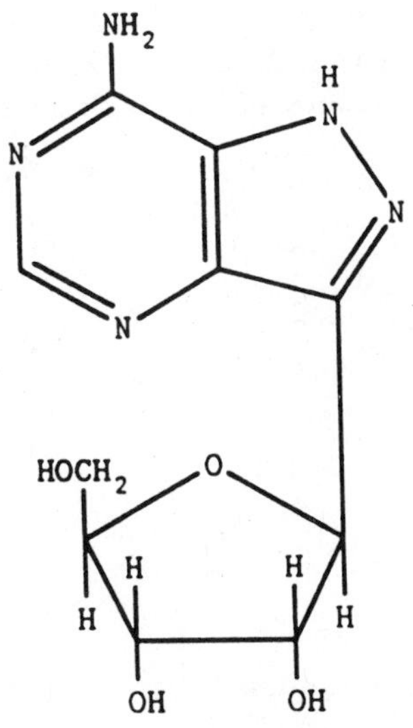

43, Formycin

The absence of glycosidic bond cleavage that would otherwise produce strong $BH^{\ddagger}$ or BH_2^+ ions, the absence of S^+-related ions, and the occurrence of an intense peak for the B + 30 ion in the spectrum of an unknown nucleoside are strong indications of the presence of a C-nucleoside. However, caution is advised (108) in using the intensity of the B + 30 peak alone in assigning a C-nucleoside structure, because there are exceptions to this and other general statements. For example, the base peak in the spectrum of 1-deazapurine riboside (109), **44**, represents the B + 30 ion (110).

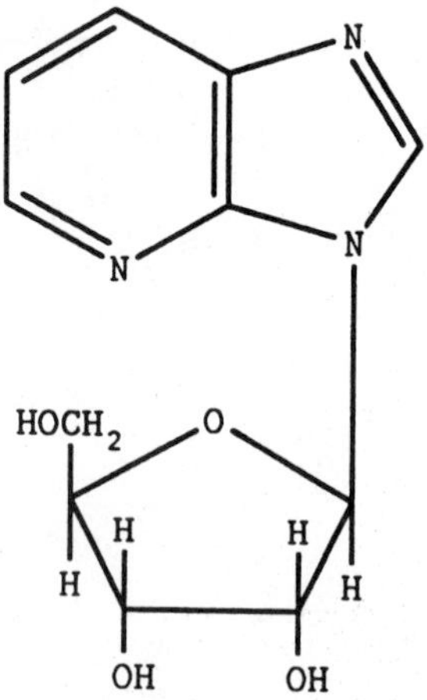

44, 1-Deazapurine riboside

B + 44 ion: The B + 44 ion contains the 1′ and 2′ carbon atoms and the substituents attached to these carbons. The B + 44 ion, observed at *m/z* 155 in the spectrum of uridine, has the following structure:

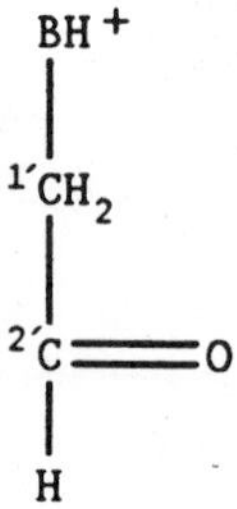

B + 44

Substitution of any of the elements comprising this ion are reflected in a shift in the mass of this ion. For example, 2′-deoxynucleosides have a peak in their mass spectra corresponding to a B + 28 ion rather than the B + 44 ion in the ribosides, showing the absence of the 2′ oxygen; methylation of the 2′-position produces a B + 58 ion, reflecting a shift of 14 u for the "B + 44 ion."

B + 60 Ion: The B + 60 relates structurally to the B + 44 ion, but, in addition, contains the sugar ring ether oxygen:

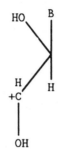

B + 60

By a close examination of the previously mentioned ions, considerable information can be gained concerning the nature of the heterocyclic base and modifications to the 1′, 2′, and sugar ring oxygen positions. Subtle differences in ion abundances, especially in the case of epimeric or anomeric analogs, are observed, but direct correlation of these differences with absolute structure is not yet possible.

Other Ions of Structural Significance

M − 30: A peak corresponding to the M − 30 ion is observed in the mass spectra of purine, but not pyrimidine, nucleosides. This ion is indicative of the presence of an unmodified 5′-hydroxymethylene group and may be used in some cases to identify modifications in the 5′-position, for example, this peak is absent in the spectrum of 5′-deoxyadenosine (**45**) (105) and related analogs, that is, 5′-deoxyguanosine (111).

B + 41: A prominent peak for the B + 41 ion in the spectrum of a nucleoside strongly indicates the presence of a cytosine related base (112). As a general rule such is indeed the case, but caution is advised in assigning a cytidine-type structure based on the abundance of this ion alone, especially without exact mass data, because exceptions have been noted (113, 114). For example, the spectrum of 3-deazauridine (**46**) (114) which, in addition to having a prominent peak for the B + 41 ion, displays peaks that are isobaric with those in the spectrum of cytidine (both compounds have the same molecular weight); peak intensities are very similar to those in the spectrum of arabinosyl cytosine (**5**), with the spectra of **46** and **5** being almost superimposable.

Ions below the Base-Related Ions: Ions occurring at masses lower than the BH⁺ ion are important for identifying specific fragmentations of the base, although sugar fragmentation ions are also present. These ions are more difficult to interpret than the ions at higher mass for reasons stated previously (Section 3.1),

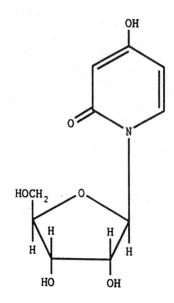

45, 5′-Deoxyadenosine   46, 3-Deazauridine

but modifications in the base will be indicated by shifts of major ions relative to those from the unmodified basic ring system.

The structural significance of the important ions in the fragmentation of a free nucleoside are summarized in the following diagram (**47**):

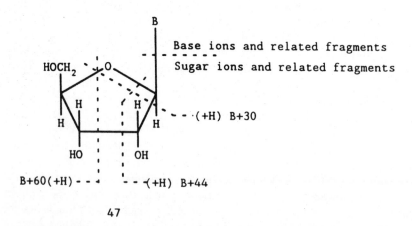

47

b. Mass Spectra of TMS Derivatives. The major reason for derivatization, as stated earlier, is to increase the volatility of the nucleoside for analysis by GC–MS. In addition, preparing and analyzing the TMS derivative of a nucleoside provides supporting and additional structural information (relative to that from the spectrum of the free compound).

In general, the peaks observed in the mass spectrum of a TMS derivative of a nucleoside have direct counterparrs in the spectrum of the free compound. The structures and mechanisms of formation of the major ions during fragmentation of the TMS derivatives of nucleosides have been investigated in detail (12) and only the major points will be presented here.

Ions in the mass spectra of nucleoside TMS derivatives providing important structural information may be divided into three major groups (12): ions related to the molecular ion (molecular ion series), ions related to the aglycone and portions of the sugar ring (base ion series), and ions derived from the sugar portion of the nucleoside (sugar ion series). The composition and structural significance of the major ions of importance in the mass spectra of the TMS derivatives of nucleosides are summarized in Tables 1–3 and are illustrated in the mass spectrum of uridine (TMS)$_4$ (**15**) shown in Fig. 2.

Recognition of the ions listed in Tables 1–3 in the mass spectrum of a newly discovered nucleoside should provide at least tentative information concerning its

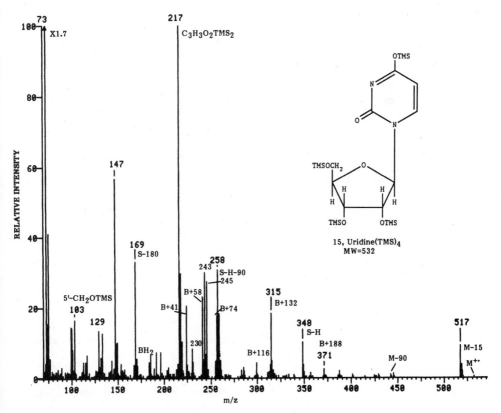

Fig. 2. Electron-impact (70-ev) mass spectrum of uridine(TMS)$_4$. The structural significance of the labeled ions is described in Tables 1–3.

TABLE 1

Ions of the Molecular Ions Series and their Structural Significance[a]

Ion	Structural Significance and Comments
M^{+}	Molecular weight of intact molecule. Use of ^{2}H-labeled reagents will permit determination of the number of TMS groups added to the free nucleoside. High-resolution data important for elemental composition of intact molecule.
$M - 15$	Permits ready identification of the molecular ion. If ratio of $M/M - 15 > 1$, guanosine may be present, but exceptions have been noted (114).
$M - 90$	TMSOH lost is exclusively from $O - 2'$.
$M - 103$	Loss of the 5'-position as CH_2OTMS. Indicator of the 5'-position.
$M - 105$	$M - 15 - 90$. No additional structural information.
$M - 118$	$M - 90 - CO$. CO lost primarily from the $O - 4'$ position.
$M - 131$	Loss of $C - 1'$, $C - 2'$, $O - 2'$, and $O - 4'$.
$M - 180$	$M - 90 - 90$. Useful in recognizing C-nucleosides.

[a]Based on data in Ref. 12.

TABLE 2

Ions of the Base Ion Series and their Structural Significance[a]

Ion	Structural Significance and Comments
$B + 204$	Same as $B + 132$ but with an additional TMS group.
$B + 188$	Shifted from $B + 116$ by addition of TMS but not structurally related.
$B + 132$	Of major structural importance in locating sites of modification in the sugar. Contains $C - 1'$, $C - 2'$, $O' - 2'$, $O - 4'$, and a rearranged hydrogen. Formed by loss of the 3' through 5' positions of the sugar. Structurally related to the $B + 60$ ion of free nucleosides by addition of a TMS group to the hydroxyl group. Sugar modifications evident.
$B + 116$	Structurally related to the $B + 44$ ion of free nucleosides, but with a TMS group added to the hydroxyl group. Sugar modifications evident.
$B + 100$	Formed from $B + 116$ by loss of CH_4.
$B + 74$	Related to the BH^{+} ion, but with a TMS group transferred from the sugar during glycosidic bond cleavage, instead of a hydrogen. Identification of base confirmed.
$B + 58$	Formed from $B + 74$ by loss of CH_4.
$B + 41$	Characteristically abundant in cytidine analogs.
$B + 30$	Same as in free nucleosides. Modifications to sugar ring ether oxygen or substitution at $C - 1'$ evident. Often a strong ion in the purine nucleosides. B will be shifted by 72 u for each TMS added to the aglycone.
$B + 13$	Base + CH observed in some but not all pyrimidine nucleosides. Absent in purine nucleosides.
BH_2, BH	Base ions. Establish nominal mass and elemental composition, with high resolution, of B, the aglycone. Shift of base ion series with ^{2}H-labeled reagents dependent on number of TMS groups added to base.

[a]Based on data from Ref. 12.

TABLE 3

Ions of the Sugar Ion Series and their Structural Significance[a]

	Structural Significance			
Ion	Ribose	Deoxyribose	2'-O-methyl	Comments
S	349	261	291	Direct indicator of sugar
S − H	348	260	290	modifications. Isomers and epimers not distinguished with any confidence. Differentiation of α from β possible if both available. Also useful for establishing identity of base-related ions.
S − 32	—	—	259	From O-methylated sugars only.
S − 90	259	171	201	Loss of TMSOH.
S − H − 90	258	170	200	
S − H − 103	245	157	187	Loss of ·CH$_2$OTMS. If abundant, suggests unmodified 5'-position.
S − 16 − 90	243	155	185	
C$_4$H$_4$O$_2$TMS$_2$	230		230	
C$_5$H$_7$O$_2$TMS	—	—	172	
C$_3$H$_3$O$_2$TMS$_2$	217	—	217	
C$_4$H$_6$O$_2$TMS	—	—	159	
S − 180	169	81	—	
CH$_2$OTMS	103	103	103	Suggestive of unmodified 5' position, but not definitive.

[a]Based on data from Ref. 12.

structure. Additional information and experiments are needed, however, before a definitive structure can be assigned. A general strategy (10) includes the preparation of stable isotope-labeled derivatives, acquiring high-resolution data for exact mass assignment (elemental composition), and comparing, if possible, the mass spectral and chromatographic characteristics of the unknown with those of a reference material. Also, as in any structure elucidation problem, advantage should be taken of any and all analytical data that are available, and the information from different techniques, for example, NMR, MS, or chromatography, must be consistent and complementary if the assigned structure is correct.

3.2.2. GENERAL STRATEGY FOR THE STRUCTURE ELUCIDATION OF AN UNKNOWN NUCLEOSIDE

The general approach used to establish the structure of an unknown nucleoside will be illustrated using a recent example from the author's laboratory (115). During the analysis of the HPLC-purified, nucleoside-containing fraction of human urine, an unidentified component was detected which produced the mass spectrum shown in Fig. 3, for which no acceptable library match was found using either our local library or other reference materials (69). A tentative molecular weight of 556 u was assigned based on a weak peak at m/z 556 accompanied by a peak at m/z 541 for the M − 15 ion. The library search located two spectra, those of inosine (TMS)$_4$ (**48**) and its pyranosyl analog (**49**), with molecular weights of 556 u; neither spectrum provided a good match with the unknown. Closer inspection of the spectrum of the sample revealed the absence of ions characteristic of a ribose sugar, for example, S (m/z 349), S − H (m/z 348), S − 90 (m/z 259), or S − H − 103 (m/z 245), but the presence of peaks at m/z 260 (S − H) and 171 (S − 90) suggesting a deoxyriboside. The absence of an intense peak at m/z 103 was, however, confusing since this suggested a 5′-deoxynucleoside which, at the time, was unknown in human urine. Correlations between other ions in the spectrum led to the tentative conclusion that the heterocyclic component of the compound was xanthine, a suspicion strengthened by a

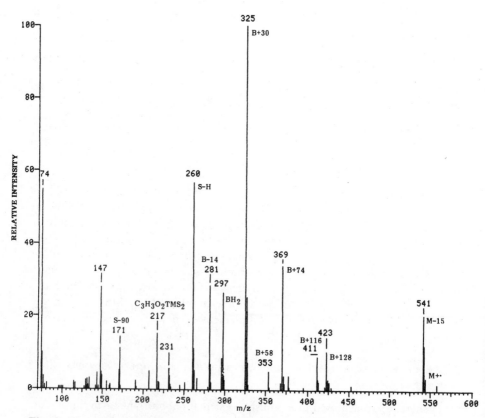

Fig. 3. The mass spectrum of an unknown nucleoside identified in an HPLC-purified fraction of human urine. Ion designations were assigned as described in the text.

48, Inosine(TMS)₄   49

comparison of the sample spectrum with that of xanthosine $(TMS)_5$ (**50**) (69). Ions common to both the unknown and **50** included (with structural assignments) m/z 297 (BH_2), 325 (B + 30), 353 (B + 58), 369 (B + 74), and 411 (B + 116). This base ion series, in addition to indicating the identity of the base as xanthine, supported the tentative assignment of the sugar as being a 5'-deoxypentose, since only this configuration would show ions in common with ribose which contains the 2'- and 3'-hydroxyl groups.

Additional information on the structure of the unknown was then obtained by use of chemical ionization, which confirmed the molecular weight assignment of 556 u, and by preparation of the TMS $(^2H_9)$ analog. The observed shift of the M − 15 ion of the labeled compound to m/z 574 indicated the addition of four TMS groups to the molecule. Shifts in the base ion series confirmed that two TMS groups had been added to the base and, thus by difference, two TMS groups were added to the sugar, which was also evident in the appropriate mass shift in the ions assigned to the sugar. Based on the above data, a tentative structure of 5'-deoxyxanthosine (**51**) was assigned to the sample.

However, at the time this work was in progress, only one 5'-deoxynucleoside, 5'-deoxyadenosine, was known to be naturally occurring, although a number of 5'-deoxynucleosides had been made synthetically. Unfortunately, 5'-deoxyguanosine, the compound needed to easily prepare a reference standard of **51**, was not readily available synthetically, but could be prepared biochemically. Efforts along this line were fruitful and a reference standard of **51**, produced by enzymatic deamination of 5'-deoxyguanosine, was obtained and shown to have

50, Xanthosine(TMS)$_5$ 51, 5′-Deoxyxanthosine(TMS)$_4$

identical mass spectral and chromatographic properties. Finally, the high-resolution mass spectrum of the urinary component and reference material confirmed the proposed elemental composition of the major ions. Thus, combining the principles of mass spectrometry and biochemistry made it possible to establish the structure of this newly discovered nucleoside in human urine.

As a final note, during the experiments to prepare the reference sample of **51**, a report of the identification of another 5′-deoxynucleoside, 5′-deoxyinosine (**52**), appeared in the literature (116) that, when the sugar ion series were compared, showed identical m/z values and, in most instances, very similar relative intensities.

3.2.3. MODIFIED NUCLEOSIDES IDENTIFIED IN RNA AND DNA

Of the more than 80 different bases and nucleosides identified to date in RNA and DNA, a significant number were characterized in part or totally by mass spectrometry. As the structures of these new nucleosides become more complex and the amount of material available for analysis gets smaller, the problems in characterization become more difficult. However, the general approach (9, 10) to solving the structure of a new nucleoside is still based on the use of low- and high-resolution EI mass spectrometry on a sample purified either using GC separation or by prior isolation using HPLC or TLC. The use of FAB and direct LC–MS analysis of tRNA hydrolysates are also becoming more important and provide data complementary to the EI mass spectrum. Two examples of newly identified

52, 5′-Deoxyinosine

nucleosides, one from tRNA and the other from DNA will be used to illustrate the general approach to this type of problem.

Elucidating the structure of a modified nucleoside, designated N, which replaces ribosylthymine in over half of the tRNA of archaebacteria, illustrates the power of mass spectrometry in solving such problems (73). The characterization of this nucleoside was achieved using a total of 7 μg of sample and was based almost exclusively on interpretation of the low- and high-resolution mass spectral data, chromatographic retention time, and comparison with data obtained from analysis of a synthetically prepared reference sample.

The sample was isolated from unfractionated tRNA from the cells of *Halococcus morrhuae* and further purified by Sephadex G-100 column chromatography. Fractions corresponding to the 4 S fraction were pooled and the tRNA precipitated, dried, and hydrolyzed to the mononucleotides using nuclease P_1. The hydrolysate was then fractionated using two-dimensional paper chromatography where pN partially overlapped with UMP. The spot containing pN and UMP was cut, eluted with water, and treated with alkaline phosphomonoesterase to provide the nucleosides. The nucleoside mixture was further purified using HPLC, which afforded nearly complete separation of N from uridine. The isolated nucleoside N was then analyzed using mass spectrometry, both as the free compound and as the TMS derivative.

Principal ions of structural significance in the low-resolution mass spectrum of the TMS derivative indicated a mixture of the TMS_3 and TMS_4 derivatives with molecular weights of 474 and 546 u, respectively. Abundant ions representing the loss of one and two molecules of TMSOH suggested the presence of a C-nucleoside, which was further supported by the absence of strong base- and sugar-ion series peaks. Exact mass measurements provided three rational compositions for the molecular mass, one of which, $C_{10}H_{11}N_2O_6$ (TMS)$_3$, corresponded to a methylated uridine. Location of the methyl group in the aglycone was established using the B + 30 ion, which was 14 mass units higher than free uracil and indicated that the sugar elements lost were indicative of an unmodified ribose.

The mass spectrum of the free nucleoside displayed ions with an abundance pattern similar to that of pseudouridine, but with m/z values shifted to higher mass by 14 u in the base-related ions. The BH, BH$_2$, S, and related ions were substantially reduced in intensity relative to those for the same peaks in the spectrum of uridine. Furthermore, the base peak of the spectrum represented the B + 30 ion, and peaks representing sequential water losses were prominent, all characteristics strongly indicating the presence of a C-nucleoside. In addition, the operation of a retro-Diels-Alder fragmentation, which specifically requires a cyclohexene-type structure for the aglycone, allowed the site of methylation to be assigned to the N − 1 position. Confirming the tentative structure was made possible by comparing the chromatographic behavior and mass spectra of nucleoside N with those of a synthetically prepared reference sample of 1-methylpseudouridine. Thus, the structure of nucleoside N was established as 1-methylpseudouridine (53) and this report is the first identification of 53 in RNA. The biochemical significance of the modified nucleosides in the tRNA of archaebacteria, and methods for their analysis, were recently reviewed (117).

In contrast to the extensive modifications observed in the bases found in tRNA, relatively few (118), only 16 (16), modified nucleic acid bases have been identified in DNA, and, until recently, hypermodification of purines was unknown. However, bacteriophage Mu encodes a protein that modifies approximately 15% of DNA adenine residues. In order to elucidate the nature of this

53, 1-Methylpseudouridine

modified adenine residue, DNA from the bacteriophage is enzymatically degraded to deoxynucleosides and the products fractionated by HPLC (119). A sample, 2–3 μg, of the modified nucleoside, designated dA$'_x$, is converted to the TMS derivative and subjected to mass spectral analysis. The low-resolution spectrum shows peaks at m/z 596 and 581 representing the M‡ and M − 15 ions, respectively. A peak at m/z 668 is observed occasionally that indicates the inconsistent incorporation of an additional TMS function. Peaks indicative of an unmodified deoxyribose group are observed at m/z 170, 155, and 103, but the S$^+$ ion (m/z 261) is not abundant. The mass difference between M‡ and S$^+$ gives a weight for the base fragment of 335 mass units, confirmed by the presence of a peak at m/z 336 for the BH ion. Exact mass values are obtained and lead to the conclusion that the sample is deoxyadenosine with the addition of the elements of $C_2H_2NOSi(CH_3)_3$. The site and arrangement of the substituents on the adenine ring are deduced as follows: (1) Substitution at either the 2 or 8 positions of the adenine ring is ruled out on the basis of earlier work; (2) expulsion of the elements $CONHSi(CH_3)_3$ from the molecular ion produces a prominent peak at m/z 481. Three structures, **54**, **55**, and **56**, are considered potential candidates on the basis of these data:

Structure **55** could produce the ion of mass 481 by the cleavage shown, but this structure would likely add only one TMS group to the base, not the required two as is observed. Further consideration of **55** is thus eliminated. Structure **56**, while adding the required two TMS groups to the aglycone, should produce an ion of mass 494, based on analogy to the structurally related mt⁶A, but this is not observed. The evidence thus leads to the most probable structure for dA′ₓ as being **54**. Since further structural details are not available from the mass spectrum, a sample of the proposed compound was synthesized and the chromatographic and mass spectral characteristics compared. These data provide the final proof that **54** is indeed the correct assignment. With the proof of structure complete, additional experiments were conducted which established that an earlier assigned structure for this DNA-modified purine as N^6-carboxymethyladenine(dA_x) was, in fact, a product of acidic hydrolysis. The preceding work provided proof of the first known hypermodified purine in DNA.

Differences in posttranscriptional modification of isoaccepting tRNAs may also be determined directly from the enzymatic hydrolysates using high-resolution mass spectrometry. For example, the same primary sequence is observed between $tRNA_1^{Lys}$ and $tRNA_3^{Lys}$ from *B. subtilis* purified by HPLC, but these isoaccepting tRNAs differ in their posttranscriptional modifications in the anticodon loop, and these differences can be detected by high-resolution mass spectrometry (120). Using this approach in the analysis of the TMS derivative of the $tRNA_1^{Lys}$ hydrolysate, the presence of both (t^6A) (**57**) and (ms^2t^6A) (**58**) was

57, t^6A; R — H
58, ms^2t^6A; R — CH_3S-

detected, while the published sequence of this tRNA contained only ms^{2}t^{6}A. Thus, high-resolution mass spectrometry applied directly to tRNA hydrolysates may be used to confirm the composition of tRNAs determined using more classical methods.

Additional examples of modified bases in RNA and DNA are found in the general references cited in the Introduction.

3.2.4. DNA ADDUCTS

Another area of considerable interest is in the characterization of the adducts formed in the reaction of various organic molecules with DNA. Investigations of this type follow in close parallel those used in the characterization of modified nucleosides derived from tRNA and urine, as described above, and recent reviews on this omportant topic are available (8, 121). Because the mass spectral approach to the analysis of these carcinogen/organic molecule/drug–DNA complexes has shifted from the classical EI approach to the use of FAB and LC–MS, further discussion on this topic will be deferred until later.

3.2.5. NUCLEOSIDE ANTIBIOTICS

Because of the small quantity of material isolated from fermentation broths, mass spectrometry is useful in elucidating the structure of newly discovered nucleoside antibiotics. As in the cases mentioned previously, the antibiotic is isolated by some form of chromatography followed by derivatization and low- and high-resolution mass spectrometry. However, as the following example illustrates, the sample must be prepared with caution to avoid degradation. An additional difficulty in the characterization of nucleoside antibiotics is that, in contrast to nucleic acid components, considerable variation may occur, not only in the aglycone, but also in the sugar portion of the nucleosides, thus adding considerable complexity to the problem.

Two nucleoside antibiotics were recently isolated from the fermentation broth of a *Streptomyces* strain (122). Converting the purified compounds to their TMS derivatives results in essentially identical mass spectra, both of which are identical to that previously reported for antibiotic AT-265 (**59**, where R = H). Examining the FAB mass spectra of the two samples reveals that dealanylascamycin (antibiotic AT-265) is, in fact, a degradation product of ascamycin (**59**) formed by quantitative hydrolysis of 5′-*O*-sulfonamide bond with loss of the alanyl group. The difference in mass between the MH$^+$ ions of **59** and dealanylascamycin, determined using FAB and exact mass measurements, indicates the loss of a C$_3$H$_5$NO residue from the latter compound during the derivatization reaction. The EI mass spectrum (16) shows an isotope pattern characteristic of mono-chlorination, the absence of substitution at the 1′ and 2′ positions of the ribose ring and identification of the base as a chlorinated adenine, indicated by the base ion series. The identity of 2-chloroadenine as the aglycone was ultimately proved by hydrolysis of the glycosidic bond and comparing the resulting heterocycle with a known sample of 2-chloroadenine. The position of the alanylsulfamoyl group at

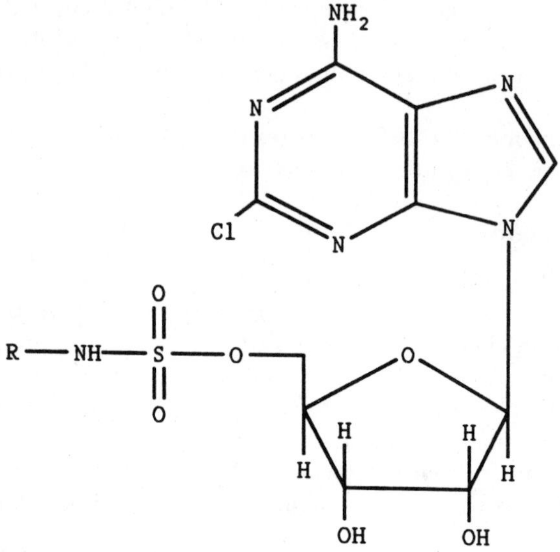

59, Ascamycin

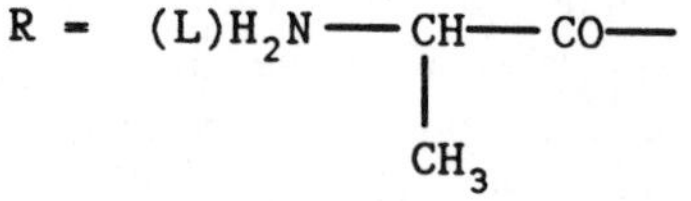

$$R = (L)H_2N - CH - CO -$$
$$\qquad\qquad\quad |$$
$$\qquad\qquad\quad CH_3$$

the 5' position of the sugar was deduced from the + and − FAB spectra and deuterium exchange experiments.

Many other examples of the use of mass spectrometry to establish the structure of nucleoside antibiotics are available, and reviews of this subject have appeared recently (8–10, 16).

3.3. Nucleotides

Applications of EI mass spectrometry to the analysis of nucleotide structure is limited because of the highly polar nature and thermal instability of these compounds under the conditions required for their volatilization. Identifying and quantitating nucleotides is best handled by conversion to the nucleoside or base stage, since, even with formation of derivatives, the nucleotides are not readily amenable to GC separation. A few reports use EI for identification or quantitation of nucleotides, for example, cAMP (123–125), or to study the fragmentation patterns of nucleotide analogs, that is, nucleoside phosphordiamidates (126). However, this sample class is now best handled using FAB, although FD has some value (127) in the mass spectral analysis of this compound class.

4.   CHEMICAL IONIZATION

The major utility of chemical ionization in the analysis of nucleic acid components falls into two categories. First, for structure elucidation, CI plays a complementary role to EI in providing a protonated molecule, MH^+, of sufficient abundance to establish with certainty the molecular weight of the sample. Because CI is a "soft" ionization technique, the extent of fragmentation is significantly less than is observed in the EI spectrum and, therefore, the amount of structural information in a CI spectrum is decreased; the extent of fragmentation can, however, be controlled by selection of the reagent gas. The second aspect of CI utility is found in studies aimed at the quantitation of nucleic acid components used as chemotherapeutic agents. In this case, advantage is taken of the significant amount of total ion current carried by the MH^+ ion to decrease detection limits, an important consideration in the quantitation of low quantities of a drug in, for example, a plasma sample.

4.1.   Chemical Ionization Spectra of Nucleosides

The appearance of the CI spectrum is primarily dependent on the structure of the nucleoside and the reagent gas used for ionization. The CI spectrum of adenosine (**60**) obtained using methane (CH_4) is shown in Fig. 4. Although differences in intensities of the peaks are obvious when spectra obtained with different reagent gases are compared, the majority of the ion current is carried by the MH^+ and BH_2 ions, which is a general characteristic of the CI spectrum of a nucleoside (128). Use of an even more basic reagent gas, for example, trimethylamine, produces a spectrum in which the $\%\Sigma_{total}$ MH^+ can reach 95%, compared to

60, Adenosine

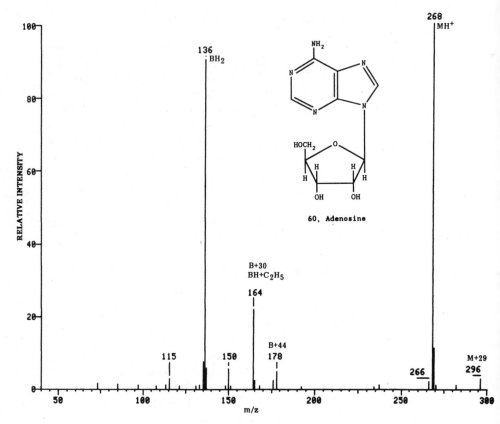

Fig. 4. CI mass spectra of adenosine using methane as the reagent gas.

34% and 66% for CH_4 and NH_3, respectively (69). Thus, if molecular weight identification or confirmation is the objective of the experiment, NH_3 or an even more basic reagent gas should be used. On the other hand, the spectrum obtained using CH_4 provides some structural information along with easy identification of the MH^+ ion. Using the more energetic reagent gas CH_4 produces a spectrum that appears to contain peaks for some of the base ion series, for example, $B + 30$ and $B + 44$, providing important structural information. However, the $B + 30$ ion, m/z 164, is actually a mixture of the $B + 30$ ion and an adduction of $BH + C_2H_5^+$, the relative contributions of which are highly dependent on the experimental conditions (128). The $B + 44$ ion, m/z 178, is, however, real and contains the same structural elements as observed using EI, but the mechanism of formation is different between the ionization modes. Other features of the CI spectra of nucleosides that deserve comment include the following two points. (1) The spectra of pyrimidine nucleosides will, in many cases, provide strong sugar ions, while the purine nucleoside spectra generally do not. This is a consequence of differences in the proton affinity of the two-ring systems. (2) The spectra of the pyrimidine nucleosides may show an ion at MH^{+2} resulting from saturation of the 5,6-double bond. Because formation of the saturated analog is time dependent, use of the MH^{+2} ion to determine isotope contributions should be performed with caution.

No systematic studies of the use of CI for the analysis of volatile derivatives of nucleic acid bases, nucleosides, or nucleotides are available. CI was used in the author's laboratory as an aid in identifying the TMS derivatization products of AMP (**61**), tricyclic nucleoside monophosphate (**62**) and 2'-deoxy-5-fluorouridine monophosphate (FdUMP) (**63**) (129), with the samples being introduced by direct probe. The spectra produced when NH_3 was used as the reagent gas were dominated by peaks for the MH^+ ion and showed essentially no fragmentation. A mixture of TMS derivatives was evident from the spectra of **62** and **63** indicating that these two compounds did not react quantitatively with the silylating reagents to form a single TMS product.

Using $CI(CH_4)$ makes it possible to identify and quantitate a number of nucleic acid base and nucleoside antitumor agents, as their permethyl derivatives (85). The CI spectra of the permethyl derivatives are dominated by a peak for MH^+ and show little evidence of fragmentation.

In summary, few systematic studies have been conducted in the use of CI for the analysis of nucleic acid components or volatile derivatives of this compound class. The major utility of CI for structural work is in establishing the molecular weight of a compound.

61, AMP(TMS)$_5$

62, TCNMP(TMS)$_5$

63, FdUMP(TMS)$_4$

4.2. Applications of CI

4.2.1. DETERMINATION OF THE RELATIVE GLYCOSYL BOND STRENGTH OF NUCLEOSIDES

Determining the strength of the base–sugar bond of nucleosides is of interest from both a clinical and a biochemical standpoint. Nucleoside analogs used as chemotherapeutic agents undergo "lethal synthesis" to the nucleotide, which in many instances, is the active form of the drug. If the glycosidic bond of nucleosides is unstable to physiological conditions, activation may not proceed. The classical method of determining glycosyl bond strength is to follow the hydrolytic cleavage by UV detection. However, using CI makes it possible to determine the relative glycosyl bond strength between isomeric pairs of nucleosides, for example, adenosine (**60**) versus 7-(β-D-ribofuranosyl)adenine (**64**) (130). Comparing the MH^+/BH_2 intensity ratios of the isomeric pairs of nucleosides and correlating the mass spectrometry data with rate coefficients determined from solution experiments gives the relative strength of the glycosidic bond. In all cases, the glycosidic bond strength of the 7-isomer is less than that of the 9-isomer. CI mass spectrometry is more simple and requires less sample than the classical method. However, volatility limitations of the free nucleosides is a limiting factor in extension of this technique to other, less volatile, nucleosides.

64, 7-(β-D-ribofuranosyl)adenine

4.2.2. STUDIES ON 5-FLOUROURACIL, RELATED ANTITUMOR AGENTS, AND OTHER CLINICAL APPLICATIONS

5-Flourouracil(5-FU) (**14**) is widely used clinically for the treatment of a variety of cancers (131). In addition to 5-FU, a number of its analogs are also of interest because they are either antitumor agents themselves, for example, ftorafur(Ft) (**65**) and 2'-deoxy-5-fluorouridine (FUdR) (**66**) or are metabolites of **14**, for example, 5-fluorouridine (FUR) (**67**), 5,6-dihydro-5-fluorouracil (**68**), and FdUMP (**63**), the later compound being the active form of **14** which inhibits thymidylate synthetase. 5-FU undergoes an extremely complex metabolism and highly sensitive detectors are needed to develop pharmacokinetic profiles of this

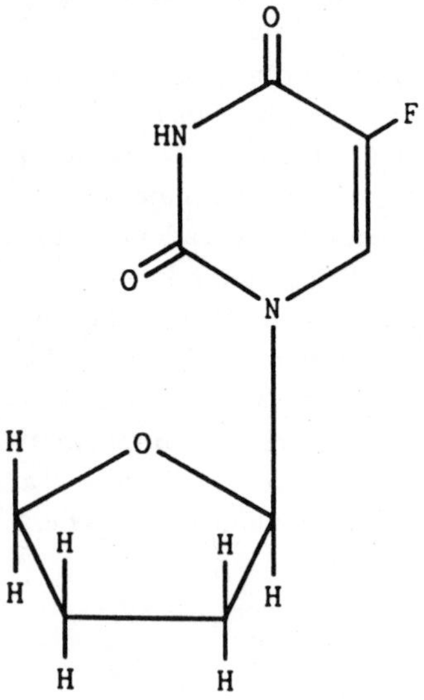

65, Ftorafur (FT)

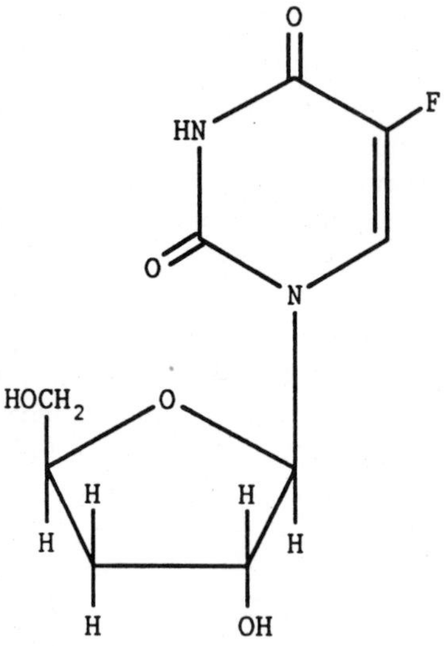

66, FUdR

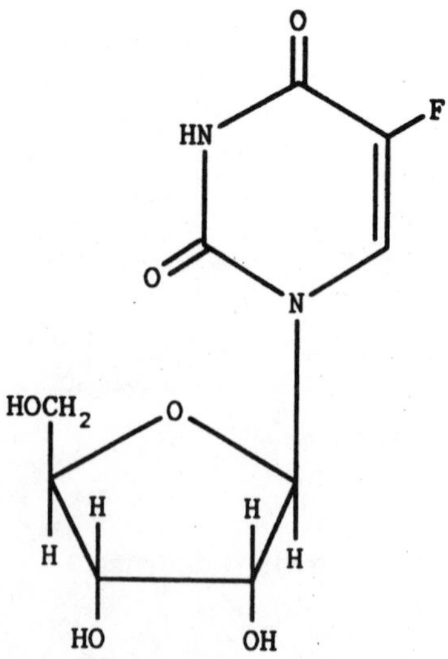

67, FUR

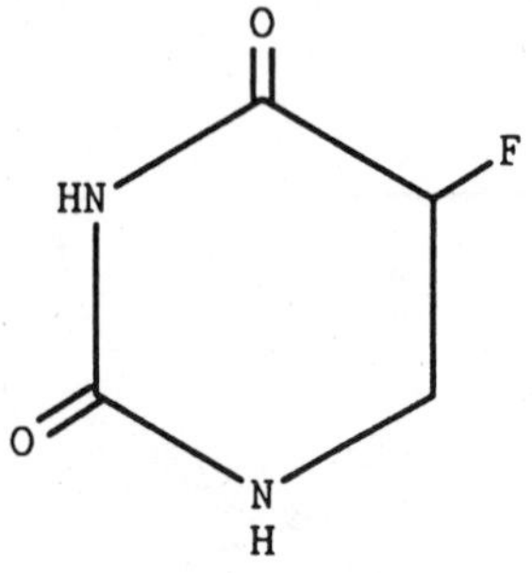

68, 5,6-Dihydro-5-FU

compound. Because of the importance in thoroughly understanding the metabolism and distribution of **14**, a number of GC–MS assays for 5-FU and the related compounds mentioned are available.

CI is the method of choice in many, but not all, of the procedures described in the literature because the greatest sensitivity possible is needed to quantitate the low levels of the drug in patient samples. Because Ref. 8 contains a review of the literature on the use of GC–MS in this area the following discussion will be limited to more recent work.

Of the many methods reported (59, 132–135) for the GC–MS quantitation of **14** (5-FU), by far the lowest detection limits are realized using negative CI(NH$_3$) for detection of the pentafluorobenzyl derivative of 5-FU(132). In this study, 5-chlorouracil, the internal standard (IS), is added to the patient's plasma sample and the buffered solution extracted with 2-propanol-diethyl ether (22 : 78, v/v). The IS and **14** are then back extracted, derivatized using pentafluorobenzyl bromide in chloroform(CHCl$_3$), with reextraction occurring during derivatization. Quantitation of **14** is performed by monitoring the M-C$_7$H$_2$F$_5^-$ ion of **14** and ion current at m/z 309 and 325 for the IS by negative ion detection in the CI mode. Using this procedure allows one to detect 50 femptograms (fg) and to monitor plasma concentrations for at least 8 h after drug administration.

Both EI and positive CI are used in the quantitation of **14** and for the identification and quantitation of **68**, a metabolite of **14**. 5-Bromouracil is used as the internal standard and the samples are analyzed as their di-n-pentyl derivatives. EI analysis allows one to detect 10 ng/mL and 80 ng/mL for **14** and **68**, respectively, while lower levels of **68**, to 10 ng/mL, require the use of CI.

CI can be used to quantitate **66** in the plasma of patients (136) and to identify and quantitate **67** in patient samples following administration of either **14** or **66** (137). In the first study, samples of **66** and the IS, 1-(2-deoxy-β-D-lyxofuranosyl)-5-fluorouracil, an epimer of **66**, are permethylated and quantitated by monitoring the MH$^+$ ion at m/z 289, the base peak in the spectra of both compounds using NH$_3$ as the reagent gas, with a detection limit of 1 ng/mL. Quantitating **67** as its permethyl derivative established that only minor quantities of 5-FU or FUdR are converted to this metabolite.

69, BEDU, R – ribose
70, BEDU metabolite, R – H

During investigations into the metabolism and pharmacokinetics of 5-(2-bromo-E-ethenyl)-2′-deoxyuridine(BEDU) (**69**), an antiviral agent used in the treatment of Herpes viruses, a major metabolite was detected during HPLC analysis of plasma extracts (138). In order to characterize the metabolite, an isobutane CI mass spectrum was obtained on a purified sample of the metabolite. The mass spectrum shows a doublet of peaks at m/z 217/219, with an isotope ratio suggesting the presence of a bromine atom, and a base peak at m/z 137, corresponding to the loss of HBr. Comparing the spectrum of the metabolite with that of the starting nucleoside establishes the identity of the metabolite as **70**, the pyrimidine base arising from cleavage of the glycosidic bond.

4.2.3. DNA MODIFICATIONS

Chemical ionization used in conjunction with HPLC purification, isotope dilution and tandem mass spectrometry can be used to identify and quantitate methylation sites in DNA following exposure to N-methyl-N-nitrosourea (MeNU) (139) and methyl methanesulfonate (140). Following exposure of the DNA to the methylating agent, for example, MeNU, the DNA is enzymatically degraded to the deoxynucleoside level and the components purified and collected using HPLC. Known quantities of synthetically prepared C^2H_3-labeled internal standards are added to the mixture of nucleosides prior to HPLC separation to provide a basis for quantitation. The individual fractions are then introduced by direct probe and analyzed in the CI mode with isobutane (C_5H_{10}) as the reagent gas. The methylated bases are identified by the appearance of abundant MH^+ ions. (Heating the probe to volatilize the underivatized samples results in the facile cleavage of the glycosidic bond and allows one to identify the mass of the aglycones.) Potential interference from isomeric products, which could produce MH^+ ions at the same m/z values, were previously established to be separated by the HPLC conditions used in this experiment. On the basis of the mass spectrometry, and with the use of radioactive labels, five methylated bases, derived from deoxynucleosides of DNA, were identified and quantitated: 7-methylguanine (**71**), 1-methyladenine (**72**), 3-methylcytosine (**73**), 3-methylthymine (**74**) and O^4-methylthymine (**75**). The data showed that the N-7 position of

71, 7-Methylguanine   72, 1-Methyladenine

73, 3-Methylcytosine

74, 3-Methylthymine

deoxyguanosine is the predominate site of modification, with 99% of the total methylated species being assigned to **71**. The other four minor components are **74** (0.5%), **73** (0.4%), and 0.1% each of **72** and **75**.

Attempts to quantitate O^6-methylguanine (**76**) using normal scanning methods were not successful because of the poor signal to noise ratio in detecting MH^+. However, reanalysis of the sample using tandem mass spectrometry (MS/MS), in this case a triple quadrupole instrument, illustrated the significant increase in both sensitivity and specificity available with this technique. Using model samples of **76** and its C^2H_3-internal standard, the first quadrupole is used to select the MH^+ ion, m/z 166 (aglycone), followed by fragmentation in the second quadrupole and separation of the daughter ions with the third quadrupole. The daughter ion spectrum displays peaks for ions of interest at m/z 166, 149 (100%), 134, and other, lower masses. A similar experiment with the labeled compound shows a spectrum which is essentially identical except for the $+3$ u shift due the deuterium label. Thus, MS/MS can provide a means of identifying a compound, even when the sample cannot be detected using normal scanning methods.

75, 4-Methylthymine

76, O^6-Methylguanine

4.3. Desorption Chemical Ionization

The analysis of nucleosides, especially 2'-deoxynucleosides, nucleotides, or oligonucleotides is difficult because of the highly polar nature of these compounds. Because EI and CI require prior volatilization of the sample, decomposition of the nucleic acid components during vaporization is a common observation, as noted above in the analysis of the methylated components isolated from DNA. A number of approaches have been explored in efforts to overcome these volatility limitations including derivatization (discussed previously) and the use of desorption techniques, such as FAB, plasma desorption (PD), and FD (discussed subsequently). One technique that has been available for a number of years, but which has not been extensively applied to the analysis of nucleic acid components, is desorption chemical ionization or DCI (141).

A major advantage of DCI, relative to other methods, like FD, is the simplicity of the technique. The sample is placed on an emitter wire at the tip of a direct exposure probe and inserted into the normal probe lock, and a current is passed through the emitter wire. The sample is desorbed and ionized by the CI reagent gas plasma, or in a variation of the method, an electron beam, the latter producing an EI-type spectrum (DEI). (See Ref. 142 for a review of desorption from extended probes and Ref. 143 for optimum operating conditions for performing DCI experiments.) The earliest reports on the application of DCI to nucleic acid components describe the direct analysis of guanosine, deoxyguanosine, cyclic AMP (144–146) and other nucleosides, including a series of pyridinium nucleoside salts (146). These are not systematic studies; a variety of reagent gases and operating conditions were used. These experiments do, however, establish that DCI mass spectrometry is a useful tool for samples intractable to the standard EI and CI methods. In general, the spectra provide discernible peaks for the MH^+ ion, fragments useful for identifying the aglycone, the BH_2 ion, and ions related to the sugar moiety. The spectrum is, however, highly dependent on the operating conditions (143). A typical spectrum, for example, that of guanosine obtained using NH_3 as the reagent gas (146), shows the following peaks (m/z, intensity): $[M + NH_4]$ (m/z 301, 3%), [MH] (m/z 284, 17%), $[BH_2]$ (m/z 152, 47%), $[B + NH_4]$ (m/z 169, 64%), $[S - H]$ (m/z 132, 7%), and $[S - H + NH_4]$ (m/z 150, 100%). Analysis of guanosine by DEI, interestingly reported earlier than the DCI method, shows a molecular ion peak at m/z 283 (6%) and a base peak at m/z 151 (BH) (147). More recent reports describe a systematic study of DCI in the analysis of the pyrolysis products of DNA (148) and DCI with MS/MS provides for the characterization and quantitation of an alkylated dinucleotide (149).

5. DESORPTION METHODS OF IONIZATION

Although EI remains the most important ionization technique for the identification or structure elucidation of nucleic acid components, two limitations of classical mass spectrometry, that is, volatility and mass range, are a characteristic of this ionization mode. Volatility limitations are overcome by the formation of derivatives, but a number of hypermodified nucleosides and, most especially, nucleotides and oligonuclotides remain, in general, intractable to analysis by EI. In addition, formation of the derivative requires an additional sample preparation step and can, in some instances, result in modifications to the structure of the sample. Thus, the analysis of nucleic acid components is best performed on the underivatized sample, if possible directly in the biological matrix. This ideal is beginning to be realized and advances in instrumentation and the development of new techniques in mass spectrometry have moved the "impossible" into the category of "let's try it and see."

5.1.   Fast Atom Bombardment (FAB)

Two concurrent developments occurred in the early 1980s that revolutionized the application of mass spectrometry to the analysis of heat labile, highly polar and/or high-molecular-weight nucleic acid components. These advances, the introduction of FAB (2) as an ionization technique and the availability of mass spectrometers with mass ranges exceeding 5000 daltons, provided, for the first time, the capability for the mass spectral analysis of nucleosides, nucleotides, and oligonucleotides in a simple and reproducible manner without (1) the need for derivatization, (2) the application of heat to vaporize the sample, and (3) any particular concern for the molecular weight of the sample. For example, the analysis of hypermodified nucleosides can be performed on the free sample without having to prepare a derivative or heat the sample, which could alter the structure of the nucleoside. Likewise, the analysis of free nucleotides and nucleotide polymers containing two, three, or even more residues was realized for the first time. The introduction of FAB and the high-mass instruments thus opened completely new areas for investigation of nucleic acids and their components by mass spectrometry. Elemental compositions can be obtained on thermally labile and high-molecular-weight samples and fragmentation routes established, which are of value, for example, in the sequencing of oligonucleotides. Also the FAB process generates normally abundant MH^+ ions, with only a few fragments. The application of MS/MS techniques to mixture analysis thus becomes possible and holds promise for the analysis of nucleic acid components directly in the biological sample. Finally, the application of FAB to all classes of nucleosides, nucleotides, and oligonucleotides is generally successful. Free nucleosides that, prior to the introduction of FAB, had been difficult or impossible to analyze by mass spectrometry proved to be readily amenable to FAB ionization. For example, guanosines, deoxyguanosines, cytidine analogs, and all classes of nucleotides can be handled routinely and compounds such as mesoionic nucleosides (150), nucleosides with amino acid side chains, for example, polyoxins (151), ribosyl diphthamide (152), cysteine adducts of deoxycytidine (153), alkylated purine nucleosides and nucleotides (154–158), and nucleic acid adducts (159, 160), among others, have been successfully analyzed using FAB.

Because of the considerable interest in the analytical potential of FAB for the analysis of nucleic acid components, recognized by mass spectroscopists and basic, applied, and clinical researchers alike, the literature on the subject is extensive. Recent reviews, or in-depth discussions, on the mass spectral analysis of nucleic acid components by FAB are available (7–10, 16, 19–21), to which the reader is directed.

5.1.1. NUCLEOSIDE SPECTRA AND APPLICATIONS

The FAB mass spectrum of a nucleoside is very simple, compared to the EI spectrum; it more closely resembles a spectrum obtained using CI (161). As shown in Fig. 5, the general features of the FAB spectrum include the presence of intense MH^+ and BH_2 ions, which establish the molecular weight of the intact nucleoside and permit identification of the aglycone, and the absence of sugar-

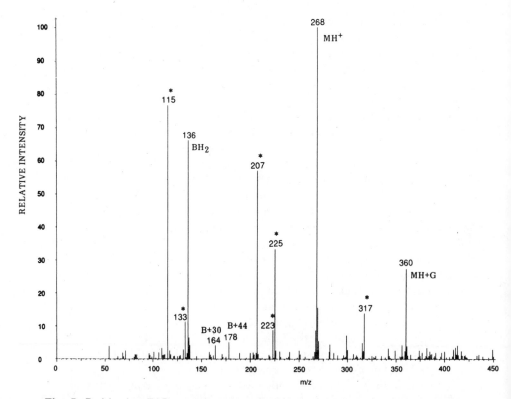

Fig. 5. Positive-ion FAB mass spectrum of adenosine obtained using glycerol as the matrix. Ions related to the matrix are indicated with an asterisk (*) and are assigned as follows: m/z 115, glycerol(G) + Na^+; m/z 133, Cs^+ from cesium ion gun used in this liquid SIMS experiment; m/z 207, 2G + Na^+; m/z 225, G + Cs^+; m/z 317, 2G + Cs^+. Other peaks, none of which are sample related, remain unassigned. Sample concentration is approximately 500 ng/μL.

related ions. A glycerol adduct is commonly formed, which gives a peak 92 mass units above the MH^+ ion and dimers, M_2H^+, are often also observed.

Because fragment ions in both CI and FAB arise from the protonated molecule, the structures and mechanisms of ion formation in FAB are thought (161) to be analogous to those proposed for CI (128), and the similarity in the spectra appear to support this idea. However, compared to the EI spectrum, the FAB spectrum shows a net loss in structural information, although the gross features of nucleoside structure are clearly reflected in the FAB spectrum.

One approach to regaining some of the structural information lost in the FAB analysis of free nucleosides is to prepare the TMS derivative of the sample (162). Using this technique, a substantial increase in the number of structurally significant fragment ions is realized, with 8 of the 10 sugar- and 13 of the 16 base-series ions being present; in this regard, the FAB spectrum is similar to the EI spectrum of the TMS derivative of adenosine. The FAB mass spectrum of the TMS derivative of adenosine, Fig. 6, indicates that a significant amount of the sample is present as the $(TMS)_3$ derivative, while most is present as the $(TMS)_4$ analog. Analyzing the same sample by EI indicates formation of the full TMS

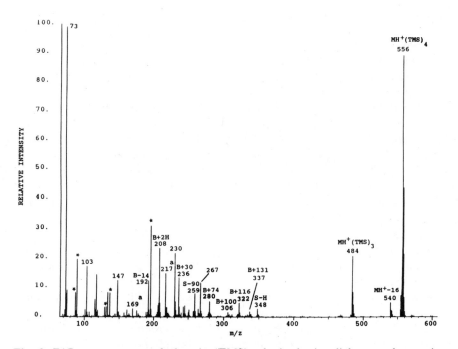

Fig. 6. FAB mass spectrum of adenosine$(TMS)_4$ obtained using diglyme as the matrix. Matrix associated ions are identified by an asterisk. Ions with a superscript [a] are common to both the matrix and sample. Analysis of the TMS derivatives of nucleosides provides a significant increase in number of structurally relevant fragments compared to analysis of the free compound by FAB.

derivative, TMS_4, so hydrolysis of one of the derivative functions, probably from the exocyclic amino group occurs during FAB ionization. The spectrum shown in Fig. 6 is obtained without heating of the probe.

Of interest in this spectrum is the presence of many odd-electron ion species presumably formed by free radical mechanisms, possibly due to the presence of silicon or the matrix used in these experiments. The TMS derivatives of nucleotides give similar, but not as dramatic, results.

Collisionally induced dissociation (CID) provides a more sophisticated means of enhancing the fragmentation of MH^+ from free nucleosides and nucleotides during FAB analysis (21). A number of experimental variables in the use of MS/MS for the analysis of nucleic acid components were examined including a comparison of spectra with and without CID, and using both positive- and negative-ion detection. Comparing the spectra with and without CID shows a significant increase in the abundance of the structurally relevant B + 30 and B + 44 ions, in the CID mode, permitting recognition of modifications at the 1' or 2' positions or the O-4' ring oxygen. Comparison of the + vs − ion detection mode shows the data were complementary. In general, the positive-ion spectrum shows a greater number of fragments, although all major features are also observed in the negative-ion mode. Using both detection methods is therefore recommended because, in at least one case, additional structural information is obtained in the negative-ion mode that permits differentiation of isomers of the aglycone. Also of importance is that the negative-ion spectra, but not the positive, show the retro-Diels-Alder expulsion of HNCO from pyrimidine nucleosides. This reaction is of considerable importance in locating modifications in the C-2, O^2, and N-1 positions of the pyrimidine ring.

As significant as the increase in structural information is the ability, using CID–MS/MS, to obtain a mass spectrum of the sample without the presence of interfering ions from the matrix. When a FAB spectrum is obtained using the normal operating mode, the presence of matrix ions makes identification of sample-related ions somewhat difficult. In addition, if the structure of the nucleic acid component is unknown, there is a danger that the sample ions will be masked by the matrix ions. The normal procedure is to reanalyze the sample in a second matrix that, by producing different matrix ions, should permit identification of the sample ions. However, using the CID–MS/MS technique avoids this problem because only sample-related ions are selectively transmitted to the collision cell by the first MS stage, and the mass spectrum of fragments (daughters) obtained by the second MS stage.

As already mentioned, the analysis of a nucleoside by FAB–MS is a simple and straightforward process; results can generally be obtained if the quantity of material available is in the high nanogram to microgram range. Additional information may also be gained concerning the number of exchangable hydrogens in the molecule by performing the analysis in a matrix of O-perdeuterioglycerol and ^2H_2O (163, 164) where up to 97% of the 28 labile hydrogens in selected samples can be exchanged. A similar approach using ^2H-labeled 3-

nitrobenzyl alcohol (165) should extend the ability to determine the number of active hydrogens in less polar nucleic acid samples, for example, derivatized analogs.

FAB analyses require the presence of a matrix, which is both a boon and a bane. The long-lived ion currents in FAB result in continued renewal of the sample at the matrix surface. At the same time the matrix constantly contributes abundant ions to the background of the spectrum. In addition, the liquid matrix can interact with the sample or effect side reactions resulting from the FAB ionization. For example, dehalogenation reactions are observed during the FAB analysis of a number of I-, Br-, Cl-, and F-containing nucleosides (166). The order of exchange, following the same order as the electronegativity of the halogen atoms, is more extensive in the positive-ion detection mode and is a major process in the eight nucleosides examined. Therefore, the FAB mass spectrum of a nucleic acid sample suspected of containing halogen atoms should be interpreted with caution.

Some difficulty may also be encountered in detection of $M + 2$ stable isotopes using low-resolution FAB data, which are based on the abundance of the MH^+ ion. A study (167) of the FAB spectra, obtained in variety of matricies, of a number of nucleosides shows an enhancement in the abundance of the $(M + 2H)^+$ and $(M + 3H)^+$ ions, which could be confused with the presence of sulfur atoms or affect the average molecular weight calculated for higher-molecular-weight samples. This reduction is observed in both purine and pyrimidine nucleosides and is thought to result from multiple protonation of the nucleoside followed by one and two electron reductions during desorption.

In spite of the practical difficulties in using FAB, the successful analysis of samples not possible by EI attests to the importance of the technique. For example, the analysis of the products formed between pyrrolizidine alkaloids and large number of nucleosides and nucleotides is accomplished using FAB (168, 169). These samples are refractory to analysis by EI. However, tandem mass spectrometry with CID shows (169) detailed information concerning the sites of base, sugar, and alkaloid modification. The most informative data are obtained in the positive-ion analysis of the MH^+ and $(M + K)^+$ ions, with data from negative-ion data providing only confirmatory results, except for some minor fragments indicative of the alkaloid binding site. Representative of the products are structures **77** and **78**.

An especially exciting application of FAB is illustrated by the direct analysis of the nucleoside antibiotic toyocamycin (**79**) in a fermentation broth (170) with no sample preparation. A combination of negative- and positive-ion FAB, high-resolution FAB, and MIKES (mass-analyzed ion kinetic energy spectrometry) allows one to monitor nucleoside levels at concentrations in the 600 ng/μL range. Hence FAB is an important tool for monitoring large scale fermentation processes. This application is one of the few examples of mass spectrometry being used for the detection of a compound of interest in a biological medium without any sample preparation.

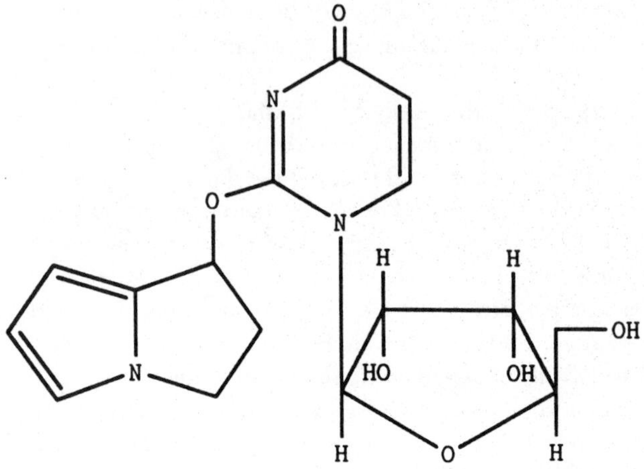

77

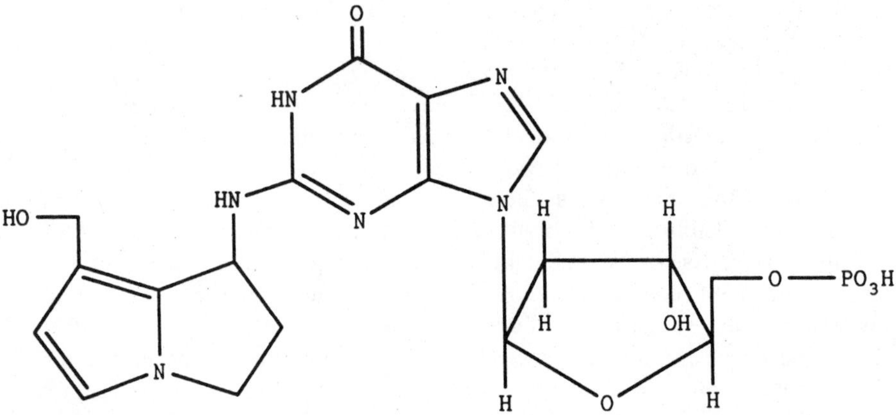

78

5.1.2. NUCLEOTIDE SPECTRA AND APPLICATIONS

Although important in the analysis of nucleosides, especially the hypermodified, highly complex components of tRNA, the mass spectral analysis of nucleotides, ranging in structure from simple mono- (171), cyclic (172), and triphosphate (173) nucleosides to more complex dinucleoside monophosphates (174–176) and trinucleoside diphosphates (177, 178) illustrates the value of FAB for the analysis of nucleic acid components not possible with any other, readily available method.

The FAB spectrum of a nucleotide, see Fig. 7, may be obtained using either the positive- or negative-ion detection mode, with most work being done with

79

negative ions because of the complexity of the positive-ion spectrum. In the positive-ion mode, the MH$^+$ ion may be represented by a minor peak because of cationization (adducts with K$^+$ or Na$^+$) of the phosphate residues. Although cation adduct peaks are somewhat useful in determining the number of exchangable phosphate hydrogens, the splitting of the ion current between the cations and MH$^+$ decreases sensitivity and adds considerable complexity to the spectrum. The BH ions are prominent and may be accompanied by the sodium ion replacement observed 22 u higher in mass for each Na$^+$ added. A number of phosphate ions are also generally observed, but do not provide any structural information. In contrast to the complexity of the positive-ion spectrum, the negative-ion FAB spectrum of nucleotides is simple with the (M − H)$^-$ and (B − H)$^-$ ions dominating the spectrum. An exception is the negative-ion spectrum of triphosphate nucleosides that can also show the presence of various numbers of metal ions (174).

Negative-ion FAB may be used to distinguish 2′,3′- from 3′,5′-cyclic monophosphates, for example, in plant materials (179). Differentiating these two nucleotides requires the use of MIKES, or a tandem instrument, for selection of the MH$^+$ ion in the positive-ion detection mode. For example, differences in fragmentation between 2′,3′-cCMP (**80**) and 3′,5′-cCMP (**81**) are most evident in cleavages across the sugar ring of **81** to provide B + 30 and B + 44 ions, with these ions being weak or absent in the spectrum of **80**. On the other hand, peak at the m/z 178 is unique to **80**. A similar pattern is observed upon analysis of the corresponding adenosine and guanosine cyclic monophosphates, that is, the 3′,5′ isomers produce the B + 30 and B + 44 ions while the 2′,3′ isomers do not.

The next level of complexity, that is, analyzing dinucleoside monophosphates (N^{1}pN^2) requires for the first time a consideration of sequence information. As

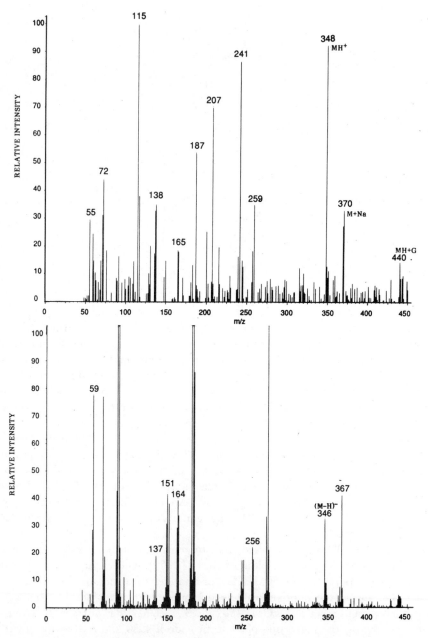

Fig. 7. Positive- (top) and negative-ion FAB mass spectra of AMP obtained using glycerol as the matrix. The top panel shows the spectrum resulting from "background subtraction," while the bottom panel displays the spectrum as obtained during the experiment. The only peaks clearly related to the sample are the M + H, M + Na, and MH + glycerol(G) peaks in the positive ion spectrum and the M − H peak at m/z 346 in the negative-ion spectrum. Sample concentration is approximately 500 ng/μL in these measurements.

266

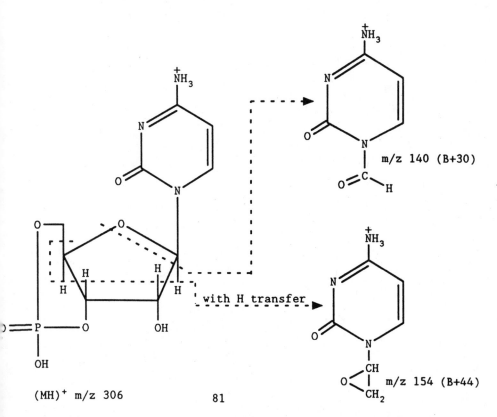

80

(MH)$^+$ m/z 306

m/z 178

with H transfer

m/z 140 (B+30)

with H transfer

m/z 154 (B+44)

(MH)$^+$ m/z 306

81

267

might be expected, the spectrum is more complex than that of the mononucleotides, but the major structural features are observed (21, 176). $(M - H)^-$
and matrix adduct ions are present, permitting assignment of molecular weight,
with the major fragmentation being cleavage of the sugar–phosphate bond to
give nucleoside monophosphate anions; cleavage of the base sugar bond is not a
prominent event, but the presence of B^- ions allow assignment of the nucleic acid
base residues. Sequence information is available from a cleavage across the 5′-
sugar residue to produce an ion unique to the mass spectrum of the 3′-end
nucleotide plus the elements of C_3H_4O, as shown for the isomeric pair ApC (**82**)
and CpA (176). The deoxy analogs undergo essentially the same behavior.

An added structural feature of dinucleoside monophosphates is also of
consequence in light of the identification of 2′,5′-linked nucleotides as natural
products. Differentiation of the isomeric 2′,5′- from the 3′,5′-linked isomers is
possible based on the appearance of $(M - H - 90)^-$ in the CID–MS/MS
spectrum, formed by a transannular cleavage of the sugar ring, as shown for

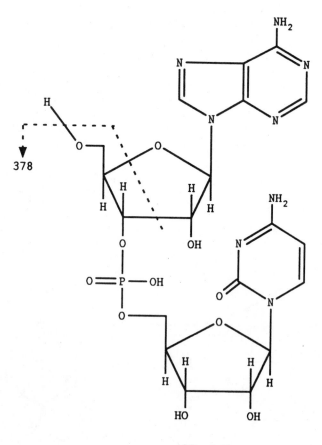

82, ApC

83, A(2',5')C

adenylyl-(2',5')-cytidine (**83**) (21); this fragment is not observed in the case of the 3',5'-linked isomer.

Not surprising is that FAB mass spectrometry can be applied to a number of important problems in the biochemical and biomedical areas. Included among these applications are the development of a method for incorporation of ^{18}O into UDP–glucuronic acid (180), the differentiation of ^{18}O-labeled UTP (181), the identification of partially protected dinucleoside monophosphates (182), and the characterization of 3-aminocarbazole adducts with d[Tp(Ap)pT] (183).

5.1.3. OLIGONUCLEOTIDES

The direct analysis of intact, free oligodeoxynucleotides containing up to 10 base residues has been reported using negative-ion FAB (184–187). The detailed analysis of the FAB spectra of smaller oligomers, in some cases either partially or completely derivatized, also has been described (176, 179, 188).

The negative ion FAB mass spectrum of a free, oligodeoxynucleotide, for example, the decamer d(GAAGATCTTC) (**84**) (184) shows an $(M - H)^-$ ion at m/z 3024, establishing the molecular weight of the sample. The main fragmentations result in formation of sequence ions arising from cleavages beginning at either end of the chain, but with the abundance of the "3'-sequence ions" being greater. Thus, the intensity of the m/z 2775, 2462, 2149, and so forth, fragments are more intense than those at m/z 2815, 2511, 2207, and so forth, shown in structure **84**. (The reader is advised that the nomenclature in this area can be confusing and attention must be paid to how terms are defined.)

Although a greater abundance of the 3'- vs 5'-sequence ions is generally observed in oligodeoxynucleotides containing at least five base residues, exceptions to this abundance rule are noted for shorter chains (176, 184, 188). The ambiguity in sequence information may be removed by either blocking the 5' end of the chain (184), which results in a defined mass shift of the 3'-sequence ions, or by using MS/MS with CID to acquire the spectrum (178). However, as the length of the chain increases to the 5- or 6-mer stage, ions representing competing pathways become less well defined and secondary fragmentations become more prominent, thus making sequence determination of an unknown more difficult (178). On the other hand, FAB has its greatest utility in confirming the sequence of a synthetic oligomer, not sequencing DNA fragments. Therefore, some structural information should be available on which to base the interpretation of the spectrum. Using negative-ion FAB provides rapid and routine method for characterizing the monomeric and oligomeric building blocks used in the phosphotriester synthesis of DNA fragments (175, 184–187). At least one free phosphate hydroxyl group must be available for anion formation, since attempts to analyze fully protected samples is unsuccessful using FAB. Once ionized, however, the partially derivatized samples show fragmentation patterns similar to those obtained with the fully deprotected oligonucleotides, except for the increased complexity of the spectrum due to extra bond cleavages next to the protecting group (186, 187). The experimental procedures used in the analysis of a large number of partially protected oligodeoxynucleotides, in some cases with modifications to the phosphate group, for example, ^{18}O or S replacing ^{16}O, are described (188).

5.2. ^{252}Cf-Plasma Desorption

^{252}Cf plasma desorption (PD) is an important alternative to FAB for the characterization of fully protected synthetic intermediates used in the synthesis of nucleic acid fragments. The advantages (23, 189–191) of PD, relative to FAB and chemical methods, for the characterization of intermediates and products of oligonucleotide synthetic procedures include (1) the capacity to directly analyze the fully protected samples without the need of deprotection steps, (2) the availability of both molecular weight and sequence information in the negative ion PD spectrum, (3) reliability and speed (the sequence of small oligomers being available in minutes), and (4) applicability to a wide variety of blocked deoxy-

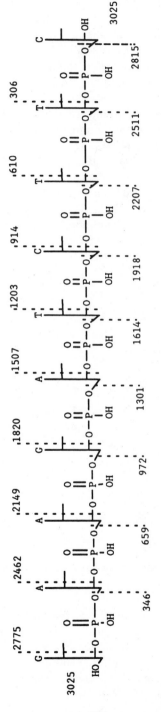

271

and ribo-oligonucleotides. Sequence information is more easily obtained using negative-ion detection, compared to the positive-ion mode, but some specific decomposition pathways are observed in the positive spectrum, which are not obvious in the negative-ion spectrum. The structural information in both modes is complementary. Of particular interest is the observation of very high mass negative ions, for example, up to m/z 4577 in the spectrum of a blocked heptamer, even though resolution was poor with the time-of-flight analyzer used in this work.

The negative-ion PD spectra of 10 underivatized trideoxynucleoside diphosphates were used to develop structure–fragmentation relationships relating the identity and position of the base residues to the intensity of the sequence ions (192). Using these data in conjunction with a computer program made it possible to rapidly and easily determine the structure and sequence of oligomers.

[252]Cf-Plasma desorption has also been used in the structure elucidation of the nucleoside antibiotic adenomycin (**85**) (193), a sample not amenable to EI, CI, or FD, and for the analysis of a series of adenosine and xanthosine derivatives being tested as adenosine agonists and antagonists (194).

85, Adenomycin

5.3. Other Desorption Ionization Techniques

5.3.1. FIELD DESORPTION (FD)

Field desorption is an important technique for the analysis of underivatized nucleic acid components, especially nucleotides, and research continues in finding ways to improve the method, for example, using laser-assisted FD improves the stability of ion currents (195). Comparing an FD spectrum to FAB spectrum of a series of pyridine nucleotides and nucleotide triphosphates suggests (195) that, while neither method is ideal, FD spectra provide molecular weight and characteristic structural information, with the absence of matrix effects. Sample requirements are an order of magnitude less than those for FAB. FAB, on the other hand, is experimentally easier, but suffers from a complex set of matrix effects. While these criticisms of FAB have validity, it should be noted that the FD spectra were all acquired in the positive-ion mode and detection limit estimates are higher by at least an order of magnitude over those commonly reported; in fact, detection of mid (196) to low (129) nanogram quantities of nucleotides are now being reported using FAB. The major limitations of FD for the analysis of nucleic acid components continue to be in the difficulty of the experimental procedure, the production of short-lived ion currents, the absence of structurally informative fragments, except those generated by thermal decomposition of the sample, and a limitation of the technique for the analysis of oligomeric samples.

In spite of the disadvantages and limitations of FD, the technique is an important alternative to FAB in cases where FAB does not work, for example, in the analysis of fully blocked monomers or products used in, or obtained from, the triester method of polynucleotide synthesis (197).

5.3.2. SECONDARY ION MASS SPECTROMETRY (SIMS)

SIMS provides another alternative to FAB analysis for fully protected oligonucleotides (198, 199). In addition to the formation of $(M + H)^+$ and cationized species, the fully protected oligonucleotides show some specific fragmentations. Fission of a C5'-O bond results in the positive charge remaining on the carbon-containing fragment, while cleavage of the C3'-O bond is not detected. Fission of the C3'-O bond results, instead, in the positive charge being retained on the phosphate-containing fragment. Examining the negative-ion SIMS spectrum shows a prominent $(M - H)^-$ ion and characteristic fragment ions formed by fission of any of the three bonds attached to the phosphate groups. Major fragments in the positive ion SIMS spectrum of fully protected CpCpC are shown in structure **86** (198).

SIMS has been applied to the analysis of free nucleosides (200) and a series of protected dinucleoside monophosphates (199). The SIMS analysis of the free nucleosides is of interest and should be considered as an alternative if FAB is not successful. The spectra are simple, showing the aglycone as the base peak of the spectrum, and the method is applicable to samples which cannot be analyzed by EI, for example, deoxycytidine and deoxyguanosine analogs. However, the very low abundance of the molecular-weight-related ions is discouraging. The SIMS spectra of the blocked dinucleoside monophosphates, however, should be of value as an important alternative to FD, PD, and FAB. The SIMS spectra yield a considerable amount of structural information, including molecular weight, identification of the nucleic acid bases, identification of the blocking groups and sequence information. In general, the spectra are very similar to those obtained using PD. An additional advantage of the SIMS method, over FD and PD, is the generation of long-lived ion currents, which can provide metastable ion data in either the positive or negative ion detection modes.

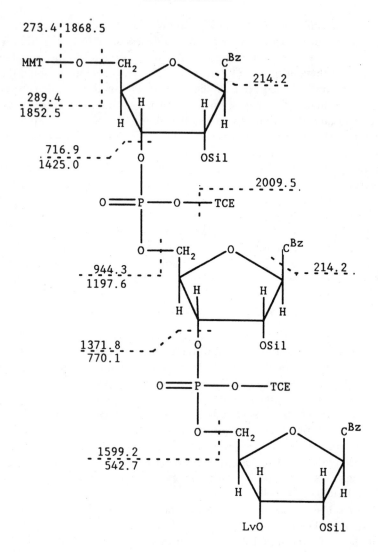

86

5.3.3. LASER DESORPTION (LD)

Using laser-desorption/Fourier-transform (FT) mass spectrometry (LD FTMS) for the analysis of biological materials, including free nucleosides, is also possible (201). The negative-ion spectra are, in most cases, dominated by the $(B - H)^-$ ions, but molecular weight and other structural information is also obtained. Positive-ion spectra display a protonated, or cationized, molecule and a BH_2 ion, but no other structural information is obvious. The intent of this report is to show the utility of the technique and additional work is warranted, especially with the potential of high-resolution, complex MS/MS studies and other specific attributes of the FT mass spectrometer.

6. LIQUID CHROMATOGRAPHY-MASS SPECTROMETRY

Liquid chromatography-mass spectrometry, of all possible techniques, holds the greatest promise for the analysis of mixtures of nucleic acid components. Probably the greatest advantage of LC–MS, relative to GC–MS or direct probe analysis, is the capability of separating and analyzing complex mixtures of components with widely differing polarities, without the need for derivatization (9, 24). Although direct analysis of mixtures is possible using MS/MS techniques, differentiating isomers still requires chromatographic separation. Because of the availability of a wide selection of stationary phases, the options available in mobile phase composition, and the capability of effecting separations in the liquid phase, HPLC has become the chromatographic system of choice for the separation of all classes of nucleic acid components. However, the greatest limitation of HPLC is the need for a sensitive, general detector; this need is met, with some current limitations, by a mass spectrometer. Likewise, the analysis of nucleic acid components using mass spectrometry is restricted by the necessity of performing the analysis in the vapor phase, a requirement with severe limitations in the nucleic acid field. Thus, the successful combination of HPLC with MS is an extremely exciting development.

The major limitations of LC–MS at the present time are (1) the absence of high-resolution capability and (2) the experimental difficulties and variables characteristic of each LC–MS technique. However, since LC–MS is still in its infancy, the limitations of the technique should be overcome with time, or at least the variables will be better understood and controlled with further experience.

Techniques for performing LC–MS as applied to the analysis of nucleic acid components include thermospray (TSP), direct liquid injection (DLI), moving belt and atmospheric pressure chemical ionization (APCI). A bibliography of recent LC–MS literature is available (202).

6.1. Thermospray

Of the methods available for performing LC–MS, the system that has been most fully investigated for the analysis of nucleic acid components is thermospray (TSP). A particular advantage of TSP over the other LC–MS methods is that, in addition to functioning as an LC–MS interface, it also serves as a unique ionization method (203) for production of ions from a nonvolatile sample.

The procedures used for the analysis of a complex mixture, that is, the separation and direct analysis of the nucleoside components of a tRNA hydrolysate, have been described (24) and illustrate the considerable potential of thermospray LC–MS in the characterization of nucleic acid components. Experimental conditions, which are somewhat critical for a successful analysis, include the temperature of the interface (240–280°C, best) and spray (275–300°C, optimum) and the use of a linear solvent gradient. Buffer selection is also important and ammonium acetate is preferred over other volatile buffers which have been investigated.

The mass spectrum of a nucleoside ionized using thermospray exhibits peaks for three principal ion species (24): (1) the protonated molecule (MH^+) represents the intact nucleoside, (2) the BH_2 ion characterizes the aglycone, and (3) a sugar-derived ion complexed with NH_4^+, which permits identification of the sugar as deoxyribose (m/z 134), ribose (m/z 150), or 2′-O-methylribose (m/z 164). In addition, exocyclic substitutions on the base may give rise to additional fragments of structural importance, although the B + 30, B + 44, and B + 60 ions observed in the EI and FAB spectra are absent. Ion abundance appears to vary with nucleoside structure, for example, cytidine provides MH^+ and BH_2 ions two to five times as abundant as from other nucleosides. Ion abundance also depends on the operating temperature of the interface; this effect differs between nucleosides. In spite of these experimental complications, which represent the major disadvantage of thermospray, the technique is very useful for the identification of both known and unidentified nucleosides in complex mixtures, especially when the TSP data are combined with information obtained using FAB and low- and high-resolution EI.

An outstanding example of the combination of all available mass spectral data to determine the structure of an unidentified nucleoside is the structure determination of a newly discovered fluorescent tricyclic nucleoside from archaebacterial tRNA (204). Analysis of the hydrolysate by HPLC indicated the presence of a highly fluorescent and previously unreported component. The direct analysis of the hydrolysate using TSP LC–MS produced peaks at m/z 350 (1%) for MH^+ and at m/z 218 (100%) for the BH_2 ion; the difference of 132 mass units suggested the presence of an unmodified ribose. No known nucleosides from RNA had a molecular weight of 349 daltons. A FAB spectrum of the unknown, isolated and collected by HPLC, showed peaks at m/z 350 (52%) for MH^+ and at m/z 218 (100%) for the BH_2 ion, confirming the TSP results. The EI spectrum of the TMS derivative of the sample showed an intense molecular ion peak at m/z 565, indicating addition of three TMS groups, all located in the sugar, and the absence of active hydrogens in the aglycone. The base-ion series lacked any evidence of a side chain and the M/M − 15 ratio suggested a guanine-type base, not alkylated at the N-7 position. High-resolution mass measurements suggested a composition corresponding to guanosine + C_5H_6. These data, along with the UV and fluorescent properties of the molecule, led to structure **87**, an analog of the aglycone of Y nucleoside. A search of the literature revealed that the aglycone had been previously prepared, so the unknown nucleoside was hydrolyzed to the base stage. A comparison of the chromatographic and mass spectrometric properties of the base derived from the unknown nucleoside and a sample of the reference material showed the two compounds to be identical.

87

Thermospray LC–MS also has been used to establish the purity of nucleoside antitumor agents (205, 206), for example, 3-deazauridine, tetrahydrouridine, and triazone and to identify a metabolite of the antiviral nucleoside analog 2′,3′-dideoxyadenosine (207).

More recently, electrochemistry/thermospray/tandem mass spectrometry has been used to study the biooxidation of purines (208).

6.2.   Direct Liquid Injection

Direct liquid injection (DLI) of the effluent from the chromatograph into the source of the mass spectrometer is of utility in a number of problems in nucleoside analysis. The initial report in this area (209) shows that mixtures of nucleosides may be separated and that the spectra produced are dominated, in most cases, by the MH$^+$ ions of the intact molecule. A number of operating restrictions, however, detract from the otherwise significant potential of the technique. Among the limitations are the formation of cluster ions by the solvent, the limitation of mobile phase to methanol and acetonitrile, both with aqueous volatile buffers, the lack of sensitivity, with 25–30 μg of sample being required for analysis and a lower mass limitation of m/z 130. Improvements to the system have been reported (210) that result in better sensitivity and a wider usable mass range. The improved interface is used for the analysis of nucleosides in human urine (211) and for the characterization of some synthetic nucleosides (212). Spectra of reference samples, obtained using the modified system, are characterized by the appearance of strong MH^+ ions, an easily identifiable S^+ ion, and ions associated with the aglycone with portions of the sugar attached, for example, the $B + 30$ and $B + 44$ ions. Thus, modifications to the base and sugar residue may be identified. Identifying pseudouridine in urine is possible, but other components present in lesser quantities that are known to be in urine are not detected, so the sensitivity of DLI remains a problem.

6.3. Atmospheric Pressure Chemical Ionization

Atmospheric pressure chemical ionization (APCI) coupled with tandem mass spectrometry has been described in the identification of radiation-induced damage to polyadenylic acid (213). This combination of a soft ionization technique with tandem mass spectrometry is shown to be superior to normal LC–MS for analysis of complex mixtures, with the production of daughter ions, containing considerable structural information, being crucial for structure elucidation. Using the normal scan mode, the nucleoside spectra are as expected using ammonia as the reagent gas, with the MH^+ ion being the most abundant ion of the spectrum and the BH_2 ion the only fragment being observed. Selection of the MH^+ ion followed by collision and scanning of the daughter ion spectrum provided a spectrum containing a mixture of ions representing both the sugar and base portions of the nucleoside; selection of either the BH_2 or S^+ ions allowed identification of the daughter ions derived from each of these species. The combination of APCI with the MS/MS capabilities of the instrument were required for the identification of the products. A limitation of this particular method is the drop in sensitivity, estimated to be 10-fold, in performing the CAD experiments.

6.4. Moving Belt

The oldest of the LC–MS interfaces, the moving belt, is a viable method for the analysis of nucleosides and, in at least one case, the analysis of a nucleotide has been reported (214, 215). The spectra of the nucleosides are essentially the same as those observed in the DLI and APCI interface, all are CI (ammonia) spectra, with the MH^+, BH_2, and $(S + NH_4)^+$ ions being easily recognized, although some abundance differences are evident in data collected with the three interfaces. Since the moving belt has not been applied to the analysis of mixtures, its potential in this regard is difficult to judge. The major limitation of the moving belt, at least in the past, has been the requirement for volatility of the sample, an obvious deficiency. However, the recent report (216) of the combination of direct FAB ionization using a moving belt interface could make this combination potentially the most powerful of the LC–MS methods. Although no nucleic acid components have been analyzed using the FAB moving-belt system, the potential of the combination is exciting, since none of the other systems provide mass spectra of nucleotides.

Finally, a method for dynamic analysis using FAB, the continuous-flow FAB probe (217, 218), also holds considerable promise for the analysis of nucleic acid components, although the system has not yet been used for the analysis of this compound class.

7. CONCLUDING REMARKS

There is no doubt that mass spectrometry has played, and will continue to play, an important role in the analysis of nucleic acid components. Historically, the major application of mass spectrometry has been in determining the structures of modified nucleosides and nucleic acid bases contained in various samples of biochemical and biomedical interest. This role is unlikely to change, since new nucleosides may be expected to be identified in various RNA and DNA species, new drugs (belonging to the antimetabolite class) for the treatment of cancer and viral infections, for use as antibiotics, and in the treatment of AIDS will be introduced, and new nucleoside antibiotics with complex structures will continue to be produced by fermentation methods. Use of mass spectrometry in the preceding areas will provide, as examples, a better understanding of the structure–function relationships of modified nucleosides in RNA and provide important qualitative and quantitative data for improving the clinical efficiency and design of antitumor, antiviral, and anti-AIDS drugs. Capabilities of providing important information in these areas currently exist, as demonstrated earlier in this chapter.

Research efforts in the biotechnology area will also benefit with the application of FAB, PD, SIMS, and, possibly FD, to the analysis of synthetic and genetically engineered products. The direct monitoring of fermentation broths to optimize production of scarce nucleoside antibiotics is a good example of the potential of mass spectrometry in this area.

The potential of LC–MS is obvious, but additional research is needed to better define the experimental variables and, if possible, make LC–MS a more routine technique. Two areas that need to be investigated are the use of moving-belt FAB and continuous-flow FAB. Both of these techniques can be coupled to essentially any mass analyzer, but coupling with a magnetic instrument could provide high-resolution capabilities not currently available on LC–MS instruments and could expand the mass range available for the analysis of high-molecular-weight samples.

Mixture analysis using MS/MS, possibly applied directly to crude biological samples, should also be explored, especially in the clinical area. Applications of MS/MS, using either hybride, triple quadrupole, or multisector magnetic instruments should be an area of exciting research of benefit to all areas of nucleic acid chemistry.

The next few years should see many of the frontier experiments of today become more routine, with a significant expansion of the applications of mass spectrometry to biochemical and biomedical problems spreading to a larger

number of laboratories with greater capabilities. The future role of mass
spectrometry in the nucleic acid field is assured and may be expected to be as
exciting and challenging as its past.

ACKNOWLEDGMENTS

The author would like to thank the members of his research group for their
assistance in preparing the figures and structures for this manuscript and for
offering helpful comments on various aspects of this work. Thanks to Peter Baker,
Tom McClure, Vicky Mykytyn, Mark Reimer, Stacy Tryon and Bill Hammargren. Financial support from NIH grants CA 42309 and CA 43068 for portions of
this work is gratefully acknowledged.

References

1. K. Biemann and J. A. McCloskey, *J. Am. Chem. Soc.* **84**, 2005 (1962).

2. M. Barber, R. S. Bordoli, R. D. Sedgwick, and A. N. Tyler, *Nature (London)* **293**, 270 (1981).

3. C. R. Blakley, J. J. Carmody, and M. L. Vestal, *Anal. Chem.* **52**, 1636 (1980).

4. J. A. McCloskey, "Mass Spectrometry," in P.O.P. Ts'o, Ed., *Basic Principles in Nucleic Acid Chemistry*, Academic Press, New York, 1974, Vol. I, p. 209.

5. C. Hignite, "Nucleic Acids and Derivatives," in G. R. Waller, Ed., *Biochemical Applications of Mass Spectrometry*, Wiley-Interscience, New York, 1972, Chapter 16.

6. C. Hignite, "Nucleic Acids and Derivatives," in G. R. Waller and O. C. Dermer, Eds., *Biochemical Applications of Mass Spectrometry, First Supplimental Volume*, Wiley-Interscience, New York, 1980, Chapter 16.

7. A. L. Burlingame, D. Maltby, D. H. Russell, and P. T. Holland, *Anal. Chem.* **60**, 294R–342R (1988).

8. K. H. Schram, "Purines and Pyrimidines," in A. M. Lawson, Ed., *Mass Spectrometry: Applications in Clinical Biochemistry*, Walter de Gruyter and Co., Berlin, 1988, Chapter 10, pp. 507–570.

9. J. A. McCloskey, "Experimental Approaches to the Characterization of Nucleic Acid Constituents By Mass Spectrometry," in S. J. Gaskell, Ed., *Mass Spectrometry in Biomedical Research*, Wiley, Chichester, 1986, Chapter 6.

10. J. A. McCloskey, "Techniques for the Structure Elucidation of Complex Nucleosides by Mass Spectrometry," in F. C. Alderweirldt and E. L. Esmans, Eds., *Proceedings of the 4th International Round Table on Nucleosides, Nucleotides and Their Biological Applications*, University of Antwerp, Antwerp, 1982, p. 47.

11. K. H. Schram and J. A. McCloskey, "Nucleosides and Nucleotides," K. Tsuji, Ed., in *GC and HPLC Determination of Therapeutic Agents*, Marcel Dekker, New York, 1979, Chapter 33.

12. H. Pang, K. H. Schram, D. L. Smith, S. P. Gupta, L. B. Townsend, and J. A. McCloskey, *J. Org. Chem.* **47**, 3923 (1982).

13. M. A. Quilliam, K. K. Ogilvie, K. L. Sadana, and J. B. Westmore, *Org. Mass Spectrom.* **15**, 207 (1980).

14. R. G. Teece and K. H. Schram, "Preparation and Gas-Phase Analysis of Permethylated Nucleosides," in L. B. Townsend and R. S. Tipson, Eds., *Nucleic Acid Chemistry: Improved and New Synthetic Procedures, Methods and Techniques*, Wiley, New York, 1986, p. 311.

15. W. A. Koenig, L. C. Smith, P. F. Crain, and J. A. McCloskey, *Biochemistry* **10**, 3968 (1971).

16. J. A. McCloskey, "Mass Spectrometry of Nucleic Acid Constituents and Related Compounds," in A. L. Burlingame and N. Castagnoli, Eds., *Mass Spectrometry in the Health and Life Sciences*, Elsevier Amsterdam, 1985, p. 521.

17. A. M. Lawson, W. A. Koenig, L. C. Smith and J. A. McCloskey, *Adv. Mass Spectrom.*, 5, 753 (1971).

18. A.L Burlingame, K. Straub, and T. Baille, *Mass Spectrom Rev.* 2, 331 (1978).

19. K. H. Schram, *Trends in Anal. Chem.* 7, 28 (1988).

20. D. L. Slowikowski and K. H. Schram, *Nucleosides Nucleotides* 4, 309 (1985).

21. F. W. Crow, K. B. Tomer, M. L. Gross, J. A. McCloskey, and D. E. Bergstrom, *Anal. Biochem.* 139, 243 (1984).

22. H. R. Schulten, *Int. J. Mass Spectrom. Ion Phys.* 32, 97 (1979).

23. C. J. McNeal, K. K. Ogilvie, N. Y. Theriault, and M. J. Nemer, *J. Am. Chem. Soc.* 104, 981 (1982).

24. C. E. Edmonds, M. L. Vestal, and J. A. McCloskey, *Nucleic Acids Res.* 13, 8197 (1985).

25. J. A. McCloskey and S. Nishimura, *Accounts Chem. Res.* 10, 403 (1977).

26. R. E. Summons, C. C. Duke, J. V. Eichholzer, B. Entsh, D. S. Letham, J. K. MacLeod, and C. W. Parker, *Biomed. Mass Spectrom.* 6, 407 (1979).

27. K. Nakano, K. Shindo, T. Yasaka, and H. Yamamoto, *J. Chromatogr.* 33s, 127 (1985).

28. H. A. Kirst, D. E. Dorman, J. L. Occolowitz, N. D. Jones, J. W. Paschal, R. L. Hamill, and E. F. Szymanski, *J. Antibiotics* 38, 575 (1985).

29. T. Marunaka, Y. Umeno, and Y. Minami, *J. Chromatogr.* 190, 107 (1980).

30. J. L. Chabard, C. Lartigue-Mattei, F. Vedrine, J. Petit, and J. A. Berger, *J. Chromatogr* 221, 9 (1980).

31. A. H. Van Gennip, J. Grift, and E. J. Van Bree-Blom, *J. Chromatogr.* 163, 351 (1979).

32. M. Desage, J. Soubeyrand, A. Soun, and J. L. Brazier, *J. Chromatogr.* 336, 285 (1984).

33. C. Lartigue-Mattei, J. L. Chabard, H. Bargnoux, J. Petit, and J. A. Berger, *J. Chromatogr.* 229, 211 (1982).

34. S. Floberg, P. Hartvig, B. Lindstrom, and G. Lonner-Holm, *J. Chromatogr.* 225, 73 (1981).

35. J. M. Rosenfeld, V. Y. Taguchi, B. L. Hillcoat, and M. Kawai, *Anal. Chem.* 49, 725 (1977).

36. A. L. Harris, C. Potter, C. Bunch, J. Boutagy, D. J. Harvey, and D. G. Grahame-Smith, *Br. J. Clin. Pharmac.* 8, 219 (1979).

37. J. Boutagy and D. J. Harvey, *J. Chromatogr.* 156, 153 (1978).

38. H. Pang, D. L. Smith, P. F. Crain, K. Yamaizumi, S. Nishimura, and J. A. McCloskey, *Eur. J. Biochem.* 127, 459 (1982).

39. *Transfer RNA: Biological Aspects*, D. Soll, J. N. Abelson, and P. R. Schimmel, Eds., Cold Spring Harbor Laboratory, 1980.

40. I. Jardine and M. M. Weidner, *J. Chromatogr.* 182, 395 (1980).

41. M. Dizdaroglu, *J. Chromatogr.* 367, 357 (1986).

42. P. F. Crain and J. A. McCloskey, *Anal. Biochem.* 132, 124 (1983).

43. R. W. Ruddon, Ed., *Biological Markers of Neoplasia: Basic and Applied Aspects*, Elsevier, New York, 1978.

44. G. Nass, Ed., *Recent Results in Cancer Research: Modified Nucleosides and Cancer*, Springer-Verlag, Berlin, 1983.

45. G. C. Mills, F. C. Schmalstieg, and R. M. Goldblum, *Biochem. Med.* 34, 37 (1985).

46. F. Esposito, T. Russo, A. Ammendola, A. Duilio, F. Salvatore, and F. Cimino, *Canc. Res.* 45, 6260 (1985).

47. E. Borek, O. K. Sharma, F. L. Bushman, D. L. Cohn, K. A. Penley, F. N. Judson, B. S. Dobozin, C. R. Horsburgh, Jr., and C. H. Kirkpatrick, *Canc. Res.* 46, 2557 (1986).

48. C. W. Gehrke, K. C. Kuo, G. E. Davis, R. D. Suits, T. P. Waalkes, and E. Borek, *J. Chromatogr.* **150**, 455 (1978).

49. M. Usiel, L. H. Smith, and S. A. Taylor, *Clin. Chem.* **22**, 1451 (1976).

50. C. Y. Ip, D. Ha, P. W. Morris, M. L. Puttemans, and D. L. Venton, *Anal. Biochem.* **147**, 180 (1985).

51. J. Greenhut and F. B. Rudolph, *J. Chromatogr.* **319**, 461 (1985).

52. G. Apell, F. L. Bushman, and O. K. Sharma, *J. Chromatogr.* **374**, 149 (1986).

53. T. P. Wallkes, C. M. Gehrke, R. W. Zumwalt, S. I. Chang, D. B. Lakings, D. C. Tormey, D. I. Ahmann, and C. G. Moertel, *Cancer Res.* **36**, 390 (1975).

54. G. B. Chheda, H. B. Patrzyc, A. K. Bhargava, P. F. Crain, S. K. Sethi, J. A. McCloskey, and S. P. Dutta, *Nucleosides & Nucleotides* **6**, 597 (1987).

55. T. McClure, K. H. Schram, K. Nakano and T. Yasaka, *Nucleosides & Nucleotides*, **8**, in press (1989).

56. R. T. Markiw, *Biochem. Med.* **8**, 182 (1973).

57. J. M. Strong, L. W. Anderson, A. Monks, C. A. Chisena, and R. L. Cysyk, *Anal. Biochem.* **132**, 243 (1983).

58. C. Jakobs, L. Sweetman, W. L. Nyhan, L. Gruenke, J. C. Craig, and S. K. Wadman, *Clin. Chim. Acta* **143**, 123 (1984).

59. B. H. Min, W. A. Garland, T. M. Lewison, and B. M. Mehta, *Biomed. Mass Spectrom.* **12**, 238 (1985).

60. B. Dauphin, G. Teller, and B. Durand, *Planta* **144**, 133 (1979).

61. I. M. Scott and R. Horgan, *Biomed. Mass Spectrom.* **7**, 446 (1980).

62. J. A. McCloskey, B. Basile, K. Kimura, and T. Hashizume, *Proc. Japan Acad., Ser. B* **57**, 276 (1981).

63. H. Miyazaki, Y. Matsunaga, K. Yoshida, S. Arakawa, and M. Hashimoto, *J. Chromatogr.* **274**, 75 (1983).

64. S. E. Hattox and J. A. McCloskey, *Anal. Chem.* **46**, 1378 (1974).

65. E. White, P. M. Krueger, and J. A. McCloskey, *J. Org. Chem.* **37**, 430 (1972).

66. A. M. Lawson, R. N. Stillwell, M. M. Tacker, K. Tsuboyama, and J. A. McCloskey, *J. Amer. Chem. Soc.* **93**, 1014 (1971).

67. D. R. Hunt, C. E. Hignite, and K. Biemann, *Biochem. Biophys. Res. Commun.* **33**, 378 (1968).

68. J. A. McCloskey, R. N. Stillwell, and A. M. Lawson, *Anal. Chem.* **40**, 233 (1968).

69. B. Basile, M. F. Scott, F. F. Hsu, and J. A. McCloskey, *Mass Spectra of Bases, Nucleosides, Nucleotides and Their Derivatives*, Department of Medicinal Chemistry, University of Utah, Salt Lake City, UT, 1981.

70. M. Dizdaroglu, *Anal. Biochem.* **144**, 593 (1985).

71. P. L. Stetson, J. Maybaum, U. A. Shukla, and W. D. Ensminger, *J. Chromatogr.* **375**, 1 (1986).

72. L. M. S. Palni, S. A. B. Tay, and J. K. MacLeod, *Plant Physiol.* **84**, 1158 (1987).

73. H. Pang, M. Ihara, Y. Kuchino, S. Nishimura, R. Gupta, C. R. Woese, and J. A. McCloskey, *J. Biol. Chem.* **257**, 3589 (1982).

74. For brevity, $O^4,2',3',5'-O$-tetrakis(trimethylsilyl)uridine is referred to as uridine(TMS)$_4$. If the position of the added derivative group is not obvious from the structure of the free nucleoside, the sites containing the TMS functions will be indicated.

75. D. L. von Minden, R. N. Stillwell, W. A. Koenig, K. J. Lyman, and J. A. McCloskey, *Anal. Biochem.* **50**, 110 (1972).

76. K. H. Schram, Y. Taniguchi, and J. A. McCloskey, *J. Chromatogr.* **155**, 355 (1978).

77. U. Krahmer, J. G. Liehr, K. J. Lyman, E. A. Orr, R. N. Stillwell, and J. A. McCloskey, *Anal. Biochem.* **82**, 217 (1977).

78. D. L. von Minden and J. A. McCloskey, *J. Am. Chem. Soc.* **95**, 7480 (1973).

79. G. R. Pettit, P. Brown, J. J. Einck, K. Yamauchi, and R. M. Blazer, *Synthetic Comm.* **7**, 449 (1977).

80. G. R. Pettit, J. J. Einck, and P. Brown, *Biomed. Mass Spectrom.* **5**, 153 (1978).

81. G. R. Pettit, R. M. Blazer, J. J. Einck, and K. Yamauchi, *J. Org. Chem.* **45**, 4073 (1980).

82. J. J. Einck, G. R. Pettit, P. Brown, and K. Yamauchi, *J. Carbohydrates Nuclosides Nucleotides* **7**, 1 (1980).

83. R. G. Teece, D. Slowikowski, and K. H. Schram, *Biomed. Mass Spectrom.* **10**, 30 (1983).

84. R. P. Panzica, L. B. Townsend, D. L. von Minden, M. S. Wilson, and J. A. McCloskey, *Biochim. Biophys. Acta* **331**, 147 (1973).

85. C. Pantarotto, A. Martini, G. Belvedere, A. Bossi, M. G. Donelli, and A. Frigerio, *J. Chromatogr.* **99**, 519 (1974).

86. C. F. Gelijkens, D. L. Smith, and J. A. McCloskey, *J. Chromatogr.* **225**, 291 (1981).

87. E. Schubert and K. H. Schram, unpublished results.

88. L. M. S. Palni, S. A. B. Tay, and J. K. MacLeod, *Plant Physiol.* **84**, 1158 (1987).

89. C. H. Hocart, O. C. Wong, D. S. Letham, S. A. B. Tay, and J. K. MacLeod, *Anal. Biochem.* **153**, 85 (1986).

90. M. A. Quilliam, K. K. Ogilvie, K. L. Sadana, and J. B. Westmore, *J. Chromatogr.* **194**, 379 (1980).

91. M. Ludewig, K. Dorffling, and W. A. Konig, *J. Chromatogr.* **243**, 93 (1982).

92. R. M. Kok, A. P. J. M. DeJong, C. J. Van Groeningen, G. J. Peters, and J. Lankelma, *J. Chromatogr.* **343**, 59 (1985).

93. G. B. Mohamed, A. Nazareth, M. J. Hayes, R. W. Giese, and P. Vouros, *J. Chromatogr.* **314**, 211 (1984).

94. D. E. G. Shuker, E. Bailey, S. M. Gorf, J. Lamb, and P. B. Farmer, *Anal. Biochem.* **140**, 270 (1984).

95. Q. N. Porter, *Mass Spectrometry of Heterocyclic Compounds, Second Edition*, Wiley-Interscience, New York, 1985.

96. Q. N. Porter and J. Baldas, *Mass Spectrometry of Heterocyclic Compounds*, Wiley-Interscience, New York, 1971.

97. C. Finn, H.-J. Schwandt and W. Sadee, *Biomed. Mass Spectrom.* **6**, 194 (1979).

98. M. Dizdaroglu, *BioTechniques* **4**, 536 (1986).

99. M. Dizdaroglu and M. G. Simic, *Int. J. Radiat. Biol.* **46**, 241 (1984).

100. W. P. Tong and D. B. Ludlum, *Canc. Res.* **41**, 380 (1981).

101. S. K. Sethi, C. F. Gelijkens, J. A. McCloskey, R. Shapiro, and B. A. Brandes, *Biomed. Mass Spectrom.* **10**, 665 (1983).

102. E. H. Pfadenhauer, C. S. Bankert, J. Jensen, C. E. Jones, E. E. Jenkins, and J. A. McCloskey, *Drug Metab. Dispos.* **12**, 280 (1984).

103. R. E. Vestal, K. E. Thummel, B. Musser, S. G. Jue, G. D. Mercer, and W. N. Howard, *Biomed. Mass Spectrom.* **9**, 340 (1982).

104. Ion designations are similar to those used in Ref. 4.

105. S. J. Shaw, D. M. Desiderio, K. Tsuboyama, and J. A. McCloskey, *J. Am. Chem Soc.* **92**, 2510 (1970).

106. J. M. Rice and G. O. Dudek, *Biochem. Biophys. Res. Commun.* **35**, 383 (1969).

107. L. B. Townsend and R. K. Robins, *J. Heterocycl. Chem.* **6**, 459 (1969).

108. P. F. Crain, J. A. McCloskey, A. F. Lewis, K. H. Schram, and L. B. Townsend, *J. Heterocycl. Chem.* **10**, 843 (1973).

109. I. Antonini, G. Cristalli, P. Franchetti, M. Grifantini, S. Martelli, and F. Petrell, *J. Pharm. Sci.* **73**, 366 (1984).

110. A. M. Reddy, K. H. Schram, M. Grifantinii, and G. Cristalli, unpublished results.

111. M. Reimer, T. McClure, and K. H. Schram, *Biomed. Environ. Mass Spectrom.*, **18**, 533 (1989).

112. J. G. Liehr, D. L. von Minden, S. E. Hattox, and J. A. McCloskey, *Biomed. Mass Spectrom.* **1**, 281 (1974).

113. M. Sochacki, E. Sochacka, and A. Malkiewicz, *Biomed. Mass Spectrom.* **7**, 257 (1980).

114. K. H. Schram and D. Prince, *Biomed. Mass Spectrom.* **10**, 34 (1983).

115. T. D. McClure, K. H. Schram, K. Nakano, and T. Yasaka, *Nucleosides & Nucleotides*, **8**, in press (1989).

116. G. B. Chheda, H. B. Patrzyc, A. K. Bhargava, P. F. Crain, S. K. Sethi, J. A. McCloskey, and S. P. Dutta, *Nucleosides & Nucleotides* **6**, 597 (1987).

117. J. A. McCloskey, *System. Appl. Microbiol.* **7**, 246 (1986).

118. J. Singer, W. C. Schnute, Jr., J. E. Shively, C. W. Todd, and A. D. Riggs, *Anal. Biochem.* **94**, 297 (1979).

119. D. Winton, S. Hattman, P. F. Crain, C.-S. Cheng, D. L. Smith, and J. A. McCloskey, *Proc. Natl. Acad. Sci. USA* **80**, 7400 (1983).

120. B. S. Vold, D. E. Keith, Jr., M. Buck, J. A. McCloskey, and H. Pang, *Nucleic Acids Res.* **10**, 3125 (1982).

121. K. M. Straub and A. L. Burlingame, *Biomed. Mass Spectrom.* **8**, 431 (1981).

122. K. Isono, M. Uramoto, H. Kusakabe, N. Miyata, T. Koyama, M. Ubukata, S. K. Sethi, and J. A. McCloskey, *J. Antibiotics* **37**, 670 (1984).

123. L. P. Johnson, J. K. MacLeod, C. W. Parker, and D. S. Letham, *FEBS Lett.* **124**, 119 (1981).

124. L. P. Johnson, J. K. MacLeod, R. E. Summons, and N. Hunt, *Anal. Biochem.* **106**, 285 (1980).

125. R. P. Newton, N. Gibbs, C. D. Moyse, J. L. Weibers, and E. G. Brown, *Phytochem.* **19**, 1909 (1980).

126. J. Tamas and J. Tomasz, *Biomed. Mass Spectrom.* **12**, 489 (1985).

127. H.-R. Schulten and H. M. Schiebel, "Mass Spectrometry of Pyridine Nucleotides," in D. Dolphin, R. D. Poulson, and O. Avramovie, Eds., *Pyridine Nucleotide Coenzymes: Chemical, Biochemical and Medical Aspects,* Wiley, New York, 1987, Vol. 2A, Chapter 8.

128. M. S. Wilson and J. A. McCloskey, *J. Am. Chem. Soc.* **97**, 3436 (1975).

129. W. Hammargren, Q.-M. Weng, K. H. Schram, C. Borysko, L. Wotring, and L. B. Townsend, *Anal. Biochem.*, **178**, 102 (1989).

130. J. A. McCloskey, J. H. Futrell, T. A. Elwood, K. H. Schram, R. P. Panzica, and L. B. Townsend, *J. Am. Chem. Soc.* **95**, 5762 (1973).

131. F. Valeriote and G. Santelli, *Pharmac. Ther.* **24**, 132 (1984).

132. R. M. Kok and A. P. J. M. DeJong, *J. Chromatogr.* **343**, 59 (1985).

133. T. Marunaka and Y. Umeno, *Chem. Pharm. Bull.* **30**, 1868 (1982).

134. C. Aubert, J. P. Sommadossi, P. Coassolo, J. P. Cano, and J. P. Rigualt, *Biomed. Mass Spectrom.* **9**, 238 (1982).

135. M.-C. Cosyns-Duyck, A. A. M. Cruyl, A. P. DeLeenheer, A. D. Schryver, J. V. Huys, and F. M. Belpaire, *Biomed. Mass Spectrom.* **7**, 61 (1980).

136. C. F. Gelijkens, A. P. DeLeenheer, and P. Sandra, *Biomed. Mass Spectrom.* **7**, 572 (1980).

137. C. F. Gelijkens, P. Sandra, F. Pelpaire, and A. P. DeLeenheer, *Drug Metabol. Disposit.* **8**, 363 (1980).

138. Y. Robinson, N. Gerry, R. D. Brownsill, and C. W. Vose, *Biomed. Mass Spectrom.* **11**, 199 (1984).

139. D. J. Ashworth, W. M. Baird, C.-J. Chang, J. D. Ciupek, K. L. Bush, and R. G. Cooks, *Biomed Mass Spectrom.* **12**, 309 (1985).

140. C.-J. Chang, D. J. Ashworth, I. Isern-Flecha, D. Y. Jiang, and R. G. Cooks, *Chem.-Biol. Interactions* **57**, 296 (1986).

141. M. A. Baldwin and F. W. McLafferty, *Org. Mass Spectrom.* **7**, 1353 (1973).

142. R. J. Cotter, *Anal. Chem.* **52**, 1589A (1980).

143. N. Takeda, K.-I. Harada, M. Suzuki, and A. Tatematsu, *Org. Mass Spectrom.* **20**, 236 (1985).

144. D. F. Hunt, J. Shabanowitz, and F. K. Botz, *Anal. Chem.* **49**, 1160 (1977).

145. R. J. Cotter and C. Fenselau, *Biomed. Mass Spectrom.* **7**, 287 (1979).

146. E. L. Esmans, E. J. Freyne, J. H. Vanbroeckhoven, and F. C. Alderweireldt, *Biomed. Mass Spectrom.* **7**, 377 (1980).

147. M. Ohashi, K. Tsujimoto, and A. Yasuda, *Chem. Lett.* 439 (1976).

148. H. Virelizier, R. Hagemann, and K. Jankowski, *Biomed. Mass Spectrom.* **10**, 559 (1983).

149. I. Isern-Flecha, X.-Y. Jiang, R. G. Cooks, W. Pfleiderer, W.-G. Chae, and C.-J. Chang, *Biomed. Environ. Mass Spectrom.* **14**, 17 (1987).

150. E. Schubert, R. Glennon, and K. H. Schram, *J. Heterocycl. Chem.* **22**, 889 (1985).

151. J. A. Chan, R. D. Sitrin, E. W. K. Yeung, G. C. Simolike, G. D. Roberts, and P. W. Jeffs, *J. Chromatogr.* **358**, 291 (1986).

152. J. B. Bodley, R. Upham, F. W. Crow, K. B. Tomer, and M. L. Gross, *Arch. Biochem. Biophys.* **230**, 590 (1984).

153. B. C. Pal, C. Ghosh, S. K. Sethi, B. E. Suttle, and J. A. McCloskey, *Nucleosides & Nucleotides* **7**, 1 (1988).

154. M. Barber, R. S. Bordoli, R. D. Sedgwick, and A. N. Tyler, *Biomed. Mass Spectrom.* **8**, 492 (1981).

155. V. T. Vu, C. C. Fensleau, and O. M. Colvin *J. Am. Chem. Soc.* **103**, 7362 (1981).

156. C. Fenselau, V. T. Vu, R. J. Cotter, G. Hansen, D. Heller, T. Chen, and O. M. Colvin, *Spectros. Int. J.* **1**, 132 (1982).

157. G. Puzo, J. C. Prome, J. P. Macquet, and I. A. S. Lewis, *Biomed. Mass Spectrom.* **12**, 552 (1982).

158. C. Fenselau, *J. Natural Prod.* **47**, 215 (1983).

159. R. K. Mitchum, F. E. Evans, J. P. Freeman, and D. Roach, *Int. J. Mass Spectrom. Ion Phys.* **46**, 383 (1983).

160. M. L. Deinzer and A. L. Burlingame, in A. L. Burlingame and N. Castagnoli, Jr., Eds., *Mass Spectrometry in the Health and Life Sciences*, Elsevier, Amsterdam, 1985, pp. 581–595.

161. D. L. Slowikowski and K. H. Schram, *Nucleosides & Nucleotides* **4**, 347 (1985).

162. K. H. Schram and D. L. Slowikowski, *Biomed. Environ. Mass Spectrom.* **13**, 263 (1986).

163. S. K. Sethi, D. L. Smith, and J. A. McCloskey, *Biochem. Biophys. Res. Commun.* **112**, 126 (1983).

164. S. Verma, S. C. Pomerantz, S. K. Sethi, and J. A. McCloskey, *Anal. Chem.* **58**, 2898 (1986).

165. A. M. Reddy, V. Mykytyn, and K. H. Schram, *Biomed. Environ. Mass Spectrom.*, in press.

166. S. K. Sethi, C. C. Nelson, and J. A. McCloskey, *Anal. Chem.* **56**, 1977 (1984).

167. R. L. Cerny and M. L. Gross, *Anal. Chem.* **57**, 1160 (1985).

168. P. P. Wickramanayake, B. L. Arbogast, D. R. Buhler, M. L. Deinzer, and A. L. Burlingame, *J. Am. Chem. Soc.* **107**, 2485 (1985).

169. K. B. Tomer, M. L. Gross, and M. L. Deinzer, *Anal. Chem.* **58**, 2527 (1986).

170. Y. Tondeur, M. Shorter, M. E. Gustafson, and R. C. Pandey, *Biomed. Mass Spectrom.* **11**, 622 (1984).

171. J. Eagles, C. Javanaud, and R. Self, *Biomed. Mass Spectrom.* **11**, 41 (1984).

172. H.-M. Schiebel, P. Schulze, W.-D. Stohrer, D. Leibfritz, B. Jastroff, and K. H. Maurer, *Biomed. Mass Spectrom.* **12**, 170 (1985).

173. A. Samdstrom and J. Chattopadhyaya, *J. Chem. Soc., Chem. Commun.* 862 (1987).

174. G. Sindona, N. Uccella, and K. Weclawek, *J. Chem. Res(S)* 184 (1982).

175. A. M. Hogg, J. G. Kelland, J. C. Vederas, and C. Tamm, *Helv. Chim. Acta* **69**, 908 (1986).

176. J. Ulrich, A. Guy, D. Molko, and R. Teoule, *Org. Mass Spectrom.* **19**, 585 (1984).

177. J. L. Aubagnac, F. M. Devienne, R. Combarieu, J. L. Barascut, J. L. Imbach, and H. B. Lazredk, *Org. Mass Spectrom.* **18**, 361 (1983).

178. R. L. Cerny, K. B. Tomer, M. L. Gross, and L. Grotjahn, *Anal. Biochem.* **165**, 175 (1987).

179. E. E. Kingston, J. H. Beynon, and R. P. Newton, *Biomed. Mass Spectrom.* **11**, 367 (1984).

180. C. Fenselau, P. C. C. Feng, T. Chen, and L. P. Johnson, *Drug Metabol. Disposit.* **10**, 316 (1982).

181. L. M. Mallis, F. M. Raushel, and D. H. Russell, *Anal. Chem.* **59**, 980 (1987).

182. A. Wolter, C. Mohringer, H. Koster, and W. A. Konig, *Biomed. Environ. Mass Spectrom.* **14**, 111 (1987).

183. J.-J. Vasseur, B. Rayner, J.-L. Imbach, S. Verma, J. A. McCloskey, M. Lee, D.-K. Chang, and J. W. Lown, *J. Org. Chem.* **52**, 4994 (1987).

184. L. Grotjahn, H. Blocker, and R. Frank, *Biomed. Mass Spectrom.* **12**, 514 (1985).

185. L. Grotjahn, R. Frank, and H. Blocker, *Nucleic Acids Res.* **10**, 4671 (1982).

186. L. Grotjahn, R. Frank, G. Heisterberg-Moutsis, and H. Blocker, *Tetrahedron Lett.* **25**, 5373 (1984).

187. L. Grotjahn and H. Steinert, "Mass Spectrometry in Molecular Design," in A. L. Burlingame and N. Castagnoli, Jr., Eds., *Mass Spectrometry in the Health and Life Sciences*, Elsevier, Amsterdam, 1985, pp. 597–615.

188. M. Panico, G. Sindona, and N. Uccella, *J. Am. Chem. Soc.* **105**, 5610 (1983).

189. C. J. McNeal, K. K. Ogilvie, N. Y. Theriault, and M. J. Nemer, *J. Am. Chem. Soc.* **104**, 972 (1982).

190. C. J. McNeal, K. K. Ogilvie, N. Y. Theriault, and M. J. Nemer, *J. Am. Chem. Soc.* **104**, 976 (1982).

191. B. Sundqvist and R. D. Macfarlane, *Mass Spectrom. Rev.* **4**, 421 (1985).

192. A. Viari, J.-P. Ballini, P. Vigny, D. Shire, and P. Dousset, *Biomed. Environ. Mass Spectrom.* **14**, 83 (1987).

193. N. Otake, T. Ogita, Y. Miyazaki, H. Yonehara, R. D. MacFarlane, and C. J. McNeal, *J. Antibiot.* **34**, 130 (1981).

194. K. A. Jacobson, L. K. Pannell, K. L. Kirk, H. M. Fales, and E. A. Sokiloski, *J. Chem. Soc. Perkin Trans. I* 2143 (1986).

195. H.-R. Schulten and H. M. Schiebel, *Fresenius Z. Anal. Chem.* **321**, 531 (1985).

196. H. Moser and G. W. Wood, *Biomed. Environ. Mass Spectrom.* **15**, 547 (1988).

197. H. Seliger, T. C. Bach, H.-H. Gortz, E. Happ, M. Holupirek, B. Seemann-Preising, H.-M. Schiebel, and H.-R. Schulten, *J. Chromatogr.* **253**, 65 (1982).

198. R. Beavis, W. Ens, M. J. Nemer, K. K. Ogilvie, K. G. Standing, and J. B. Westmore, *Internat. J. Mass Spectrom. Ion Phys.* **46**, 475 (1983).

199. W. Ens, K. G. Standing, J. B. Westmore, K. K. Ogilvie, and M. J. Nemer, *Anal. Chem.* **54**, 960 (1982).

200. S. E. Unger, A. E. Schoen, R. G. Cooks, D. J. Ashworth, J. D. Gomes, and C.-J. Chang, *J. Org. Chem.* **46**, 4765 (1981).

201. D. A. McCrery and M. L. Gross, *Anal. Chim. Acta* **178**, 91 (1985).

202. C. E. Edmonds, J. A. McCloskey, and V. A. Edmonds, *Biomed. Mass Spectrom.* **10**, 237 (1983).

203. C. R. Blakley and M. L. Vestal, *Anal. Chem.* **55**, 750 (1983).

204. J. A. McCloskey, P. F. Crain, C. G. Edmonds, R. Gupta, T. Hashizume, D. W. Phillipson, and K. O. Stetter, *Nucleic Acids Res.* **15**, 683 (1987).

205. R. D. Voyksner, F. P. Williams, and J. W. Hines, *J. Chromatogr.* **347**, 137 (1985).

206. R. D. Voyksner, J. T. Bursey, and J. W. Hines, *J. Chromatogr.* **323**, 383 (1985).

207. P. A. Blau, J. W. Hines, and R. D. Voyksner, *J. Chromatogr.* **420**, 1 (1987).

208. K. J. Volk, M. S. Lee, R. A. Yost, and A. Brajter-Toth, *Anal. Chem.* **60**, 722 (1988).

209. E. L. Esmans, Y. Luyten, and F. C. Alderweireldt, *Biomed. Mass Spectrom.* **10**, 347 (1983).

210. F. C. Alderweireldt, E. L. Esmans, and P. Geboes, *Nucleosides & Nucleotides* **4**, 135 (1985).

211. E. L. Esmans, P. Geboes, Y. Luyten, and F. C. Alderwiereldt, *Biomed. Mass Spectrom.* **12**, 241 (1985).

212. E. L. Esmans, M. Belmans, I. Vrijens, Y. Luyten, F. C. Alderweireldt, L. L. Wotring, and L. B. Townsend, *Nucleosides & Nucleotides* **6**, 865 (1987).

213. A. J. Alexander, P. Kebarle, A. F. Fuciarelli, and J. A. Raleigh, *Anal. Chem.* **59**, 2484 (1987).

214. D. E. Games, *Spectra* **9**, 3 (1983).

215. D. E. Games, DM.A. McDowall, K. Levsen, L. H. Schafer, P. Dobberstein, and J. L. Gower, *Biomed. Mass Spectrom.* **11**, 87 (1984).

216. J. G. Stroh, Jr., J. C. Cook, R. M. Milberg, L. Brayton, T. Kihara, Z. Huang, and K. L. Rinehart, Jr., *Anal. Chem.* **57**, 985 (1985).

217. R. M. Caprioli, T. Fan, and J. S. Cottrell, *Anal. Chem.* **58**, 2949 (1986).

218. R. M. Caprioli, W. T. Moore, and T. Fan, *Rapid Commun. Mass Spectrom.* **1**, 15 (1987).

Mass Spectrometry in Pharmacology

FRED P. ABRAMSON, *Department of Pharmacology, George Washington University, Washington, DC*

1. AN INTRODUCTION TO PHARMACOLOGICAL RESEARCH

Portraying the diverse role of mass spectrometry in pharmacology is made easier by dividing MS into subsections based on the types of experiments that have been carried out. The drugs themselves do not fall into categories that would provide insight into the rationale for the use of mass spectrometry, while the instrumental approach that was selected by each investigator is an integral part of the scheme of the research.

Pharmacology is defined as "the knowledge of the history, source, physical properties, compounding, biochemical and physiological effects, mechanisms of action, absorption, distribution, biotransformation and excretion, and therapeutic and other uses of drugs" (1). Coupling the definition of pharmacology with the definition of a drug as "any chemical agent that affects living processes" (1), makes the study of pharmacology exceptionally broad. Toxicology is often considered as a subdivision of pharmacology.

To delineate the roles of mass spectrometry, pharmacology may be broken down into two subdivisions: pharmacokinetics, which is the study of the absorption, metabolism, distribution, elimination and time course of drugs in the body; and pharmacodynamics, which is the study of drug effects and determination of mechanisms of action. The contributions of mass spectrometry lie mainly in its capacity to identify qualitatively and measure quantitatively drugs and their degradation products in the complex environment into which they disperse after their administration. Mass spectrometry has also impacted pharmacodynamics, but those applications are less frequently found. Therapeutic drug monitoring, which is the adjustment of doses of drugs to produce optimal efficacy based on plasma concentrations, represents an area where pharmacokinetics and pharmacodynamics overlap significantly and where mass spectrometry has had an important role.

Given the broad definition of drugs that was stated previously, one finds substantial overlap between endogenous substances and therapeutic agents. For example, when hydrocortisone (cortisol) is used to control inflammation, it is an endogenous substance being used as a drug. To provide a somewhat more managable range of subject material, the pharmacological studies of natural substances, such as l-DOPA, or pharmaceutical analogs of natural substances, such as dexamethasone, were arbitrarily excluded in favor of those chemicals that represent classes of compounds which do not have a well-known endogenous counterpart.

Method selection in pharmacological research is no different than in any other area of analysis. The technique must be compatible with the amount of the analyte, the complexity of the matrix in which it is found, its volatility, polarity, and ionization characteristics, and the precision and accuracy required, to name just a few. An advantage of most pharmacological investigations is that one is dealing with xenobiotics, so that the native concentration of the analyte is zero. Thus, the entire signal detected could be due to the added material with no direct endogenous contribution. The dark side of this advantage is that one can attempt analyses with heroic levels of sensitivity, since abundance sensitivity is less likely to limit an otherwise sensitive and selective assay. As one's detection limits go down, previously undetected problems such as adsorption to glassware, chromatographic columns, and interfaces grow.

2. STUDIES OF DRUG METABOLISM

There is a rich literature on the use of mass spectrometry in drug metabolism. Since many such studies involve identifying previously unknown molecules, the interpretive qualities of a mass spectrum makes the mass spectrometer an ideal instrument for this purpose. The variable in this type of experiment is the method used to separate the original drug and its metabolites from the biological matrix in which it is found.

Performing a drug metabolism study is a conundrum where the job is to find something whose identity is unknown. One cannot go to a library of spectra and expect to match a newly discovered compound with those that have previously been studied. There are a number of points to consider when approaching such a problem. A critical aspect is to consider adequately the chemical nature of the drug metabolites. At the simplest level, a hydroxyl group might be added, or an N-methyl group lost. More complex chemistry results when novel functional groups are produced, such as N-oxides or hydroxylamines, or uncommon elements are added, such as sulfur. The parent drug or one or more of its metabolites may be conjugated. If conjugated to a readily cleaved group such as glucuronic acid, deconjugation may be facile. Conjugations to peptides or proteins may not be detected if too limited a range of enzymatic treatments are attempted. Covalent binding to cellular macromolecules may require application of yet more complex biochemistry before a metabolite structure can be obtained.

The wide variety of functional groups that may be added to or subtracted from a drug makes separation and derivatization extremely complicated. Drug metabolites may be much smaller or larger than their parent molecules, so that selection of separation methods presents a challenge. The acid–base characteristics of the molecule may be completely changed, as may be its polarity, so that extraction and purification from its biological matrix may not be routine. Its polarity may also determine which mass spectrometric method will be successful.

Often radioactivity has been used as a tracer in metabolic studies. Those components from urine or liver enzyme preparations that contain radioactivity are isolated and introduced into the mass spectrometer. Radioactivity also permits an easy calculation of mass balance to ascertain whether all of the originally administered dose is accounted for.

2.1. Qualitative Analysis of Metabolites

The first aspect of a study of drug metabolism is to elucidate the chemical structures of the metabolites. To do this, one needs some means to recognize that one or more components of a biological mixture actually arise from metabolic modifications of the parent molecule.

Once recognized, these metabolites must be separated from their matrix and then analyzed. One can do this separation first, and then introduce the separated component into the mass spectrometer, or one can do this in a concerted fashion using a "hyphenated" method. Either way, the structural determination of the metabolites helps determine the reaction pathways that are involved in the biochemical alterations of the drug in the body.

2.1.1. USING GC–MS

In addition to the utility of radiolabeled drugs, a mass spectrometer has the power to pick out information relating specifically to the by-products of the original compound. To that end, Knapp et al. (2) synthesized trideuteronortriptyline (NT) and administered it in a 1:1 ratio with unlabeled NT. This produces a spectral feature that permits facile discrimination of metabolites, namely, a pair of peaks of equal intensity three masses apart for any metabolite that still contains the labeled methyl group. This is unusual in a mass spectrum and allows the analyst to give that component full consideration as having been formed from the original labeled mixture.

Figure 1a shows the mass spectrum of the molecular ion region of the trifluroacetylated nortriptyline molecule. The pair of peaks at m/z 359 and 362 form the basis of the identification scheme. Figure 1b shows a spectrum from one of the many chromatographic peaks found in rat urine after the 1:1 mixture was administered. The twin peaks at m/z 357 and 360 served to identify the material as a metabolite. Its structure was dehydronortriptyline, a dehydration product presumably formed from $10 - OH - NT$ during part of the derivatization or analysis. The ability to recognize the special feature of the spectrum was readily apparent. This "twin-peak" procedure continues to be an important method for identification of metabolites and is useful regardless of the type of prior separation used.

2.2.2. USING HPLC–MS

Cyclosporine (Fig. 2a) is a cyclic 11-amino-acid-containing immunosuppressive drug that has become extremely important to the success of organ transplantation. Its amino acid composition is unusual since it contains a sarcosine, both a D- and L-alanine, an α-aminobutyric acid, a valine, and an N-

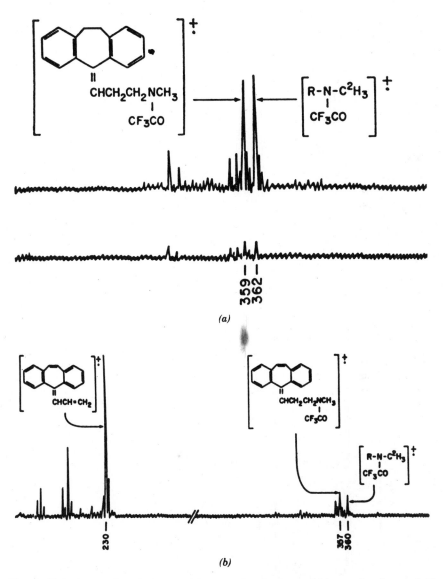

Fig. 1. Twin ion peaks associated with the molecular ions of (*a*) nortriptyline and (*b*) nortriptyline metabolite (2). Reproduced by permission from reference 2.

methylvaline, four *N*-methylleucines, and unique butenyl-dimethyl-threonine structure.

Hartman and Jardine (3) used thermospray HPLC–MS to identify some of the products of metabolism of cyclosporine. Bile was collected from rabbits who were given a tritiated cyclosporine. Comparing the HPLC chromatogram by UV

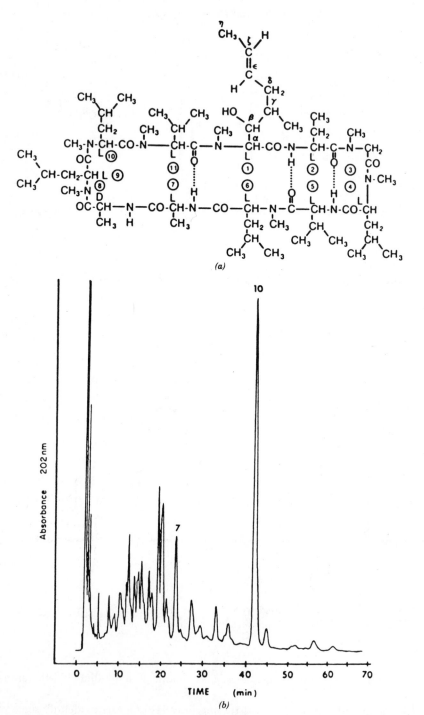

Fig. 2. (*a*) Structure of cyclosporine A: (*b*) analytical high-performance liquid chromatogram (UV detector) of rabbit biliary metabolites of cyclosporine. The numbers 7 and 10 refer to different metabolites (3). Reproduced by permission from reference 3.

294

(Fig. 2b) and radioactivity detection showed that nearly every component eluting after 10 min was radioactive and therefore a cyclosporine metabolite.

The thermospray mass spectra of metabolites 7 and 10 are presented in Fig. 3. The apparent molecular weights suggested by the natriated ions indicate dihydroxylation and oxidation of a methyl to a carboxyl, respectively. The questions of the structures of these metabolites are addressed by both partial and total hydrolyses followed by GC–MS assays. These studies show that both metabolites have oxidations on the terminal carbon of the butenyl side chain. The second site of hydroxylation in peak 7 is the tertiary carbon of one of the N-methylleucines.

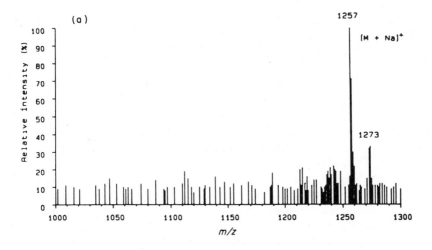

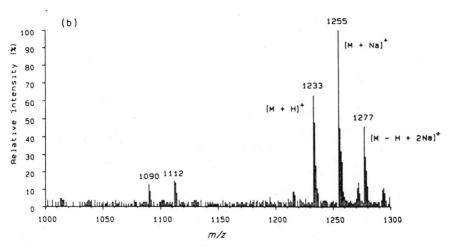

Fig. 3. Partial positive-ion mass spectra of two metabolites shown in Fig. 2b with introduction by HPLC. (a) metabolite 7; (b) metabolite 10 (3). Reproduced by permission from reference 3.

Thermospray HPLC–MS shows great promise as a tool in pharmacology research. Its virtues lie in its capacity to couple the separations from liquid chromatography with mass spectrometry in a way that does not demand that the analyte be volatile; furthermore, as a "soft"-ionization technique, thermospray provides molecular-weight information of unknown metabolites. These characteristics fit almost ideally with the current needs of drug metabolite identification.

2.1.3. USING TLC SEPARATION FOR MS

A rather facile method for obtaining purified specimens from biological systems prior to their analysis by mass spectrometry is thin-layer chromatography (TLC). The scheme of such methods is, in general, to locate whatever spots are of interest using a detection method appropriate to TLC, such as radioactivity or staining, and then scraping off equivalent regions from another plate or lane and eluting them from the silica gel in order to obtain a specimen for MS. Direct introduction of the silica is usually unsuccessful, because its large surface area promotes such violent desorption of gases when introduced into the vacuum of the mass spectrometer that the sample spurts out of the introduction probe.

There are several problems in doing a TLC–MS analysis. First, the resolution of the TLC plate may be inadequate to obtain a pure specimen, thus the resulting mass spectra will contain data from more than one compound. Second, the detection limits may be higher than expected because of background from the TLC plate itself. Indicators and other chemicals involved in the manufacture of the plates, such as plastic backings, may also contribute extensively to the signals in the mass spectrometer.

An example of TLC–MS will be presented in the context of the analysis of aflatoxins. Aflatoxins are a group of carcinogenic fungal products. Species differences in susceptibility to their effects has led to many studies of aflatoxin metabolism, since the difference likely arises from species-dependent metabolic activation. In this particular case, the production of aflatoxicol from the commonly encountered aflatoxin B1 seemed to be a good marker of susceptibility. Salhab et al. (4) examined the production of a new metabolite of aflatoxicol using this approach. These investigations yielded a band from aflatoxicol by TLC that did not correspond to any known aflatoxin metabolite.

As a class of compounds, aflatoxins are naturally fluorescent, so that each spot on a TLC plate can be identified in a nondestructive manner, scraped, and then placed in the direct introduction probe of the mass spectrometer. A key to obtaining a good spectrum with only a small amount of material was the pretreatment of the TLC plate to remove potentially interfering materials. Developing the plate twice without sample, activating it in a vacuum oven at 105°C, cooling it, and spotting it immediately thereafter dramatically reduced the large amount of hydrocarbon like material that was initially adsorbed on the plate. In fact, the solvent front from these washings was notably brown in color.

The mass spectrum of this product looked much like aflatoxicol itself, except that the masses were 16 u higher. This indicates an oxidation. As frequently occurs in mass spectrometry, the isomeric product is not identified; other methods have to be used to try to narrow the choices. The final structure proposed, as shown in Fig. 4, was aflatoxicol M_1 where the oxidation appears between the two furan rings. A synthetic standard was not prepared, but its structure was confirmed by its production from the metabolic reduction of aflatoxin M_1 that has the same hydroxy group between the furan rings, but also a keto function in the upper cyclopentene ring.

2.1.4. USING TANDEM MASS SPECTROMETRY

As described in Chapter 1, an MS/MS experiment represents the ultimate in separation. When applied to the task of identifying drug metabolites, it shows exceptional promise. Lee and Yost (5) provide a step-by-step approach to use the MS/MS technique to tentatively identify previously unknown metabolites from specimens of urine that have only been processed by deconjugation and extraction. No other separation method is necessary.

The key to the potential, and actual, success of MS/MS in such studies is that most metabolites retain a significant portion of their parent structural character, after being oxidized once or twice, dealkylated, transaminated, or conjugated, and so forth. If that is the case, then the collisionally induced dissociation (CID) spectrum of the original molecule serves as a template for the possible fragmentation pathways of the unknown metabolic products. Less frequently one sees ring opening or rearrangements to products that do not fairly well represent the structural components of the original molecule.

Therefore, the first step is to obtain a chemical-ionization (CI) spectrum of the starting drug molecule. One then selects an adduct ion and obtains the daughter ion CID spectrum, as well as parent and daughter ion scans of prominent fragment ions (if any). Using chemical ionization appears critical, since the authors could not detect metabolites using electron ionization (5). Apparently, the extensive production of nonstructurally significant ions in EI overwhelm the structurally important ions needed as precursors for CID spectra.

The analysis of a sample that contains drugs and metabolites might be as follows. Neutral loss spectra where the mass differences represent important components should be obtained. Losses of water, CO, methyl, and so forth, are less informative than those that would be more unique to the overall structure of the drug. Parent ions scans should be made for any detected fragments that were observed in the CID spectrum of the starting material. Next, one looks at the daughter spectra of the possible parent ions that have been determined in this manner. These steps can be followed iteratively to develop the optimum strategy for identifying the metabolites.

The way that four metabolites of the experimental anticonvulsant zonisamide were identified (5) puts this procedure in a more practical setting. The methane CI spectrum of zonisamide shows an abundant quasimolecular ion at m/z 213 and little fragmentation. A daughter spectrum of the ion of mass 213 shows a prominent neutral loss of 81 u, leaving a fragment of 132 u (Fig. 5). The 81 mass

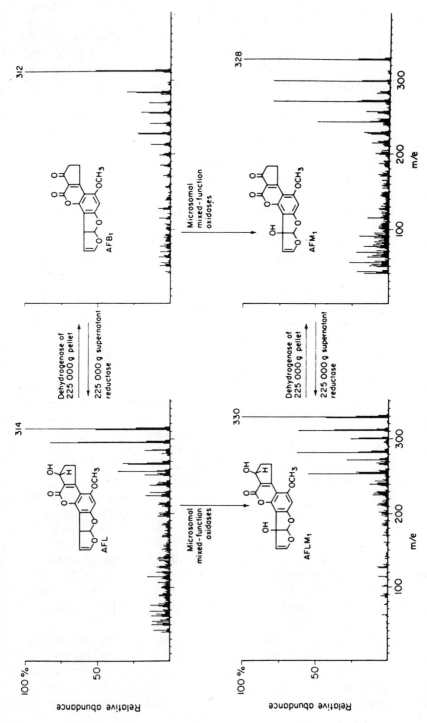

Fig. 4. Structures, metabolic interrelationships, and mass spectra of aflatoxin B₁ (AFB₁), aflatoxicol (AFL), aflatoxin M₁ (AFM₁), and aflatoxicol M₁ (AFLM₁) (4). Reproduced by permission from reference 4.

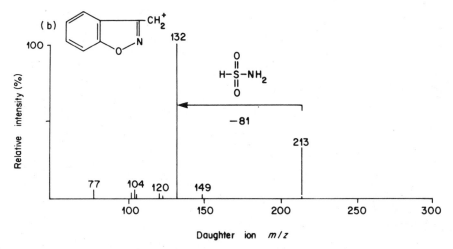

Fig. 5. Daughter spectrum of zonisamide. Positive CI-CID daughter spectrum of the protonated molecule (5). Reproduced by permission from reference 5.

neutral loss spectrum of the urine extract shows four notable ions, one from the parent compound and three others that are possibly molecular ions of metabolites. Three new parent ions generating m/z 132 are also observed (Fig. 6). Detection of each ion does not lead to a specific metabolite—some spectra do not consistently identify a particular structure—so that only four metabolites are proposed.

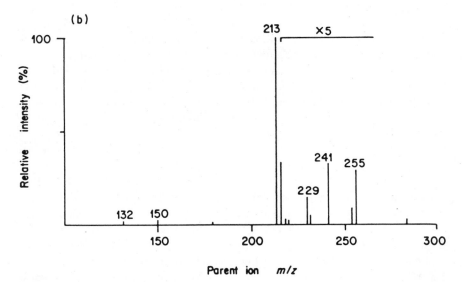

Fig. 6. Parent ion spectrum of m/z 132 from enzyme-hydrolyzed urine extract (5). Reproduced by permission from reference 5.

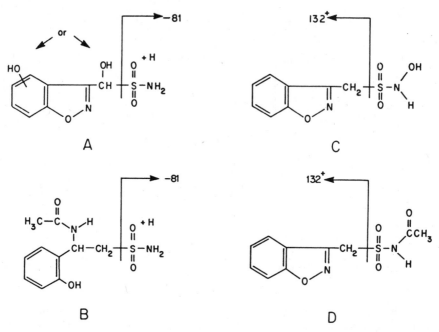

Fig. 7. Metabolites of zonisamide identified by the MS/MS technique and their characterized fragmentations observed in the daughter spectra of their $[M + H]^+$ ions (5).

These two types of experiments are complementary since a common neutral loss of 81 u implies that the sulfonamide group is intact while a common daughter, m/z 132, represents an unaltered ring structure. Thus changes to each moiety of the original molecule are facilely determined. The metabolites identified by this procedure are shown in Fig. 7. This determination was accomplished using nothing more than the spectral characteristics of the starting material. The entire analysis took only a few hours.

2.1.5. USING FAB–MS

Some drugs, and many of their metabolites, are not intrinsically volatile. For example, glucuronide conjugates, can be derivatized and analyzed by GC–MS (6) or thermospray LC–MS as discussed in Section 2.1.2. Other compounds require a technique such as fast-atom bombardment in order to provide acceptable spectra.

Among this latter group are anticancer drugs whose activity may be manifest by covalent binding to the nucleotides of DNA. While intact DNA remains beyond the capabilities of mass spectrometry, DNA hydrolysates containing individual modified nucleotides can be studied. Alternatively, studying the reactions of the drug with individual nucleotides provides better control over the reaction conditions and a better approach to the problem.

Vu et al. (7) used this approach to investigate the reaction between phosphoramide mustard, the active metabolite of the anticancer drug cyclophosphamide, and guanidine. HPLC separation showed three peaks representing what they believe to be the adducts between the drug and the nucleic acid. Three spectroscopic methods, UV, NMR, and MS, are then used to examine the structures of each adduct.

The UV spectra showed that the guanosine base is substituted in the 7 position. The NMR spectrum of adduct I shows the presence of two types of phosphorous, one from the 5'-phosphate group and the other from the phosphoramide mustard. The structures of these three adducts were finally determined by FAB–MS. The most abundant, adduct I, shows a molecular ion isotopic cluster characteristic of one chlorine (see Fig. 8a). As seen in the figure, a structure was proposed using just information from the molecular weight region, which identifies it as the covalently bound phosphoramide mustard missing one of its two original chlorine atoms. Other parts of the mass spectrum are consistent with this structure.

The FAB spectrum of the less abundant adduct II is shown in Fig. 8b. The coincidence of the apparent protonated molecule with the m/z 469/471 fragment ion cluster of adduct I, which is formed by elimination of the phosphoramide moiety, suggests that it was the adduct of guanidine with nornitrogen mustard.

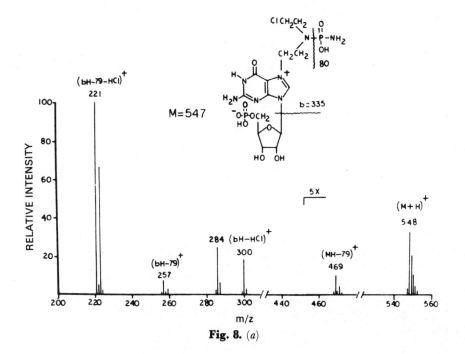

Fig. 8. (a)

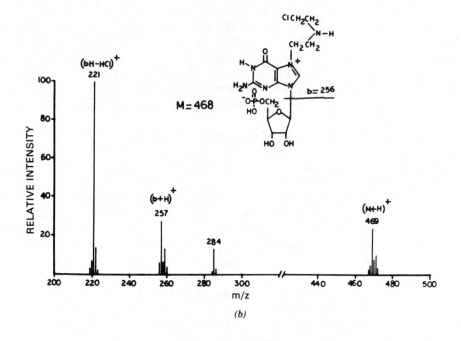

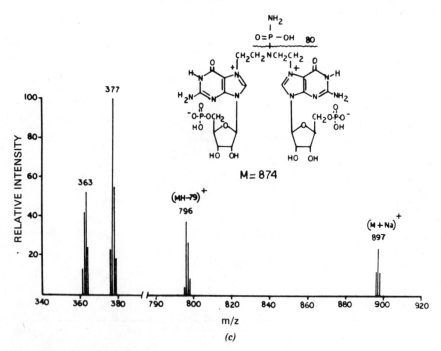

Fig. 8. Positive-ion FAB mass spectra of adducts of phosphoramide mustard with guanosine 5′-monophosphate: (*a*) adduct I; (*b*) adduct II; (*c*) adduct III (7).

Figure 8*c* shows the least abundant adduct whose molecular weight indicates a cross-linked phosphoramide mustard where each chlorine is now replaced with a 7-linked guanidine. The loss of 79 u confirms the presence of the phosphoramide group.

This research demonstrates the contributions of FAB–MS to the analyses of large, polar, and therefore thermally labile, molecules. These spectra show unusually rich fragmentation which helps to confirm the structures that are proposed from the molecular-weight information.

2.2. Quantifying the Distribution of Metabolites in a Metabolic Pathway

Once drug metabolites are identified, the next step is often to quantify those metabolites so that the fractional contribution of each can be assessed. Urine is the most commonly used biological specimen for studies of drug metabolite profiles; bile and feces are others. These sorts of studies are often considerably more difficult than qualitative ones because they are quantitative and involve numerous analytes that are likely to be of a diverse chemical nature. These studies remain important because they illuminate the metabolic pathways by which the drug is degraded, and can indicate the ways in which interactions with another drug might affect its disposition.

2.2.1. USING GC–MS

The method used in our laboratory (8) to analyze propranolol metabolites from urine is instructive in several aspects of quantitative analysis of multiple compounds which are comprised of different chemical species. Although propranolol is a lipophilic base, some of its metabolites are acidic or neutral (Fig. 9). This work was undertaken to study the effects of stimulation or inhibition of the hepatic microsomal drug metabolizing system on each specific metabolic step. To do this, each metabolite had to be quantified.

A two-step derivatization was carried out. Methylation of acidic groups with diazomethane was followed with trifluoroacetylation of alcohols, amines, and amides with trifluoroacetylimidazole (TFAI). Because diazomethane may methylate acidic hydroxy groups, each sample was also treated with just TFAI so that the endogenous methylation of hydroxylated products could be determined. Trifluoroacetylation is selected over silylation since the latter type of derivative gives ions that are less structurally significant.

Another subdivision of the analysis was carried out, namely, before and after deconjugation with β-glucuronidase/aryl sulfatase. The difference between these two assays represents the amount excreted into urine as conjugates.

Because several sample processing steps may not be reproducible, and because stable-isotope-labeled versions of the 13 compounds being determined are not available, three internal standards are used. The first of these is ICI 45,763, an analog of propranolol with a tolyloxy rather than a naphthoxy ring structure (see Fig. 9). It serves as a control for all trifluroacetylated products and is used as the

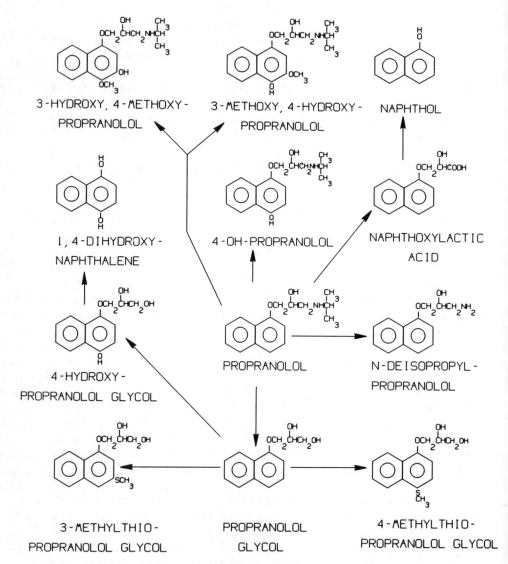

Fig. 9. Pathways of propranolol metabolism in the dog. Conjugations are not included. (9).

denominator in quantitation of all products. Phenoxyacetic acid is the internal standard for the diazomethane reaction. Observing a constant ratio between diTFA–ICI 45,763 and methyl–phenoxyacetate provides assurance that the derivatization scheme went well. Testosterone β-glucuronide is also spiked into urine so that the completeness of the deconjugation reaction could be assessed by the size of the TFA–testosterone peak.

Masses that are characteristic of each compound being quantified are selected from their spectra. This information is given in Table 1. Because a magnetic

TABLE 1

Selection of Masses for Quantitation of Propranolol and its Metabolites[a]

m/z	Structure	Compounds Identified
308	Intact propranolol side chain	ICI 45,763, propranolol, 4-OH-propranolol, and any metabolite with the intact side chain
143	Naphthoxy	Any metabolite with the intact naphthoxy ring
166	Methylphenoxyacetate	Phenoxyacetic acid
216	Methyl-α-naphthoxyacetate	α-Naphthoxyacetic acid
342	TFA Testosterone (-ketene) Methyl-TFA-α-naphthoxylactate	Testosterone, α-naphthoxylactic acid
352	DiTFA 1,4 dihydroxynaphthalene	1,4 Dihydroxynaphthalene
410	DiTFA propranolol glycol	Propranolol glycol
144 } 295 } 409 }	DiTFA N-deisopropylpropranolol	N-Deisopropylpropranolol
522	TriTFA 4-hydroxypropranolol glycol	4-Hydroxypropranolol glycol

[a]Source: Ref. 9.

scanning mass spectrometer is used for these analyses, a wide range of masses of interest could not be monitored in a selected ion recording mode, a distinct advantage for a quadrupole instrument. Full mass scans are repetitively taken and computer-reconstructed mass chromatograms are produced. An example of such a result is shown in Fig. 10. Each of the mass chromatograms $(b)-(g)$ detects one or more compound. The areas under the metabolite peaks relative to the area of the internal standard are used for quantitation.

2.2.2. USING LC–MS

Acetaminophen Metabolites in Bile. There are few examples where HPLC–MS has been used to quantify multicomponent mixtures in drug metabolism. Betowski et al. (10) describe the biliary excretion of acetaminophen and two of its conjugates.

A 5-h sampling of bile is obtained from rats that are previously dosed with acetaminophen. With no pretreatment, this bile is injected onto a reverse-phase HPLC column flowing through a thermospray interface into a mass spectrometer. The goal is to analyze acetaminophen and its glutathione and glucuronide conjugates. Knowing the structures of the three desired analytes, selected ion recordings are obtained at the three $(M + 1)^+$ ions. The intensities of the signals at the expected retention times imply that each microliter of bile contained 200 ng, 900 ng, and 1000 ng, respectively.

Analyzing this sample by FAB–MS is unsuccessful, presumably owing to the ion-suppressing effects of the complex matrix in which it is collected. Similar amounts of purified material produce intense FAB ions.

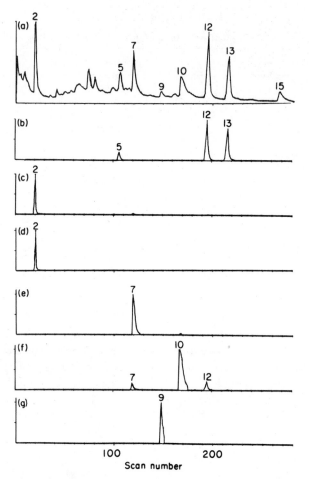

Fig. 10. Computer reconstructed ion chromatograms of a hydrolyzed urine sample from a dog receiving 180 mg/d phenobarbital chronically and a single oral 40 mg dose of propranolol. The interpretation of the masses is given in Table 1. Each number refers to a different metabolite. (*a*) Total ions; (*b*) m/z 308; (*c*) m/z 143; (*d*) m/z 240; (*e*) m/z 410; (*f*) m/z 144 + 295 + 409; (*g*) m/z 522 (8). Reproduced by permission from reference 8.

Cyclosporine Metabolites. The work of Hartman and Jardine (3), which is introduced in Section 2.1.2, presents an analytical system that is used to determine at least some of the pathways of cyclosporine metabolism. By assuming certain modifications to the parent drug, either oxidations or demethylations, selected ion chromatograms representing the new molecular species are obtained from thermospray HPLC. Figure 11, panels (*a*)–(*g*) present such data. The data in these panels show that peaks appear which are consistent with up to four levels of oxidation, as well as other combinations.

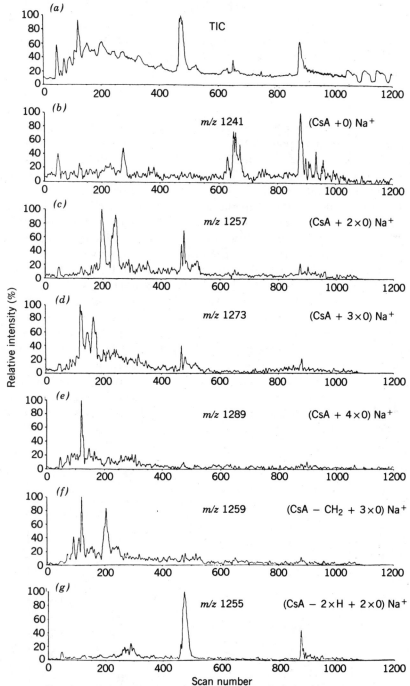

Fig. 11. Positive ion thermospray LC–MS mass chromatograms of separation of metabolites of cyclosporine A (CsA) shown in Fig. 2. (*a*) Total ions; (*b*) m/z 1241, monohydroxylated CsA; (*c*) m/z 1257, dihydroxylated CsA; (*d*) m/z 1273, trihydroxylated CsA; (*e*) m/z 1289, tetrahydroxylated CsA; (*f*) m/z 1259, trihydroxylated-*N*-demethylated CsA; (*q*) m/z 1255, carboxylated CsA (3). Reproduced by permission from reference 3.

Neither of these studies is rigorously quantitative, but the type of thermospray LC–MS data shown here suggests that it should be capable of useful quantitative work with the addition of suitable internal standards.

2.2.3. USING MS/MS

Tandem mass spectrometers are not yet used extensively for quantitative analyses, so that their potential to contribute to quantitative multicomponent analyses, such as metabolite profiles, is not well established. Work from this Department has found acceptable reproducibility and dynamic range in the determination of a drug and nine of its metabolites from mouse urine.

Hag Ali's studies on the antiparasitic drug praziquantel (PZQ), (11) include quantitative measurements of the levels of 9 of its 20 identified metabolites using MS/MS. This work was enabled by the characteristics of its collisionally induced dissociation (CID) mass spectrum, and the variety of positions in the structure that are hydroxylated. The CAD spectrum for PZQ following methane chemical ionization (see Fig. 12) shows ions representing the ABC ring structure (m/z 203), the AB ring group (m/z 132), and the D ring (m/z 83) as well as the pseudomolecular ion peak at m/z 313. If one hydroxy group is added, not only will the molecular ion shift by 16 u, but those fragments that contain the hydroxylated ring moiety will also shift by 16 u, while that portion of the spectrum that does not contain the extra oxygen will not change. For PZQ, hydroxylation on the D ring leads predominantly to dehydration so that m/z 81 is observed rather than m/z 99 when hydroxylation occurs in that ring. A similar logic can be developed for dihydroxylated metabolites. A final assumption is that a hydroxy group on the aromatic A ring never dehydrates, so that the

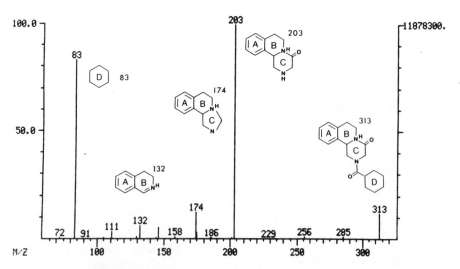

Fig. 12. Daughter ion mass spectrum of $[M + H]^+$ from PZQ (m/z 313) (11). Reproduced by permission from reference 11.

appearance of a dehydrated ion containing the AB or ABC ring structure implies a nonaromatic site of oxidation. Using this concept leads to the interpretive scheme shown in Fig. 13–14.

The analysis was carried out using mouse urine that had been pretreated by enzymatic deconjugation and clean-up on an Amberlite XAD-4 column. The sample was applied to the direct introduction probe and rapidly heated while the

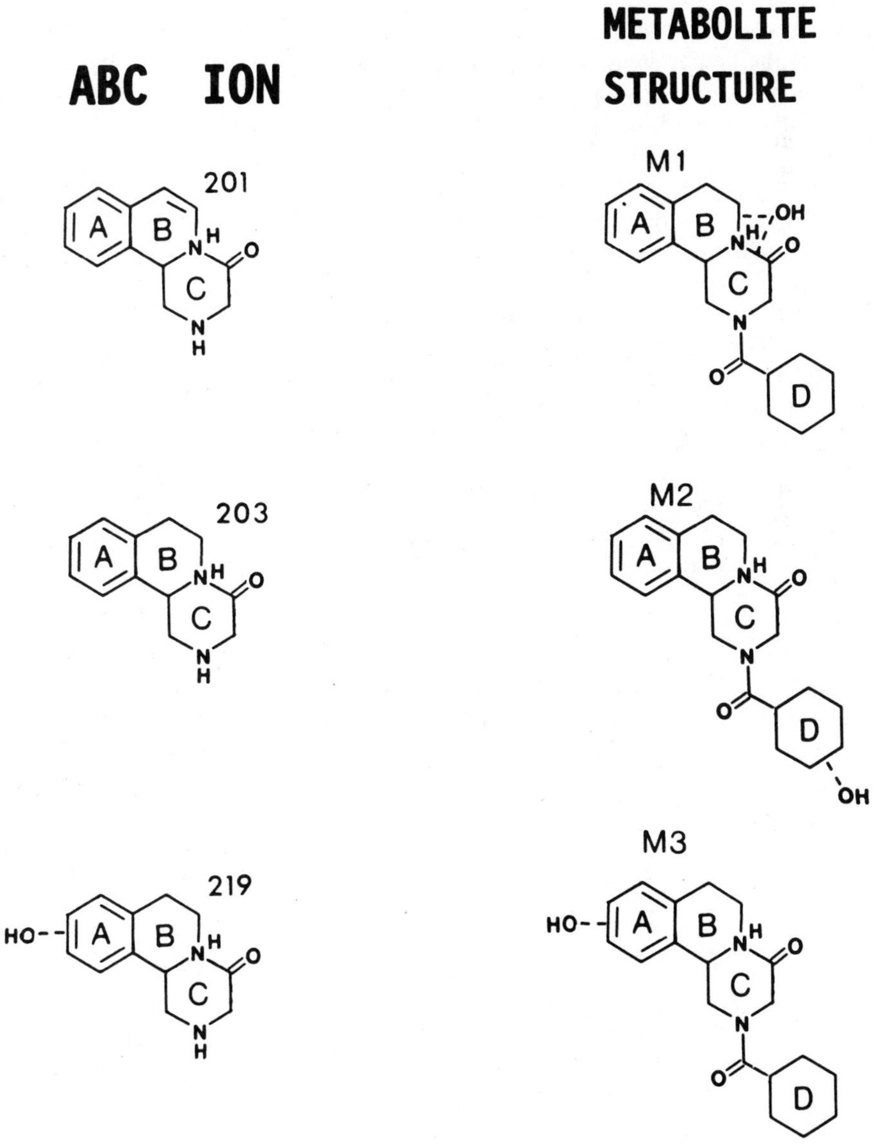

Fig. 13. Major daughter ions of PZQ and its monohydroxylated metabolites (11).

instrument was continuously acquiring data. The daughter ion spectra produced by the three possible $(M + H)^+$ ions; m/z 313 representing intact PZQ, m/z 329 representing monohydroxylated PZQ, and m/z 345, which is dihydroxylated PZQ, were obtained. Three monohydroxylated and six dihydroxylated metabolites of PZQ along with PZQ itself could be identified and quantitatively determined by MS/MS. The qualitative identification of these mono- and dihydroxylated PZQ metabolites is presented in Fig. 13-14.

The quantitation described here is for the array of hydroxylated metabolites at each level of hydroxylation. No standards for the metabolites are available, thus requiring the assumption that the relative probability of fragmentation along the desired pathway is independent of structure. If this is untrue, the absolute values for the amounts of each metabolite will change, but this will not negate the apparently good reproducibility that is observed.

Table 2 gives the values and SEMs for the metabolite profiles from nine urine specimens. The low relative errors, even for metabolites present at low levels, is indicative of the reproducibility of the method. An interesting internal check for consistency can be used here, since the determinations presented in Table 2 are based on the ABC ring ions that should be complemented by the ions found for the D ring. Obviously, if one hydroxy group is present, it is either in the ABC or D ring. In the case of the monohydroxy metabolites, the D ring data shows that 15.4% of the hydroxylation is in the D ring, a number that compares quite favorably with the 16.0% abundance of M2, the metabolite which has its hydroxy in the D ring.

Data of this type indicate that MS/MS can produce reproducible quantification of multicomponent systems. This example represents a particularly unfavorable case, since a very complex mixture was analyzed with little chemical or

TABLE 2

Quantitation of Praziquantel Metabolites using MS/MS

Metabolite	Relative Amount[a]
M1	1.7 ± 0.1
M2	16.0 ± 0.7
M3	82.3 ± 0.8
D1	8.8 ± 0.7
D2	11.3 ± 0.6
D3	2.8 ± 0.1
D4	6.4 ± 0.2
D5	57.5 ± 1.0
D6	13.2 ± 0.7

Source: Ref. 11.
[a]Means $\pm$ SE; $N = 9$. Each level of hydroxylation is normalized to 100%.

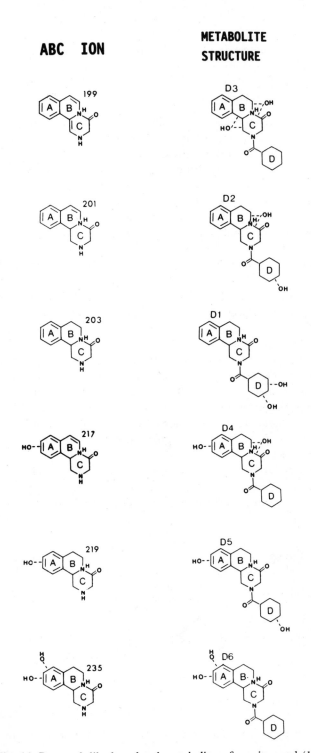

Fig. 14. Proposed dihydroxylated metabolites of praziquantel (11).

311

instrumental separation and without internal standards, just normalization of the set of selected ions.

2.2.4. REACTION INTERFACE—MS

A frequently used method for determining the metabolic profile of a drug is to radiolabel the starting material and measure the radioactivity associated with each metabolite. Recent work in this laboratory led to a technique that uses a similar philosophy, but with stable isotope-incorporated drugs (12). The reaction interface is a microwave-powered device that is placed in the gas stream between a gas chromatograph and a mass spectrometer. Eluting substances from the column enter the plasma of the reaction interface and are decomposed. The reaction products are small, polyatomic species whose mass spectra serve to monitor the elements and isotopes contained in the eluting substance. A schematic of a reaction-interface-mass-spectrometry (RIMS) apparatus is seen in Fig. 15.

The utility of this method can be illustrated with a series of chromatograms that are generated by processing urine from a dog which had been given 50 mg of $2,4,5$-^{13}C-labeled phenytoin. Following enzymatic deconjugation and extraction with XAD-2, the urine sample is ethylated and trifluroacetylated, and then injected onto a capillary GC column. With SO_2 as the reactant gas, the reaction interface produces CO_2 at m/z 44 from carbon-12 and at m/z 45 from carbon-13. Because of endogenous ^{13}C and ^{17}O, m/z 45 is a mixture of both naturally abundant isotopes and the enriched ^{13}C of the phenytoin. Based on the known natural isotope abundance and the signal at m/z 44, m/z 45 can be corrected so that it will only register a positive signal when a component containing ^{13}C enrichment elutes.

Figure 16a shows the m/z 44 chromatogram from this sample. This is a nonselective carbon signal, much as would be produced by a flame ionization detector. Panel 16b shows the gross m/z 45 signal on a somewhat expanded scale.

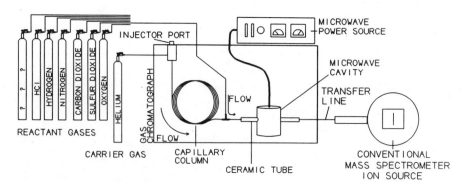

Fig. 15. Schematic of reaction interface–GC/MS (12). Reproduced by permission from reference 12.

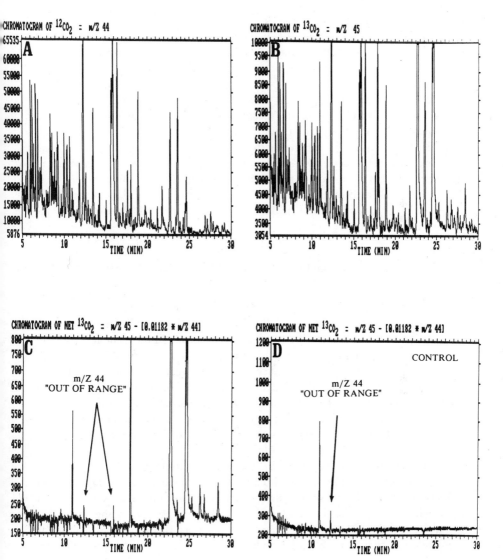

Fig. 16. Selective detection of ^{13}C-enrichment of phenytoin metabolites using reaction interface/mass spectrometry. The first three chromatograms (A)–(C) are from the same sample of extracted, ethylated dog urine. (A) m/z 44, which is unenriched CO_2 and therefore represents nonselective detection of carbon. (b) m/z 45, which is either $^{13}CO_2$ or $C^{16}O^{17}O$. Most of the signal is due to natural abundance of the two isotopes. (C) Demonstrates the improved selectivity for isotopic enrichment that is provided by subtracting from (B) the expected contributions from $^{13}CO_2$ or $C^{16}O^{17}O$ as predicted from (A). (D) Urine from a dog not receiving drug. The internal standard, ^{13}C-enriched phenobarbital, elutes at 11 min. The "OUT OF RANGE" arrows indicate artifacts where the m/z 44 trace went off scale, producing incorrect subtraction in the net chromatogram (12). Reproduced by permission from reference 12.

The substantial number of peaks is due primarily to the natural abundance of the carbon and oxygen isotopes. When they are subtracted out, the enrichment chromatogram in panel 16c is produced. The chromatogram from a control urine (panel 16d) shows no peak other than the internal standard.

In this way, a chromatogram is produced that identifies components enriched in ^{13}C so that the relative peak areas can be used to quantify. Like using radioactivity selectively to identify specific components in a complex mixture, all products of the originally stable-isotope-labeled material can be detected with RIMS. Reinjecting the sample with the microwave power turned off and acquiring full mass spectra as one would normally do in a GC–MS experiment gives a total ion chromatogram much like panel 16a but the compounds of interest are indicated by the selective chromatogram 16c. These spectra are used to qualitatively identify those peaks of the metabolite profile provided by the RIMS assay.

2.3. Stereoselective Metabolism Studied by MS

Drugs are frequently synthesized in a manner that is not stereochemically specific. Consequently, a "pure" drug will actually be a racemic mixture. If the drug, and any active metabolite, is equally active in both enantiomeric forms, is removed at equal rates from the body, and is absorbed in the same fraction and rate into the bloodstream, there would be no practical problem. While it is usual that only one enantiomer is pharmacologically active, it is unusual for an assay procedure to detect just the active species; generally the total amount is quantified. The ratio of the active and inactive enantiomers will not be constant if there are stereochemically sensitive aspects of a drug's disposition and there will be an error in these measurements that will grow with time after the drug is administered.

With the use of stable isotopes, "pseudoracemates" may be prepared by mixing an unlabeled enantiomer with a labeled antipode. If the label is placed in a metabolically stable position, the biotransformation products of the labeled enantiomer will retain the label and be differentiable from the unlabeled metabolites that came from the other enantiomer. In this way, questions about stereoselective metabolism can be studied.

Propranolol. Propranolol is a beta-adrenergic-blocking drug whose interesting pharmacology has prompted many studies of its metabolism. It is a racemic mixture so that questions of its stereoselective metabolism are best answered with isotopic pseudoracemates. Using this approach, Walle et al. (13) prepared four different pseudoracemate mixtures: d_2-(ring)-$(+)/d_0$-$(-)$, and and d_6-(isopropyl)-$(+)/d_0$-$(-)$; as well as their reverse-labeled counterparts, d_0-$(+)/d_2$-(ring)-$(-)$, and d_0-$(+)/d_6$-(isopropyl)-$(-)$ propranolol (see Fig. 9). Two different labeling sites are required since the known sites of metabolism (see Fig. 17) may affect one or the other portion of the molecule, and the reverse racemates are employed to check for isotope effects.

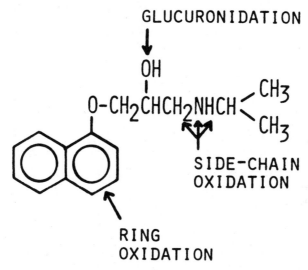

Fig. 17. Primary pathways of propranolol metabolism (13).

Figure 9 shows the metabolite pattern for propranolol in the dog. The stereochemical specificity of each of these pathways is assessed by examining the isotopic composition of each metabolite. Table 3 summarizes the findings. The $(-)/(+)$-enantiomer ratio indicates whether one or another stereoisomer is preferentially metabolized. If this ratio is near unity, metabolism is not stereoselective. In fact, most of the metabolites are formed by stereoselective mechanisms. Glucuronidation and ring oxidation are favored by the $(-)$-configuration while side chain oxidations are favored by the $(+)$-isomer.

Beyond the basic pharmacological information this sort of study provides, the significance in the case of propranolol rests in the facts that (1) it is administered as a $(+)/(-)$ mixture, (2) only the $(-)$-enantiomer is pharmacologically active, and (3) some hydroxylated metabolites have pharmacological activity comparable to the parent compound. An error in quantitative measurements of plasma levels of propranolol without regard to the specific isomeric content arises after oral administration because of a shift in the original 50/50 ratio of the $(+)$ to $(-)$ content of propranolol following the more extensive metabolism of the active $(-)$-species in passing from the intestinal tract through the liver before reaching the systemic circulation.

Norketamine. In another study, Leung and Baillie (14) investigated the stereoselective metabolism of norketamine, the N-demethylated metabolite of the anesthetic agent, ketamine. Using microsomal preparations and a pseudoracemic mixture containing (R)-norketamine and (S)-norketamine-d_2, they evaluated the production of two hydroxylated metabolites, 4- and 6-hydroxynorketamine.

In their GC–MS scheme, they monitor two fragment ions that represent the two starting materials [m/z 306 and 308 for the unlabeled-(R)-enantiomer and

TABLE 3

Stereochemical Composition of Propranolol Metabolites in the Urine of Dogs Receiving Single Oral Doses of Deuterium-Labeled Pseudoracemic Propranolol

	$(+)/(-)$ Enantiomer Ratio[a]
Unchanged propranolol	0.52 ± 0.03^b (0.54)
Glucuronidation	3.5 ± 0.5^b (3.0)
Side chain oxidation	
N-deisopropylpropranolol	0.35 ± 0.03^b (0.41)
N-deisopropylpropranolol-glucuronide	0.43 ± 0.06^b (0.38)
Propranolol glycol	0.37 ± 0.02^b (0.40)
Propranolol glycol-glucuronide	0.45 ± 0.04^b (0.53)
α-Naphthoxylactic acid	0.47 ± 0.03^b (0.49)
Isopropylamine	0.74 ± 0.09^b (0.67)
Ring oxidation	
Hydroxypropranolol	1.49 ± 0.08^b (1.69)
Hydroxypropranolol-glucuronide	1.46 ± 0.04^b (1.5)
Hydroxypropranolol-sulfate	1.04 ± 0.04 (1.14)
Ring + side chain oxidation	
Hydroxypropranolol glycol glucuronide	0.75 ± 0.04^b (0.80)
Hydroxypropranolol glycol sulfate	0.88 ± 0.06 (0.91)

Source: Ref. 13.

[a]Mean $\pm$ SE; $N = 4 - 8$. Numbers within parentheses are from a dog given reverse-labeled pseudoracemate.

[b]Significantly different from 1; $p < 0.05$.

the dideutero-(S)-enantiomer, respectively], and two fragment ions that were characteristic of the hydroxylated metabolites of either the unlabeled or dideuterated starting materials (m/z 304 and 306). Figure 18 shows the three selected ion recordings from one chromatographic analysis. The m/z 304 channel shows the presence of both 4- and 6-OH-norketamine, while the m/z 306 channel shows only the 6-OH isomer along with the unlabeled starting material. Little, if any, of the 4-OH isomer was observed.

It is obvious that the formation of 4-OH-norketamine is stereoselective, with the (R)-enantiomer being the preferred substrate. While not obvious from Fig. 18, evaluating the enantiomeric composition of the hydroxylated metabolites shows that 6-OH-norketamine is enriched in the (S)-enantiomer.

2.4. Isotope Effects in Drug Metabolism

While the use of stable isotopes can be of extraordinary value, it can also produce problems. If the label is not placed in a metabolically inert position, the label can be lost, and the profile of metabolites will be incomplete. Furthermore, the label may lead to isotope effects which significantly alter the profile and extent of metabolism. The deuterium isotope presents the largest effect; isotopes of carbon,

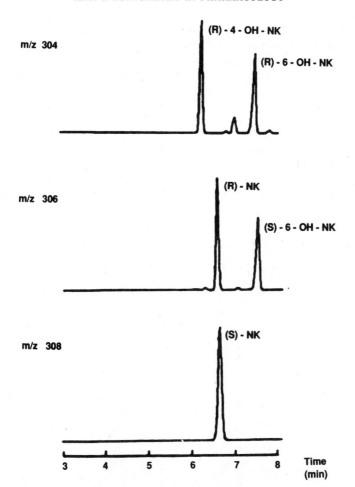

Fig. 18. Selected ion monitoring GC–MS analysis of incubation of pseudoracemic norketamine in rat liver microsomes. Ions monitored were m/z 304, (R)-4-OH-norketamine and (R)-6-OH-norketamine; m/z 306, (R)-norketamine and (S)-6-OH-norketamine; m/z 308, (S)-norketamine (14). Reproduced by permission from reference 14.

nitrogen, or oxygen differ so little from their natural counterparts that isotope effects are not observed.

One of several mechanistic aspects of the metabolism of N-methylformamide (NMF) reported by Threadgill et al. (15) is a marked kinetic isotope effect. The question they investigated was how the metabolism of NMF was associated with its toxicity. They used unlabeled NMF to which was added

$$\overset{\text{D}}{\underset{|}{\text{O=CNHCH}_3}} \quad \text{or} \quad \overset{\text{D}}{\underset{|}{\text{O=CNHCD}_3}}.$$

The NMF isotopomers were administered to mice who were sacrificed 4 h later. Their bile was obtained and examined for the presence of a glutathione conjugate. A method based on secondary ion mass spectrometry from a liquid matrix (liquid SIMS or FAB, see "desorption ionization" in the first chapter) was used to detect this product after cleanup and derivatization. By using a mixture of

$$\overset{\displaystyle H}{\underset{\displaystyle O=CNHCH_3}{|}} \quad \text{and} \quad \overset{\displaystyle D}{\underset{\displaystyle O=CNHCH_3,}{|}}$$

they were able to determine that the carbonyl hydrogen was lost in the formation of the glutathione adduct, thus establishing the position of the linkage.

When a mixture of

$$\overset{\displaystyle H}{\underset{\displaystyle O=CNHCH_3}{|}} \quad \text{and} \quad \overset{\displaystyle D}{\underset{\displaystyle O=CNHCD_3}{|}}$$

were given to the mice, the mass spectrum shown in Fig. 19 was obtained. After

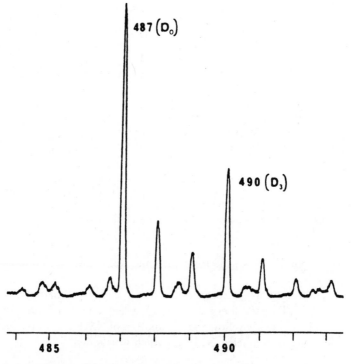

Fig. 19. The $[M + Na]^+$ region of the liquid SIMS spectrum of fully derivatized S-(N-methylcarbamoyl)glutathione isolated from the bile of mice that had received a mixture of $OHCNHCH_3$ and $ODCNHCD_3$ (15). Reproduced by permission from reference 15.

adjusting for the original composition of the mixture, which

$$
59\% \ \underset{\text{H}}{\underset{|}{\text{O=CNHCH}_3}}, \quad 18\% \ \underset{\text{D}}{\underset{|}{\text{O=CNHCD}_3}}, \quad \text{and} \quad 23\% \ \underset{\text{H}}{\underset{|}{\text{O=CNCD}_3}}
$$

which is a by-product in the synthesis of

$$
\underset{\text{D}}{\underset{|}{\text{O=CNHCD}_3}},
$$

a kinetic isotope effect of 7 was found. This meant that the hydrogen was seven times more likely to be lost than the deuterium. Such an observation places that specific hydrogen at a critical step of the metabolism for that pathway, since an isotope effect is only observed when the difference in zero-point energy between H and D is important.

2.5. Establishing Metabolic Pathways with MS

The profile of the metabolic products for a drug may be known, but it is often important to determine the reaction pathway by which each of the metabolites is produced. Frequently, these studies are done with *in vitro* systems where the concentrations are higher and the interferences lower than when studied *in vivo*. The application of mass spectrometry to such a problem is illustrated below.

Valproic acid (VPA, see Fig. 20) is an anticonvulsant drug that occasionally shows hepatotoxicity. Animal studies implicate one of its metabolites, Δ^4-VPA, as the species responsible for the liver damage, although the metabolic pathway for its formation shown in Fig. 20 involves a rather novel step, namely, the unsaturation of a nonactivated carbon. To investigate the metabolism of VPA, Rettie et al. (16) incubated VPA *in vitro* with liver microsomes from phenobarbital-pretreated rats; phenobarbital induces the hepatotoxicity of VPA, presumably by inducing the cytochrome P-450 system. Analyzing the metabolites requires a mass spectrometer, since the metabolites are produced at low levels.

Normally, full mass spectra are used to provide qualitative identification of a compound. When the amount of the compound falls below the level at which full mass spectra can be obtained, a product can be identified with a set of criteria appropriate to selected ion monitoring (see the first chapter, Section II D). As explained in the legend of Fig. 21, these are: the coincident appearances of peaks in the ion current profiles at three values of the mass spectrum of the Δ^4-VPA, their agreement with the retention time of the authentic material, and the proper ratio of responses. This is how Rettie et al. (16) identified the metabolite of VPA. The three masses are shown in the three rows of the figure, while the columns represent three different experimental conditions. These data show the formation of Δ^4-VPA only when the microsomal drug metabolizing system is complete thus proving that desaturation is mediated by cytochrome P-450.

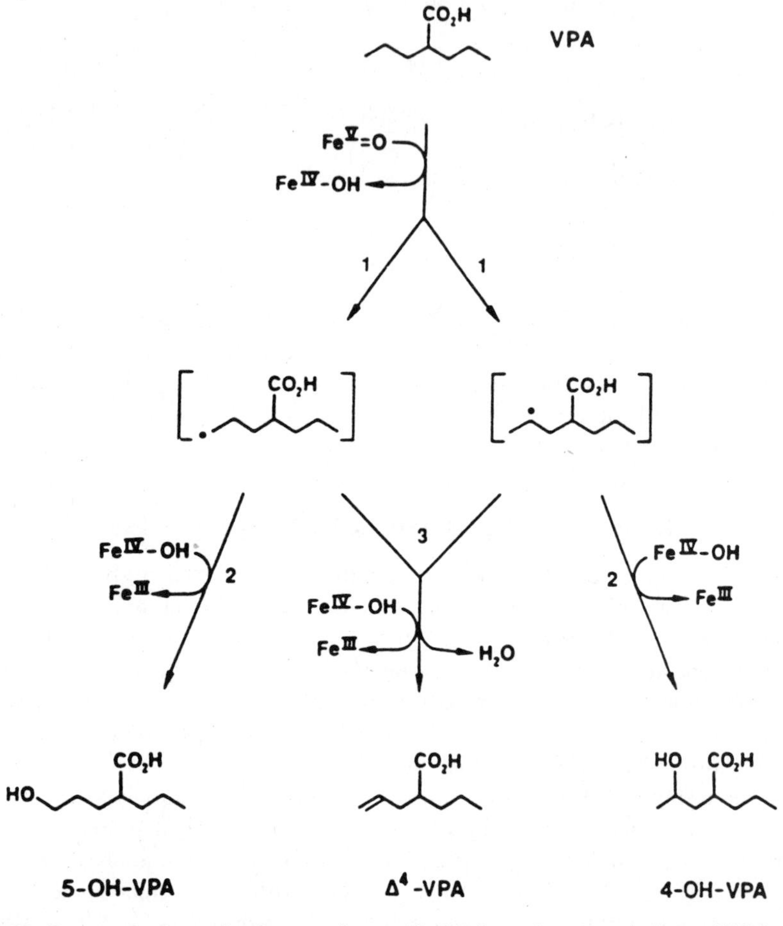

Fig. 20. Proposed scheme for the cytochrome P-450-dependent metabolism of VPA to 4-OH, 5-OH, and Δ^4-VPA (16).

2.6. Drug Metabolism Studies that Measure CO_2 in Breath

A noninvasive method for measuring the rate of metabolism has been developed which recognizes that the final product of demethylation reactions is CO_2. Aminopyrine, a little-used analgesic drug, is one of the standard substrates to assay for the hepatic microsomal cytochrome P-450 enzyme system. It contains a dimethylamino group that is oxidatively demethylated by the P-450 system. If one or both of these methyls are labeled with ^{13}C, the isotopic enrichment of the expired CO_2 serves to monitor the rate of this demethylation. Interpreting the results of this assay system requires more assumptions than measuring the appearance of the demethylated metabolite in plasma, since the ultimate

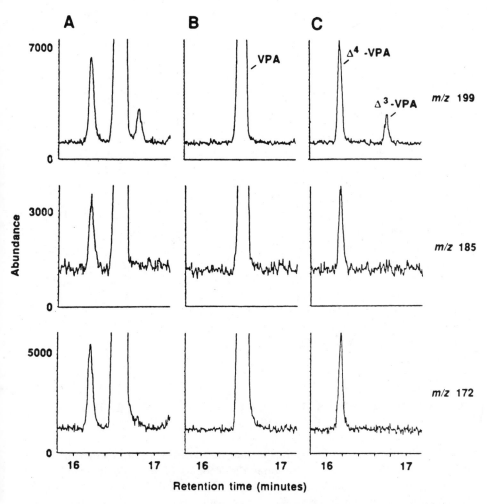

Figure 21. Detection of Δ^4-VPA as a microsomal metabolite of VPA. (A) VPA was incubated with hepatic microsomes from phenobarbital-treated rats and metabolites were extracted and analyzed as their TMS derivatives by GC–MS. Identification of Δ^4-VPA in these extracts was based on the following criteria: (i) coincident responses were observed in the ion current chromatograms corresponding to three characteristic fragments in the mass spectrum of Δ^4-VPA (namely, at m/z 199, 185, and 172); (ii) these responses occurred at the exact retention time (16.2 min) of the TMS derivative of Δ^4-VPA; and (iii) the ratios of responses in the three ion current chromatograms (2.19:1.00:1.74) were almost identical to those obtained from the authentic reference material (2.29:1.00:1.80). (B) Microsomal incubations were carried out under conditions identical to those of (A), except for the omission of reduced nicotinamide cofactors. (C) An authentic sample of Δ^4-VPA–TMS was analyzed to determine accurately the retention time of the compound and also to establish the ratios of ion current intensities at m/z 199, 185, and 172 (16). Reproduced by permission from reference 16.

production of CO_2 involves a series of metabolic steps beyond the cytochrome P-450 system.

The $^{13}CO_2$ breath test uses mass spectrometric determination of the m/z 45/44 ratio. Shulman et al. (17) use this technique to follow the development of the P-450 system in infants between the ages of 1 and 38 weeks. The obvious advantage of the $^{13}CO_2$ test is that it does not involve the administration of radioactive substrates, as do other breath tests.

Shulman et al. (17) fit the infants with masks and collect their expired gases. The total CO_2 is measured by gas chromatography and an isotope-ratio mass spectrometer was used to measure the m/z 45/44 ratio. Sampling CO_2 every 30 min following oral administration of the N,N-^{13}C-dimethyl-labeled aminopyrine allows them to determine the metabolic rate. They find a substantial increase, ~ 2–3 fold, in the production of $^{13}CO_2$ in infants 16–36 weeks old compared to those less than 8 weeks old. This finding is consistent with the generally observed immaturity of the drug metabolizing activity of newborns and the relatively rapid rate at which the system develops.

The material discussed in Sections 2.3–2.6 represents some of the most creative uses of mass spectrometry in pharmacology. These four sections emphasize stable isotopes in pharmacology as studied by mass spectrometry. Baillie's 1981 review (18) of this subject is an excellent resource that details the origins of each type of stable-isotope application, as well as presenting a much more in-depth review of applications than is presented here.

3. QUANTITATIVE ANALYSIS OF BLOOD CONCENTRATIONS OF DRUGS

Pharmacologists often need to know the pharmacokinetic profile of a drug in the blood stream, that is, its concentration in the blood as a function of time after its administration. This profile requires a determination of the fraction of the drug that has been absorbed, a term called *bioavailability*, the speed of the absorption process, the rate of metabolism or excretion, and the volume into which the drug appears to distribute. This information is required by the Food and Drug Administration as a prerequisite to a company's being given approval to market a particular drug.

Moreover, a knowledge of the pharmacokinetics of a drug provides a rational basis on which to develop dosing schemes. Since many drugs are given repetitively, knowing its half-life permits repeating the dose at a time when an appropriate amount of the drug is removed. If too much disappears between dosing intervals, the drug will have limited efficacy. If too little is eliminated, then the second dose may nearly double the blood concentrations and the third may nearly triple them. Continued administration of the drug may lead to toxic blood levels. Thus, dosing regimens must be carefully developed from a knowledge of the time course of a drug's concentrations in the blood.

Quantitative information about the concentration of a drug is also important to predict its pharmacological activity. Although few drugs act within the bloodstream itself, the actual site of activity, whether the brain, heart, or kidney, and so on, receives drug via the blood supply. For most drugs, there is a linear relationship between the amount of drug in a target tissue and the concentration in the blood. Because of this relationship, one can predict the activity of a drug based on its blood concentration.

The most familiar example of this principle is the blood alcohol concentration, which is used to charge automobile operators with driving while intoxicated. The site of alcohol's action is in the brain, but the equilibrium that exists between the brain and blood concentrations permits the blood concentration to predict the level of intoxication.

This strategy is also used in the hospital setting to assess the probability that a particular set of symptoms is due to an excess amount of a drug that has been taken by the patient, rather than some other underlying condition that might be unrelated to drugs and might require other treatment. In Section 5.4.1 the use of mass spectrometry to identify drugs in the comatose patient is discussed.

A more frequent use of quantitative drug assays is to optimize therapy. This is called therapeutic drug monitoring. When a drug is initially studied, the blood concentrations are measured in a large group of patients and correlated with the observed beneficial or untoward effects. From this correlation, the optimal range for blood drug concentrations is determined. Subsequent patients will have their blood concentration measured and will have their dose adjusted, if necessary, to provide blood concentrations in this desired range. Mass spectrometry is infrequently used for the routine determinations, those are usually carried out with immunological or chromatographic methods. However, when a drug is first being investigated, the high sensitivity and selectivity of mass spectrometry may make it the method of choice.

The superiority of mass spectrometric detection for the quantitative analysis of drugs is summarized in a review by Garland and Powell (19) in which a variety of GC, HPLC, and GC–MS methods for quantifying amitriptyline are compared. There is an approximately five-fold sensitivity advantage for GC–MS, which could be useful if sample sizes are limited. When stable-labeled isotopic analogs were used as internal standards, the GC–MS methods also demonstrate a four-fold better precision. Thus, the inherent qualities of the mass spectrometer make it a more sensitive detector, while its ability to use an ideal internal standard greatly improves its analytical performance.

3.1. Pharmacokinetics Studies

3.1.1. DIETHYLSTILBESTROL

Diethylstilbestrol (DES) is a synthetic estrogen that has been widely used as a feed additive to increase yield in meat-producing livestock. Less well known is its frequent use as a treatment for prostate cancer. Although it has been in use since 1941, its human pharmacokinetics had never been adequately characterized.

In 1985, we developed a GC–MS method for measuring DES in the plasma of patients with prostate cancer, as well as from blood and tissues of experimental animals (20). Developing an assay requires a derivatization scheme appropriate to the structure of DES (Fig. 22), a minimization of interferences to provide the most sensitive and specific method possible given the available mass spectrometer, and an appropriate internal standard.

The acidic character of the phenolic groups in DES permits derivatization in a variety of ways. On the other hand, it was thought that the presence of high levels of free fatty acids in plasma could make derivatization by alkylation or trimethylsilylation less desirable, since these endogenous acids may interfere in the chromatography and analysis. We chose acylation with trifluoroacetic anhydride, since it would not produce stable derivatives of the fatty acids but readily produces the bistrifluoroacetyl-DES that chromatographs well and following electron-impact ionization has its base peak at m/z 460, representing the molecular ion. Good chromatographic behavior and an abundant structurally specific ion are important considerations when choosing among derivatization schemes.

Despite these advantages, the selected ion current profile (chromatogram) for m/z 460 is not sufficiently selective for DES when the chromatography is carried out on a packed column. Endogenous substances are found coeluting with DES. Consequently, we switched from a packed to a capillary chromatographic system and produced a much more sensitive and selective analysis. Choosing the internal standard is not difficult, since there are few choices. The homolog dimethylstilbestrol (DMS, Fig. 22) is available, while the more desirable isotopically labeled DES analogs were not available at that time.

Three selection ion current channels are used. In addition to m/z 460, the mass spectral peak at m/z 431 represents loss of one ethyl group from DES and is also reasonably abundant. This provides a measure of confirmation regarding the identity of DES in this complex system. As long as the intensities at m/z 460 and m/z 431 maintain their proper relationship, significant interferences could be discounted, since it is unlikely that the mass spectrum of an interfering substance would have these two peaks at similar relative intensities. The internal standard is monitored at m/z 432, representing its molecular ion.

Trans(E)-dimethylstilbestrol bis(trifluoroacetate)

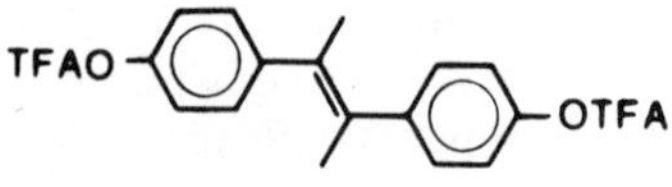

Trans(E)-diethystilbestrol bis(trifluoroacetate)

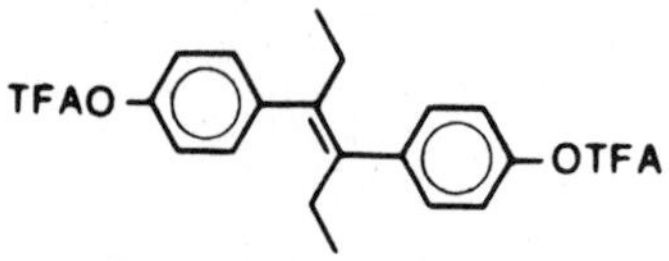

Fig. 22. Structures of diethylstilbestrol and dimethylstilbestrol as their TFA derivatives (20).

Figure 23 shows chromatograms from two blood samples from rats. The left three traces are from a rat that was given no DES and demonstrate the specificity of the method. The two peaks seen in the m/z 432 trace are from the *trans* and *cis* isomers of the internal standard. The right three traces show DES at a concentration of 9 ng/mL from a rat that had been dosed with DES. DES also exists in two isomeric forms, so that two peaks are seen in the m/z 460 and 431 channels.

The limit of quantitation for this method is 0.3 ng/mL from 1 mL plasma samples. In addition, samples from animal tissues such as prostate, liver, and muscle could be analyzed with similar sensitivities.

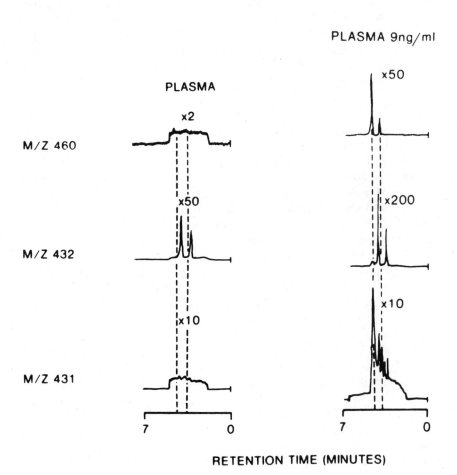

Fig. 23. Selected ion current profiles (chromatograms) detecting DES (m/z 460 and 431) and DMS (m/z 432). Panels on left are from control rat plasma (not receiving DES), while the right-hand panels are from plasma obtained 5 h after a 1.2 mg/kg DES dose. The dashed lines show the expected retention times for DES isomers (20). Reproduced by permission from reference 20.

We were able to show with this method that the plasma decay of DES in man has a $t_{1/2}$ of 80 min during a 4-h period of observation (21). We also were able to examine an alternative dosing form for DES. Rather than the conventional oral dosing at 1–5 mg/d, some urologists report greater success using 1000 mg infusions of stilphostrol, a water-soluble product, which is converted to DES in the body by dephosphorylation. Plasma samples from these patients show 1000-fold larger plasma DES concentrations, perhaps explaining the improved results.

3.1.2. FLURAZEPAM

Far more sensitivity is possible if one can take advantage of those drugs that natively capture electrons. Electron capture negative ionization (ECNI) (see Negative Ion Formation in the first chapter) of such specimens produces a large signal and a low background relative to less selective forms of ionization. Derivatizations to yield an electron-capturing species can be carried out, but the demand on chemical and physical separations becomes greater since endogenous materials may also be converted.

Miwa, Garland, and Blumenthal (22) follow this strategy to produce an assay for flurazepam which has a sensitivity limit of 12 pg/mL. Flurazepam has one chlorine and one fluorine atom in its structure, as well as central ring structure that itself captures electrons. Owing to the high extent of metabolism and the large volume of distribution, plasma levels of flurazepam during therapy are near 1 ng/mL and quickly decay with a half-life of 2–3 h. This means that kinetic studies will need sensitivity near 10 pg/mL. Examining the details of the work of Miwa et al. (22) exemplifies many of the problems and some possible solutions to assays in the subnanogram per milliliter range. The principles are not just applicable to drugs but are useful in a general sense.

The major problems in high-sensitivity analyses are background, nonlinearity, and carryover. Miwa et al. (22) use a three-stage solvent extraction scheme to purify their plasma samples. This appears adequate for their needs. Nonlinearity at low levels is due to many factors, but the best known are adsorption to glassware and to GC columns. A similar approach is used to deal with both of these. Not only is silanization of the glassware and columns carried out, but another substance is added to all samples to overwhelm adsorptive sites without interfering with the analysis, that is, a carrier. This molecule is like flurazepam except it has its chlorine replaced with hydrogen, hence its chemical nature was similar to flurazepam, but its retention time and mass spectrum do not cause interferences. The 2 μg of this material that are spiked initially into each 2 mL of plasma saturates the adsorptive sites so effectively that the subnanogram per milliliter amounts of the analyte are protected.

To deal further with adsorption on the column, yet another structural analog, this time one with a fluorine replaced with a hydrogen, was used along with a silanizing agent to "prime" the column. To avoid carryover or "ghost" peaks, they also use this compound to tune the instrument and thereby avoid injection of unusually large amounts of flurazepam that would carry over into subsequent

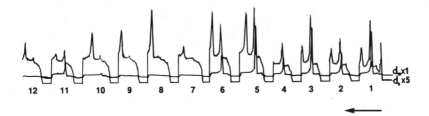

Fig. 24. Selected ion current profiles (chromatograms) showing the effect of the addition of carrier substance, compound III, on the recoveries of flurazepam (m/z 387) and flurazepam-d_{10} (m/z 397). Selected ion current profiles 1–6 are from the analysis of 1 mL of plasma sample spiked with 1 ng of flurazepam, 5 ng of flurazepam-d_{10}, and 2 μg of compound III. Selected ion current profiles 7–12 are from the analysis of 1 mL of plasma sample spiked only with 1 ng of flurazepam and 5 ng of flurazepam-d_{10} (22). Reproduced by permission from reference 22.

analyses. They comment that this "priming" method improves their transmission of flurazepam by 1000-fold. Historically, experimenters use labeled internal standards as carriers to accomplish the same goals. In this case, the internal standard, $^2H_{10}$-flurazepam, is added in only 5 ng/mL amounts. However, using $^2H_{10}$-flurazepam as a carrier would require much higher levels and would have led to off scale signals for the internal standard since sensitivity of the method is so good.

The efficiency of the 2 μg/mL carrier molecule is demonstrated in Fig. 24. The chromatograms labeled 1–6 included this carrier while the last six did not. Several things can be noted from these tracings. Most obviously, little or no flurazepam at 1 ng/mL is detected when the carrier is absent. Even the 5 ng/mL internal standard is not detected well. Although traces 1–6 show substantial variability in absolute height, the variations appear accurately dealt with by the internal standard. In fact, the coefficient of variation from replicates of a pooled plasma sample containing 135 pg/mL of flurazepam is 4%.

Miwa et al. (22) also note the superior sensitivity of ECNI versus positive-ion chemical ionization. After optimization under both conditions, they find that ECNI is 50 times more sensitive than positive ion CI. This is expected, since, under CI conditions, there are far more low-energy electrons available for attachment to yield negative ions than there are high-energy electrons to ionize the CI gas by impact and produce positive ions.

3.1.3. AUTOINDUCTION OF CARBAMAZEPINE

An important aspect of pharmacokinetics, which is elegantly and uniquely studied by using stable isotopes and mass spectrometry involves changes in the kinetics of a drug when it is given chronically. The time course of some drugs might be altered by changes in, for example, drug metabolizing capacity brought on by the drug's own activity. The kinetics of a tracer dose given during a chronic period of dosing can be compared to the drug's kinetics after just one dose to see whether changes have occurred. This particular strategy closely mimics the use of mass spectrometry in biochemical studies where a labeled pulse of an endogenous substance is used to assess its turnover rate. Here, the chronically maintained drug concentration is analogous to the endogenous production of a biochemical substance and the tracer can be used without disturbing the ongoing process.

The antiepileptic drug carbamazepine is known to induce its own metabolism in animals, yet induction in man is uncertain. Bertilsson et al (23) address this question by adding $^2H_4$-labeled carbamazepine (CBZ) to unlabeled CBZ upon initiating therapy and at three other times through 5 months of chronic treatment. Using a GC–MS method that had been developed for general clinical pharmacokinetic studies (24) gave them the requisite data.

This assay demonstrates how the selectivity of mass-spectrometric detection facilitates the overall analytical scheme. Palmer et al. (24) uses the most straightforward possible components of a GC–MS method to produce the assay: no derivatization, packed column chromatography, an analog (10,11-dihydroCBZ) as an internal standard, electron ionization, and only two monitored ion currents, one each for the CBZ and the internal standard. When using the $^2H_4$-labeled CBZ, a third ion current channel had to be examined.

The simplicity of the method permits 80–100 analyses per day, since the total running time for each injection was 5 min. The detection limits, 50 ng/mL from a 0.5 mL sample, are quite adequate with respect to the therapeutic concentrations of CBZ that are in the microgram per milliliter range. While a 50 ng/mL detection limit is relatively high for mass-spectrometric methods, it is consistent with a method that does not require special chromatographic or mass spectrometric techniques to attain selectivity from interfering materials. Such problems emerge as the detection limits reach the low or subnanogram per milliliter levels.

The pharmacokinetic study is able to show clearly that CBZ enhances its own metabolism (23). After 20–30 days of dosing, the rate of clearance of CBZ averages twice that observed early in the course of treatment. This means that doses which provide effective concentrations during the first week or two of therapy are too low once this autoinduction phenomenon levels out.

3.1.4. QUATERNARY AMMONIUM MUSCLE RELAXANTS

The quantitative analysis of two quaternary ammonium neuromuscular blocking agents described by Castagnoli and coworkers (25) contains several points of interest, although there are only a few drugs that would be amenable to their approach which includes ion-pair extraction and pyrolysis.

Pancuronium and vercuronium are neuromuscular blocking agents that are used during surgery. Charged molecules such as these quaternary amines are usually unsuitable for most mass-spectrometry methods except FAB or thermospray where their ionic character is advantageous. This work takes advantage of this ionic character in other ways. Quaternary amines are extracted from plasma in different ways than almost any other molecule, and the pyrolytic conversion of the quaternary ammonium salt into the volatile tertiary amine provides selectivity.

Ion-pair extraction is used to select lipophilic ionic substances and back-extraction is used to remove whatever neutral lipid molecules are extracted in the first step. Thus, an extracted sample should only contain lipophilic ions. An aliquot of this extract is then placed on a direct introduction probe and heated to just below the pyrolysis point of the drug. This volatilizes many impurities so that when the temperature reaches the point that the pancuronium or vercuronium is pyrolized and thereby volatilized, a selective and sensitive determination is possible using isobutane chemical ionization and deuterated internal standards. Detecting the decomposed drug at a high mass, m/z 543, where relatively few interferences would be expected, improves the success of their analysis.

This method produces linear quantitation over the range of 1–500 ng/mL of plasma. It is reproducible with coefficients of variation of less than 6% at the 25 ng/mL level. Using this method enables the pharmacokinetic study of either drug.

3.1.5. VOLATILE ANESTHETICS

The volatile anesthetics, which are used in surgery, are also drugs, just as the other chemicals included in this chapter. Their volatility leads to an aspect of the use of mass spectrometry in pharmacology that is substantially different than those discussed elsewhere.

Continuous monitoring the blood gases of anesthetized patients allows one to measure the dissolved levels of the anesthetic along with the partial pressures of oxygen and carbon dioxide. Although rational, this might not be cost effective if only one patient is monitored by one mass spectrometer. However, Ozanne et al. (26) describe a manifolding system that permits one central mass spectrometer to serve each of 10 operating rooms. While the details of their apparatus are not important here, the type of measurements they made is of interest.

Four anesthetic agents were considered, nitrous oxide and three halogenated anesthetics: halothane, enflurane, and isoflurane. Nitrous oxide and carbon dioxide both have molecular ion peaks at m/z 44, but the contribution to m/z 44 from CO_2 can be computed from the m/z 12 signal, the C^+ fragment from CO_2, and subtracted to yield an N_2O-specific signal. The other three agents are monitored individually by signals at the same two masses. The mass spectral peak at m/z 51 represents CF_2H^+ and that at m/z 67 represents $CHFCl^+$. These fragments are common to each anesthetic, but they can be differentiated on the basis of the ratio of peak intensities at m/z 51 and m/z 67. In this way, the anesthesiologist can observe the actual levels of anesthetic, and adjust its administration to maintain safety and efficacy.

3.1.6. STAGGERED STABLE ISOTOPE ADMINISTRATION

Pharmacokinetic studies are usually done by giving a dose of a drug at one specified time and taking samples at suitable times afterwards in order to examine the time dependence of the drug. An alternative procedure is the staggered stable isotope administration (27), which may be used if repeated samples are difficult to obtain, as might be the case at the time of a biopsy or from a spinal tap. In this experiment, two or more isotopically labeled forms of a drug are given intravenously at intervals appropriate to the kinetics expected for the drug. The one sample that is obtained carries in it the time history of the two or more injections. The mass spectrometer can quantify each isotopic form of the drug that permits an evaluation of the kinetics from the single sample.

An application of this staggered method (27) is in a dog that was given three doses of phenobarbital: one labeled with five deuterium atoms, one labeled with two ^{15}N atoms and one ^{13}C atom, and one unlabeled. The second dose was administered 10 min after the first and the third dose was administered 15 min after the second. To evaluate how well a single sample might compare with the conventional sampling scheme, five cerebrospinal fluid (CSF) samples were taken over a 90-min period. The kinetics of uptake were evaluated over the entire 90 min sampling period using the concentration of the unlabeled drug, and at each of three different time points after all three isotopic species had been introduced. By the conventional time-dependent kinetic calculation, the entry half-life for phenobarbital in CSF was 18 min. The staggered isotope method gave half-lives of 22–24 min indicating that it may provide valid kinetic parameters.

In theory, this technique opens up many new types of kinetic experiments, particularly when a tissue sample can be obtained during a biopsy or a surgical procedure. Its obvious limitations relate to the general lack of availability of multiple isotopically labeled drugs and their attendant expense. The use of high-resolution mass spectrometry might provide some assistance, because a drug containing only a single heavy atom of hydrogen, carbon, nitrogen, or oxygen might be resolvable from one another. The possible applications of this method would not be restricted to pharmacology, but could extend into the kinetics of endogenous substances.

3.1.7. HPLC–MS-BASED ASSAYS

It appears that most quantitative analyses of plasma drug concentrations utilize GC–MS methodology. Given the great utility of LC–MS in qualitative studies of drugs and their metabolites, and the explosive growth of HPLC-based quantitative drug measurements, it may appear surprising that very few quantitative analyses of drugs use HPLC–MS. One explanation may be that LC–MS is newer than GC–MS and insufficient time has elapsed to make its more routine use common.

A more profound explanation is offered by Covey et al. (28) who note that practical detection limits for LC–MS are 10–50-fold higher than usually obtained with GC–MS. They also note difficulties with variable responses to different analytes. Many of these difficulties should be overcome with isotopic internal standards and more reliable equipment.

3.2. Bioavailability Studies

The term bioavailability refers to the fraction of a drug that reaches the systemic circulation based on the amount actually administered. When given intravenously, a drug's bioavailability is defined as 100%, since it is directly placed in the systemic circulation, but other routes of administration, particularly oral, may have much lower values. This low bioavailability may be due to a variety of factors, one of which is the way the drug itself is compounded and manufactured. Consequently, the FDA mandates that the bioavailability be monitored carefully since unexpected alterations in bioavailability would lead to alterations in blood concentrations and effects.

The amount of drug absorbed is quantified by the area under the concentration versus time curve (AUC). For this, quantitative measurements of drug concentrations usually made over the entire duration of a drug's presence in the body. Bioavailability is determined in an absolute or a relative manner. In an absolute determination, the AUC for some alternative route of administration is compared with the AUC from an intravenous dose. In a relative determination, two nonintravenous dosing procedures are compared.

Mass spectrometry is useful in bioavailability studies simply by its being the basis for the measurement of the drug, or by its capacity to discriminate a labeled drug from an unlabeled drug if one were given by one route or dosage form and the other from another route or form. The latter capacity produces a method that is one of the most important and frequently used applications of mass spectrometry in pharmacology.

3.2.1. Absolute Bioavailability Studies

Strong et al. (29) report the first use of stable isotope methodology in bioavailability studies. Prior to this work, a bioavailability study required two separate sets of experiments, one each for each route of administration or dosage form. This means twice as many venipunctures and, sometimes, twice as many subjects. Interindividual variability requires relatively large number of experiments in order to obtain a statistically meaningful result.

What Strong et al. did was to synthesize singly ^{13}C-labeled N-acetyl-procainamide (NAPA) and to inject it intravenously into a subject who had simultaneously swallowed a capsule of unlabeled NAPA. Each blood specimen therefore contains concentrations of both labeled and unlabeled NAPA. By quantifying both the labeled and unlabeled drug, the AUCs corresponding to intravenous and oral dosing could be determined in the same individual at the same time. Selected ion monitoring of the quasimolecular ions of labeled and unlabeled NAPA (m/z 279 and 278) is carried out using methane chemical ionization. To further improve quantitation precision, an internal standard of ^{2}H$_5$-labeled NAPA is added to each specimen prior to processing. Its quasimolecular ion (m/z 283) is also monitored. After corrections for impurities and natural abundance, the mass spectrometric analysis of the 279/283 and 278/283 ratios provide the specific concentration values. Because of the economy of fewer human subjects, shorter analysis times, and greater experimental accuracy, the concept of this method has wide application.

3.2.2. RELATIVE BIOAVAILABILITY STUDIES

Two studies of relative bioavailability will be presented. Each asks a different question regarding the availability of a drug from two different orally administered forms. Nitrendipine is a drug classified as a calcium-channel blocker whose actions are beneficial in several cardiovascular diseases. Of interest is the bioavailability of nitrendipine when administered orally as solution or as a tablet. Formulating a drug in different ways affects its disintegration, and subsequent different rates of dissolution can have therapeutic consequences. Even though the total amount of drug absorbed might be the same, its onset of action and peak concentrations might be different. The object of this type of study is called *bioequivalence*, that is the attainment not only of equal AUCs between two preparations, but their equal time courses.

The second study is not of different dosing forms, but rather a comparison of a drug with another molecule which is converted to that same drug. For example, stilphostrol is the diphosphate ester of DES. In the United States, tablets of DES containing no more than 5 mg are marketed, while stilphostrol can be obtained in 50 mg tablets. Certain protocols for treating prostate cancer use hundreds of milligrams of DES so that the 5 mg tablets would be impractical. However, the relative bioavailability of DES from stilphostrol had not been determined.

Nitrendipine. For the analysis of nitrendipine, Mikus et al. (30) used a ECNI mass spectrometric method. The especially high sensitivity attainable by ECNI is essential here since the plasma concentrations are as low as 100 pg/mL. Having a nitro group, nitrendipine will effectively capture electrons and yield negative ion spectra without having to add electronegative groups via derivatization. Three isotopic forms of nitrendipine are used: unlabeled and tetra-^{13}C-labeled, which are used as the dosing forms, and octadeuteronitrendipine, which is the internal standard. In addition to an absolute bioavailability study using labeled intravenous nitrendipine and a solution of unlabeled nitrendipine as an oral preparation, the authors also compare an unlabeled tablet with an oral solution of the carbon-labeled material. They sample the subjects repeatedly for 24 h after the simultaneous ingestion of the two preparations and find that the AUC for the tablet is 82% relative to the solution. There was a significant difference in the lag time for the appearance of nitrendipine in plasma after the tablet is ingested (1.5 h) compared to the solution (0.2 h). This is an indication of the time required for the tablet to disintegrate and dissolve and indicates a difference in bioequivalence between the two preparations.

Mikus et al. (30) point out that the use of mass spectrometry provides significantly greater sensitivity than the previous analytical method. This permits quantification of plasma concentrations for up to 24 h, while previous work ran out of sensitivity by 8 h.

Diethylstilbestrol. Although the question being asked is similar, the circumstances of the DES bioavailability study is quite different. Although both DES and stilphostrol have been available for years, their therapeutic equivalence was untested. Using dogs rather than cancer patients, Abramson and Miller (21) compare the plasma concentrations of DES following 50 mg stilphostrol equivalent doses with doses of DES (31.3 mg) that could be liberated from 50 mg of stilphostrol. They use the same mass spectrometric assay that is described earlier (see Section 3.1) and that involves capillary GC separation, electron-impact ionization, and a homolog as the internal standard.

The plasma concentrations are in the 1–10 ng/mL range and show that the pro-drug was actually a better source of DES than is DES itself. Presumably DES is less soluble leading to poor absolute bioavailability while the highly water-soluble stilphostrol overcomes this deficiency. This work suggests that physicians could use a more convenient dosing form of DES, that is, stilphostrol, when higher than conventional doses are desired. The selectivity and sensitivity of the capillary GC–mass spectrometry method provides the analytical capabilities needed for accurate quantitation at low levels from plasma samples.

4. CLINICAL TOXICOLOGY, FORENSIC TOXICOLOGY, AND DRUGS AFFECTING PERFORMANCE

The definitive identification of drugs by mass spectrometry makes it an ideal tool to provide unimpeachable evidence when the data might be used in an adversarial situation. Many crime laboratories are recognizing that some of what have been their standard methods, such as a colorimetric or TLC-based screen followed by "confirmation" by GC, are not adequately specific. Consequently, mass spectrometry has become the ultimate device for ensuring the presence of abused or illicit drugs.

One frontier in which mass spectrometry has made significant advances is assisting emergency room physicians identify the causal agent when approaching a comatose patient. There its capacity to rapidly identify a wide range of drugs from complex matrices has led to such applications. If one or more drugs are detected in the patient, the course of treatment would be more accurately directed.

4.1. Drug Testing in Athletes

There has been a long-standing concern in international competition that some athletes gain a "chemical edge" owing to their use of performance-enhancing drugs. To ensure that competition is free from such improprieties, the International Olympic Committee introduced a limited amount of drug testing at the 1968 Olympics. Since then, full-scale drug testing is the norm at each Olympic competition.

The Olympic Analytical Laboratory was set up at UCLA for the 1984 Olympic Games in Los Angeles. The details of that undertaking as well as a summary of their experiences is published (31). The sheer magnitude of the analytical problem is noteworthy. In addition to less sophisticated instruments, the laboratory contains seven GC–MS units and eight GCs with N-P detectors. A staff of 24, including six mass spectroscopists and three service engineers processed approximately 100 GC–MS assays per day after screening samples by either GC, RIA, or GC–MS. All positive results from the screens were confirmed by GC–MS.

Anabolic steroids are the only class of drugs for which screening by GC–MS was employed. For this analysis, urine specimens are extracted with XAD-2, deconjugated with a *Helix Pomatia* enzyme mixture for 3 h, extracted, dried, and silylated. Using capillary GC columns interfaced to the mass spectrometer and monitoring ion current at only two m/z values for each steroid makes it possible to enhance the sensitivity. A positive sample contains the appropriate two ions in the appropriate ratio at the appropriate retention time. If steroids are detected, the assay is repeated using 20 selected ions to confirm that specific compound.

All other types of drugs whose presence is inferred by their screening procedures are confirmed by GC–MS. This test uses full-spectrum scanning and a matching algorithm based on the 100+ spectra of the banned substances contained in the computer library. In the 15 days of the Olympiad, nearly 100,000 samples were screened by one method or another, and nearly 400 were "flagged" by the screening procedure such that a confirmatory GC–MS analysis was undertaken. This protocol has proven so effective that it remains the standard for the Olympics as well as for intercollegiate athletics in the United States.

4.2. Drug Testing in Racehorses

To ensure fair competition, most drugs are banned from use in racehorses; a few are permitted with public notification and a veterinarian's prescription. It is necessary to monitor the urine from racehorses to ensure that the rules are being followed.

The Equine Drug Testing and Toxicology Laboratory at the New York State College of Veterinary Medicine is the leading laboratory in this area. Applying HPLC and tandem mass spectrometry demonstrates how well this method can work for identification of drugs in this setting (32).

Because the direct introduction of urine samples into the mass spectrometer was unsatisfactory, they introduced samples into a short HPLC column whose output was nebulized and sampled by an atmospheric-pressure chemical-ionization source attached to their MS/MS instrument. In this way, only a simple organic solvent extraction scheme provided efficient analysis.

As noted earlier (Section 2.1.4) mass spectrometry can serve to separate information from mixtures as well as to detect and identify. In this way the analyst can use much simpler, faster, and more efficient preanalysis procedures

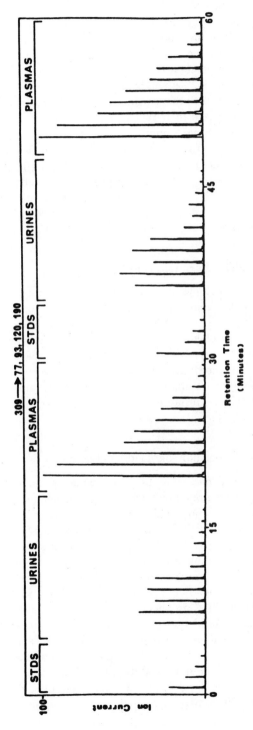

Fig. 25. One-hour 60-sample LC−MS/MS analysis of samples from a phenylbutazone pharmacokinetic study in the horse. Selected reaction monitoring of four daughter ions of phenylbutazone. Samples were injected with an autoinjector each minute. The phenylbutazone standards contained 400, 200, 100, 50, and 25 ng, respectively. All samples were analyzed in duplicate (32). Reproduced by permission from reference 32.

while maintaining the specificity of the overall method. Because the tandem mass spectrometer is capable of exceptionally high selectivity, its applications may be among the most efficient from the laboratory's standpoint.

It is just this point that Covey et al. (32) illustrate in their analytical protocol for phenylbutazone, an antiinflammatory drug known in racing circles as "Bute" after its tradename, Butazolidin. Although the sample work-up time must be considered, they describe a method that can analyze one sample per minute. The key feature is how well optimized their HPLC separation is with respect to the selectivity of the MS/MS. By using 33-mm HPLC columns, they are able to free the drug of interest from interferring components in such a way that the phenylbutazone retention time is just 1 min. A selective assay is provided by monitoring the ion current corresponding to four prominent daughter ions peaks, m/z 77, 93, 120, and 190, which arise from the quasimolecular ion, m/z 309 (see Fig. 25). Although these are summed, presumably their relative intensities could be used to confirm the presence of phenylbutazone even more specifically.

4.3. Forensic Applications

The unique capacity to obtain molecular "fingerprints" of a substance present at submicrogram levels makes mass spectrometry a critical component of a laboratory whose results might be used in court. The most obvious use is to confirm the identity of a controlled substance when material is confiscated from a suspect or a crime scene. A variety of screening procedures may be used, but only a structurally sensitive method, such as MS, NMR, or IR is capable of unambiguously confirming the result. The latter two methods cannot always be used when the amount of the substance is much below 1 mg, especially if the sample is impure or in a biological matrix.

5.3.1. CONFIRMATION OF SCREENING FOR ILLICIT DRUGS

It is now widely recognized that, while useful for screening large numbers of samples, colorimetric, chromatographic, and immunologic methods do not provide unambiguous identification of the presence of a drug of abuse. Mass spectrometry is now used routinely in many forensic toxicology laboratories. Mulé and Casella present their GC–MS procedure, which is used to confirm positive results produced by immunoassay screening (33). Separate protocols are followed for urine specimens that are immunologically positive for marijuana (as 11-nor-δ-9-tetrahydrocannabinol-9-carboxylic acid), cocaine (as benzoylecgonine), morphine and codeine, amphetamine and methamphetamine, and phencyclidine. Confirmation of identification is based on the three selected ion currents that are appropriate to each drug or metabolite being examined. If the retention time is correct to within 1% and the ratios of intensities are correct to within a 20% tolerance, the immunological drug screening test is confirmed.

Although primarily designed for definitive identification, these methods have quantitation limits near 10 ng/mL when used with an appropriate internal standard. The authors state that these methods are in routine use in their laboratory and that one trained technician can work up about 25 samples per day.

5.3.2. IDENTIFICATION OF CHINA WHITE

The screening of suspects for abused drugs is similar to the procedures used in drug overdose cases (see Section 5.4) as long as the ingested drug is one which is already catalogued. The discovery of newly synthesized materials (the so-called "designer drugs") has been enabled by mass spectrometry. The story of a designer drug named "China White" illustrates how mass spectrometry is used along with NMR and IR to identify a novel material (34).

After several initial attempts to characterize the material by NMR and electron impact mass spectrometry, chemical ionization MS is used so that a molecular weight determination might be obtained. The EI experiments (Fig. 26) show m/z 259 as the highest mass ion detected while a molecular weight of 350 was determined from the CI experiment. A loss of 91 (350 − 259) suggests a benzyl structural component, and the even molecular weight suggested an even number of nitrogens, most probably two. Searching the literature for a precedent compound, Kram et al. find 3-methylfentanyl. Its NMR spectrum did not perfectly agree with the unknown, but its similarity suggests that 3-methylfentanyl is close to the correct material.

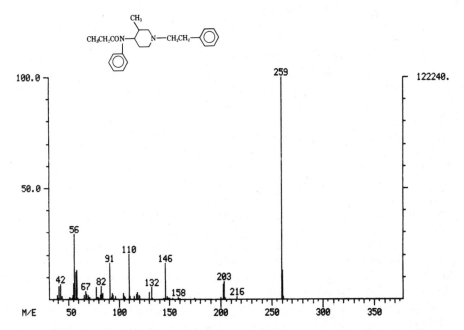

Fig. 26. Mass spectrum of "China White" and its structure (34). Reproduced by permission from reference 34.

Because the weakest aspect of identification by MS is differentiation of isomers, NMR is often used. The NMR spectrum of China White indicates that only the α- and β-methylene carbons were possible sites for the methyl group. The choice between these is based on mass-spectral characteristics. China White is identified as α-methylfentanyl (Fig. 26). The overall identification process involved GC, HPLC, NMR, IR, and MS. Because of the information content of this battery of methods, no synthesis work need be done prior to making the α-methylfentanyl whose spectra confirm the structure of China White.

5.3.3. LSD DETECTION IN URINE

Revealing the use of illicit substances provides another forensic application of mass spectrometry. In general, urine is screened by immunological methods and confirmed by GC–MS. LSD (lysergic acid diethylamide) is an exceptionally potent drug; 25 μg doses can produce psychedelic effects. This high potency necessarily leads to low concentrations in urine, since so little drug is ingested. The development of a confirmatory analysis for LSD reviews the previous difficulties associated with its assay, and presents a new method that extends the limit of detection down to 0.05 ng/mL (35).

The philosophy of the new method (35) is very similar to the quantification of flurazepam (see Section 3.1) using electron-capture negative-ionization mass spectrometry. Using a relatively large amount of labeled internal standard, and adding an analogous compound, in this case methysergide, in yet greater amounts serves as a deactivator for each sample. As did Miwa et al. (22), Lim et al. (35) showed that the sensitivity using electron ionization is much less than with ECNI.

The electron-capturing properties of LSD are enhanced by derivatization by trifluoroacetylation. The liability of derivatizations such as attempted here is that many interfering substances are also converted into readily detectable substances, thus placing more of the burden of selectivity on the clean-up and chromatography.

In addition to providing for the detection of LSD with excellent detection limits and good precision, this method also provides information regarding three metabolites of LSD. Among them, N-desmethyl LSD, had never been reported in man before, although its presence is inferred from animal experiments and from discrepancies between RIA and HPLC assays. Lim et al. (35) show that N-desmethyl LSD is present in every sample where LSD is found, although the relative amounts of the two compounds were variable. Lim et al., therefore, propose that N-desmethyl LSD be used as a confirmatory substance in the forensic identification of LSD in contrast to the usual criteria for identifying drugs for forensic purposes, namely, a full mass spectrum or, at least, the appearance of three or more selected ions relating to the compound at the appropriate retention time and in the appropriate ratios. With ECNI, fragmentation is frequently minimal, so that the ability to examine several ions is severely impeded and qualitative identification will not be possible at the lowest detection limits where those ions will have inadequate abundance.

5.3.4. DETERMINATION OF MORPHINE IN HAIR

Hair is a potential reservoir of drug history, since ingested substances are often incorporated into its structure. With vigorous extraction, these drugs can be liberated and detected. Pelli et al. (36) carried out such an investigation with hairs from two heroin addicts who died of overdoses. These workers attained high selectivity by using collisionally induced dissociation on a double-focusing mass spectrometer operating in the mass-analyzed ion kinetic energy spectrum mode (MIKES). This method uses a similar strategy as does tandem MS since the only signals detected will be linked by a particular dissociation step.

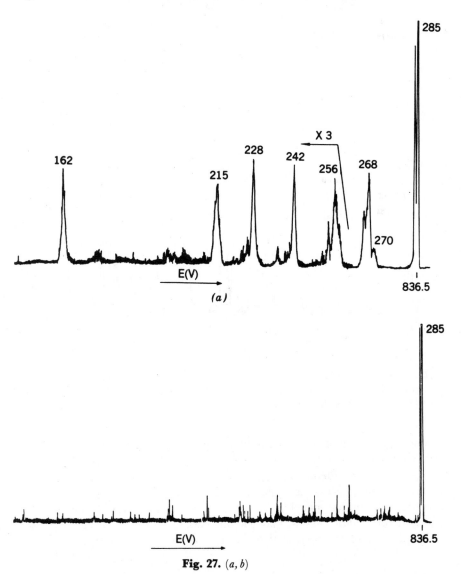

Fig. 27. (a, b)

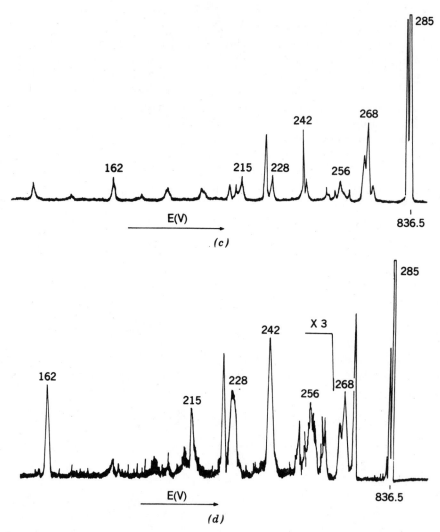

Fig. 27. Collisionally induced spectra of m/z 285. (a) From a morphine standard; (b) from hair devoid of morphine; (c) from 5 fg of morphine spiked onto hair; (d) hair from a heroin addict (36). Reproduced by permission from reference 32.

Panel (a) of Fig. 27 shows the MIKES analysis of the morphine molecular ion, m/z 285, produced upon EI of pure morphine, which was introduced into the ion source by direct introduction. Panel (b) shows results of a similar analysis of blank hair, while panel (c) shows a similar spectrum for 5 fg of morphine spiked onto blank hair. The bottom panel is the spectrum obtained from an extract of hair from a heroin addict. Hair may be increasingly used as a noninvasive, nondilutable forensic sample, thus replacing urine as a monitor of drug abuse.

4.4. Emergency Toxicology Applications

The question facing the emergency room physician attending a comatose patient is whether the condition is drug-related or is due to some other underlying problem, such as trauma or stroke. As mass spectrometry becomes more widely available, samples of blood, urine, or other fluids from such a victim could be analyzed for the presence of drugs. If a drug is found, it provides information not only on the etiology of the coma, but also on possible therapeutic interventions that might be expected to lessen the time of unconsciousness.

4.4.1. DETECTION OF DRUG OVERDOSES

A variety of approaches are used for this purpose. The example to be cited here is chosen because it was among the very first to attempt this sort of analysis, and also because it demonstrates some aspects of the use of mass spectrometry that are not described elsewhere in this chapter. In 1971, Milne, Fales, and Axenrod published their approach to identifying drugs from intoxicated patients (37). They used isobutane chemical ionization for samples placed on a direct introduction probe.

Their assumption from having done GC–MS assays in this setting is that the concentration of drugs in various body fluids is high in the case of an overdose, so that sophisticated work-ups are not necessary, and that gas chromatography would not be needed if simple mass spectra are generated. Isobutane chemical ionization is chosen since fragment ion production is suppressed. Examining the spectra of 48 drugs gives 36 with no significant fragment ions. The main fragmentation from the rest is loss of water.

Thirty of the 48 drugs have unique molecular weights, so their identification is easy. Fragmentation or isotope pattern differences resolve uncertainties of another six pairs leaving three isobaric pairs. Two of these three pairs are barbiturate isomers, whose differentiation would not likely be clinically important. The last pair, mescaline and butethal, could be differentiated by a simple extraction procedure since one is a base and the other is an acid.

Figure 28 shows the isobutane chemical ionization spectrum of a gastric aspirate sample from an overdose patient. Five drugs are identified in this spectrum. In each case, the M + 1 ion provided unambiguous determination of the drug, and the gentle butane chemical ionization keeps the spectra simple, so that it could readily be interpreted by an unskilled observer.

The initial success of mass spectrometry, particularly coupled with gas chromatography, is in identifying drugs causing coma. In many institutions, including my own, once the identity of the range of drugs likely to be encountered had been determined, gas chromatography alone, or some other method less sophisticated than mass spectrometry, is able to answer most of the analytical needs of the emergency room.

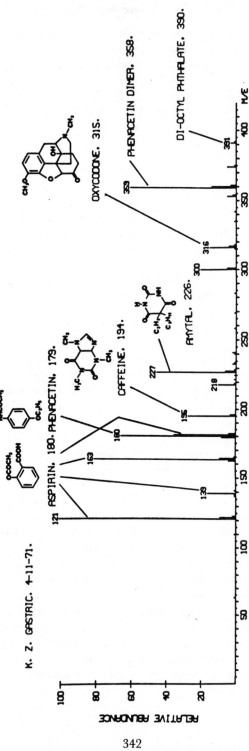

Fig. 28. Isobutane CI mass spectrum of gastric contents in an overdose case (37). Reproduced by permission from reference 37.

342

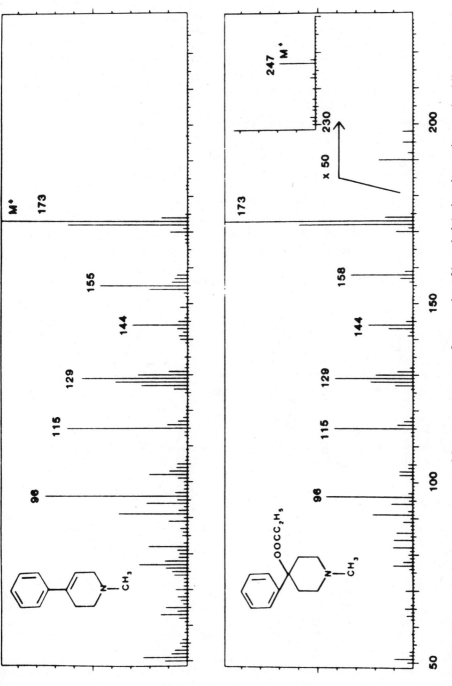

Fig. 29. Electron-ionization mass spectra of the two components of preparation of 1-methyl-4-phenyl-proprionoxypiperidine separated by gas chromatography (38). Reproduced by permission from reference 38.

4.4.2. IDENTIFICATION OF A NEUROTOXIC IMPURITY IN A SYNTHETIC NARCOTIC

Mass spectrometry played a remarkable role in the discovery of a new type of neurotoxin, 1-methyl-4-phenyl-1,2,3,6-tetrahydropyridine (MPTP). When a drug abuser who had been a patient at NIH died, his brain was found to have characteristics of Parkinson's disease. This corroborated what had been his clinical condition. The cause of this disorder seemed to coincide with ingestion of certain drug preparations which he synthesized.

GC–MS analysis of a speck of material on a vacuum desiccator from a laboratory in his home revealed the presence of two components (38). Their EI spectra are shown in Fig. 29. A proposed scheme for their mutual production is shown in Fig. 30. The desired compound has narcotic activity, but the dehydration product is a potent neurotoxin, producing a parkinsonian syndrome when given to monkeys.

Further metabolism studies indicated that when MPTP is taken up into certain brain cells it is oxidized into the 1-methyl-4-phenyl-pyridinium ion, MPP^+. Once in this quaternary ammonium form, it could not escape from the cell since it was no longer lipophilic. Figure 31 shows the CAD mass spectrum (see tandem MS/MS in the first chapter) of a sample of MPP^+ along with a spectrum from a brain tissue extract, demonstrating its presence in the target tissue. The

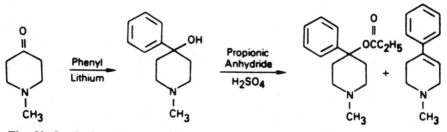

Fig. 30. Synthetic pathway used by a drug abuser chemist which resulted in MPTP contaminating the targeted meperidine analog (38).

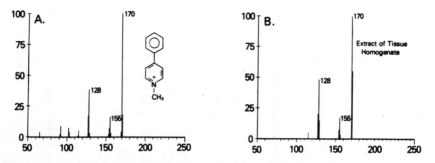

Fig. 31. MS/MS of authentic MPP^+ (*A*) and an ethanol extract of brain tissue homogenate incubated with MPTP (*B*) ionized by FAB in a secondary-emission mass spectrometer (38). Reproduced by permission from reference 38.

discovery of this general process of neurotoxicity generated substantial interest into the etiology of several neurological diseases. Other, analogous, cellular activation processes may act on chemicals in the environment to produce such symptoms.

5. CONCLUSIONS

Pharmacology dates back to Paracelsus in the 16th century, while mass spectrometry began with J. J. Thompson in 1910. Obviously, pharmacology did not need mass spectrometry to become an important medical science and to contribute to human well-being. Despite the disclaimer, this chapter demonstrates how much mass spectrometry impacts a wide variety of pharmacological problems.

Among the persistent trends in any analytical area are expansion of the scope of the materials that are able to be handled and the sensitivity/selectivity characteristics. In pharmacological research, we now see applications of mass spectrometry to assess the purity of genetically engineered insulin and other materials formerly thought too difficult to be determined by MS. The development of surface-ionization methods such as FAB or ^{252}Cf bombardment extends the range of molecules accessible to mass spectrometry. This expansion has led to refinements in mass spectrometers capable of dealing with molecules of this size.

Not long ago, any pharmacological assay that detected levels of a drug below 1 ng/mL was noteworthy. In contrast, several methods with orders-of-magnitude better sensitivity are described here, and there are many more. This improvement in sensitivity has been accomplished by improved instrument efficiency, and by appreciating the special advantage that ECNI provides in terms of absolute ion yields.

The remarkable growth of applications of tandem mass spectrometers speaks to their special characteristics. The intrinsic selectivity provided by the MS/MS method permits analyses that seem almost too good to be true. A totally untreated urine sample can be a useful sample. The structure of drug metabolites can be fairly securely determined in just a few minutes from submicrogram quantities of a biological specimen.

There is no reason to expect that applicability of mass spectrometry to pharmacological research has reached its zenith. Better instrumentation, new methodology, and more creative chemistry are always on the horizon, and these will continue to promote growth in this area.

ACKNOWLEDGMENTS

I am very grateful to the pharmacological mass spectroscopists around the country who provided reprints and preprints of their work. Part of the preparation of this chapter was supported by USPHS Grant NIH GM-36143.

References

1. L. Z. Benet and L. B. Sheiner, in A. G. Gilman, L. S. Goodman, T. W. Rall, and F. Murad, Eds., *Goodman and Gilman's "The Pharmacological Basis of Therapeutics,"* 7th ed., Macmillan, New York, 1985, p. 1.

2. D. R. Knapp, T. E. Gaffney, and R. E. McMahon, *Biochem. Pharmacol.* **21**, 425–429 (1972).

3. N. R. Hartman and I. Jardine, *Biomed. Env. Mass Spectrom.* **13**, 361–372 (1986).

4. A. S. Salhab, F. P. Abramson, G. W. Geelhoed, and G. S. Edwards, *Xenobiotica* **7**, 401–408 (1977).

5. M. S. Lee and R. A. Yost, *Biomed. Env. Mass Spectrom.* **15**, 193–204 (1988).

6. C. Fenselau and L. P. Johnson, *Drug Metab. Dispos.* **8**, 274–283 (1980).

7. V. T. Vu, C. C. Fenselau, and O. M. Colvin, *J. Am. Chem. Soc.* **103**, 7362–7364 (1981).

8. V. T. Vu and F. P. Abramson, *Biomed. Mass Spectrom.* **5**, 686–691 (1978).

9. V. T. Vu and F. P. Abramson, *Drug Metab. Dispos.* **8**, 300–304 (1980).

10. L. D. Betowski, W. A. Korfmacher, J. O. Lay, D. W. Potter, and J. A. Hinson, *Biomed. Env. Mass Spectrom.* **14**, 705–710 (1987).

11. M. Hag Ali, Ph.D. Dissertation, Department of Pharmacology, George Washington University, "The Effect of Schistosomiasis Mansoni Infection on the Toxicity and Metabolism of the Antischistosomal Drug, Praziquantel, in Mice," Washington, DC, 1986.

12. D. H. Chace and F. P. Abramson, in: T. A. Baillie and J. R. Jones (Eds.), Synthesis and Applications of Isotopically Labelled Compounds. Proceedings of the Third International Symposium, Innsbruck, Austria, 1988, Elsevier, Amsterdam, 1989, 253–258.

12a. D. H. Chace and F. P. Abramson. *Analytical Chem.* **61**, in press, 1989.

13. T. Walle, M. J. Wilson, K. Walle, and S. A. Bai, *Drug Metab. Dispos.* **11**, 544–549 (1983).

14. L. Y. Leung and T. A. Baillie, in E. F. Domino and J. M. Kamenka Eds., *Sigma and Phencyclidine-Like Compounds as Molecular Probes in Biology*, NPP Books, Ann Arbor, MI, 1988, pp. 607–617.

15. M. D. Threadgill, D. B. Axworthy, T. A. Baillie, P. B. Farmer, K. C. Farrow, A. Gescher, P. Kestell, P. G. Pearson, and A. J. Shaw, *J. Pharmacol. Exp. Therap.* **242**, 312–319 (1987).

16. A. E. Rettie, A. W. Rettenmeier, W. N. Howald, and T. A. Baillie, *Science* **235**, 890–445 (1985).

17. R. J. Shulman, C. S. Irving, T. W. Boutton, W. W. Wong, B. L. Nichols, and P. D. Klein, *Pediatr. Res.* **19**, 441–445 (1985).

18. T. A. Baillie, *Pharmacol. Rev.* **33**, 81–132 (1981).

19. W. A. Garland and M. L. Powell, *J. Chromatogr. Sci.* **19**, 392–434 (1981).

20. F. P. Abramson and M. P. Lutz, *J. Chromatogr.* **339**, 87–95 (1985).

21. F. P. Abramson and H. C. Miller, Jr., *J. Urol.* **128**, 1336–1339 (1982).

22. B. J. Miwa, W. A. Garland, and P. Blumenthal, *Anal. Chem.* **53**, 793–797 (1981).

23. L. Bertilsson, B. Hojer, G. Tybring, J. Osterloh, and A. Rane, *Clin. Pharmacol. Therap.* **27**, 83–88 (1980).

24. L. Palmer, L. Bertilsson, P. Collste, and M. Rawlins, *Clin. Pharmacol. Therap.* **14**, 827–832 (1973).

25. K. P. Castagnoli, Y. Shinohara, T. Furuta, T. L. Nguyen, L. D. Gruenke, R. D. Miller, and N. Castagnoli, Jr., *Biomed. Env. Mass Spectrom.* **13**, 327–332 (1986).

26. G. M. Ozanne, W. G. Young, W. J. Mazzei, and J. W. Severinghaus, *Anesthesiology* **55**, 62–70 (1981).

27. J. E. Evans, T. R. Browne, D. L. Kasdon, G. K. Szabo, B. A. Evans, and D. J. Greenblatt, *J. Clin. Pharmacol.* **25**, 309–312 (1985).

28. T. R. Covey, E. D. Lee, A. P. Bruins, and J. D. Henion, *Anal. Chem.* **58**, 1451A–1461A (1986).

29. J. M. Strong, H. S. Dutcher, W.-K. Lee, and A. J. Atkinson, Jr., *Clin. Pharmacol. Therap.* **18**, 613–622 (1975).

30. G. Mikus, C. Fischer, B. Heuer, C. Langen, and M. Eichelbaum, *Br. J. Clin. Pharmacol.* **24**, 561–569 (1987).

31. D. H. Catlin, R. C. Kammerer, C. K. Hatton, M. H. Sekera, and J. L. Merdink, *Clin. Chem.* **33**, 319–327 (1987).

32. T. R. Covey, E. D. Lee, and J. D. Henion, *Anal. Chem.* **58**, 2453–2460 (1986).

33. S. J. Mule and G. A. Casella, *J. Anal. Toxicol.* **12**, 102–107 (1988).

34. T. C. Kram, D. A. Cooper, and A. C. Allen, *Anal. Chem.* **53**, 1379A–1386A (1981).

35. H. K. Lim, D. Andrenyak, P. Francom, R. Foltz, and R. T. Jones, *Anal. Chem.* **60**, 1420–1425 (1988).

36. B. Pelli, P. Traldi, F. Tagliaro, G. Lubli, and M. Marigo, *Biomed. Env. Mass Spectrom.* **13**, 63–68 (1987).

37. G. W. A. Milne, H. M. Fales, and T. Axenrod, *Anal. Chem.* **43**, 1815–1820 (1971).

38. S. P. Markey, *Proc. Japan. Soc. Medical Mass Spectrom.* **9**, 3–13 (1984).

Author Index

Numbers in parentheses are reference numbers and indicate that the author's work is referred to although his name is not mentioned in the text. Numbers in *italics* indicate pages on which the complete reference appears

Subject Index

Cumulative Author Index, Volumes 1–34 and Supplemental Volume

Cumulative Subject Index, Volumes 1–34 and Supplemental Volume